The Best Ever

★ ★ ★ ★ ★

BAKING COOKBOOK

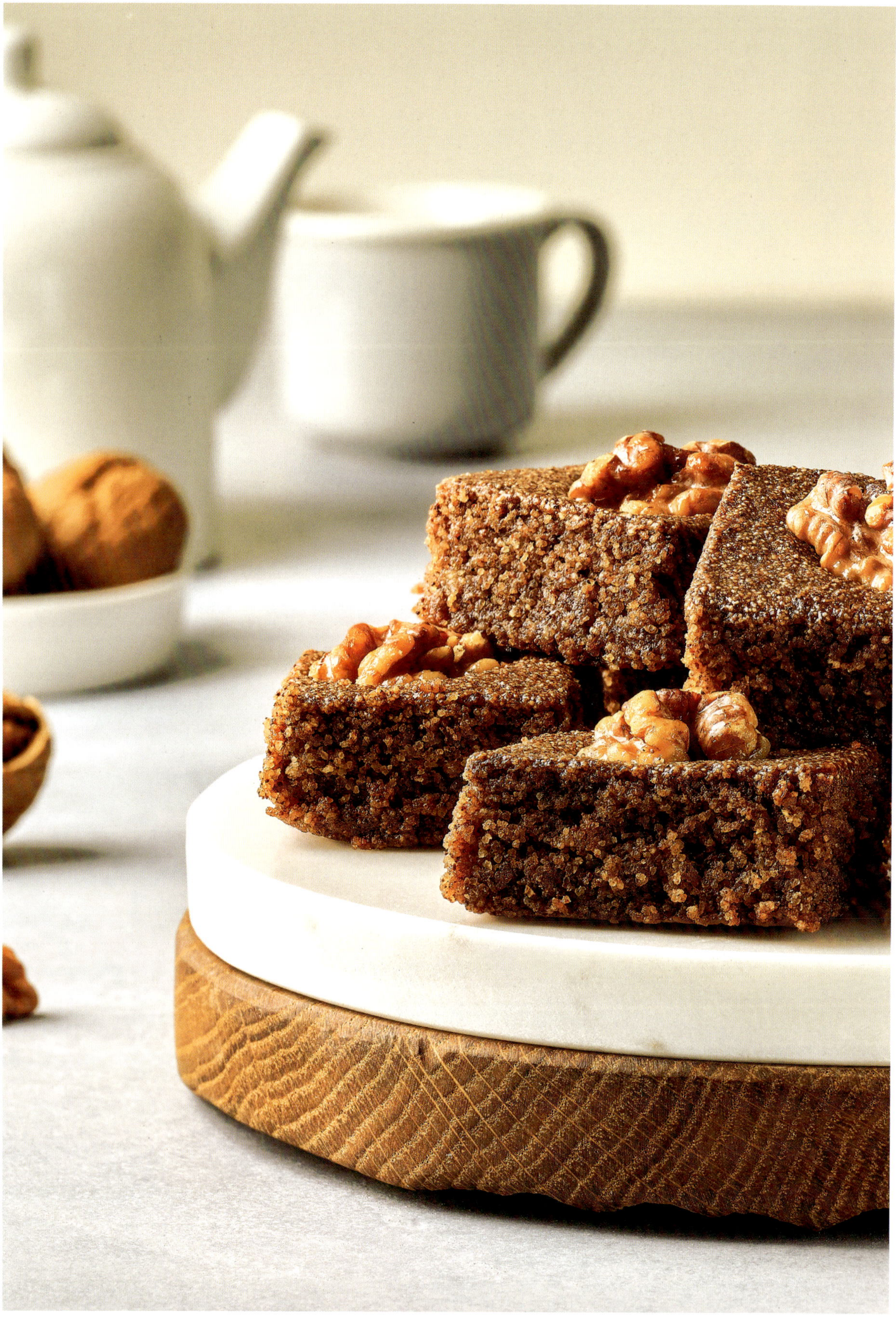

Destination Baking

Nothing beats the heady scent of home-baked treats wafting from the oven. Whether it's cakes or cookies, pies or tarts you are after, here are all the sweet and savoury, decadent and delicious recipes you need to let your inner baker run free in the kitchen.

BEST EVER BAKING – WITH 175 RECIPES TO ENJOY.

★ ★ ★ ★ ★

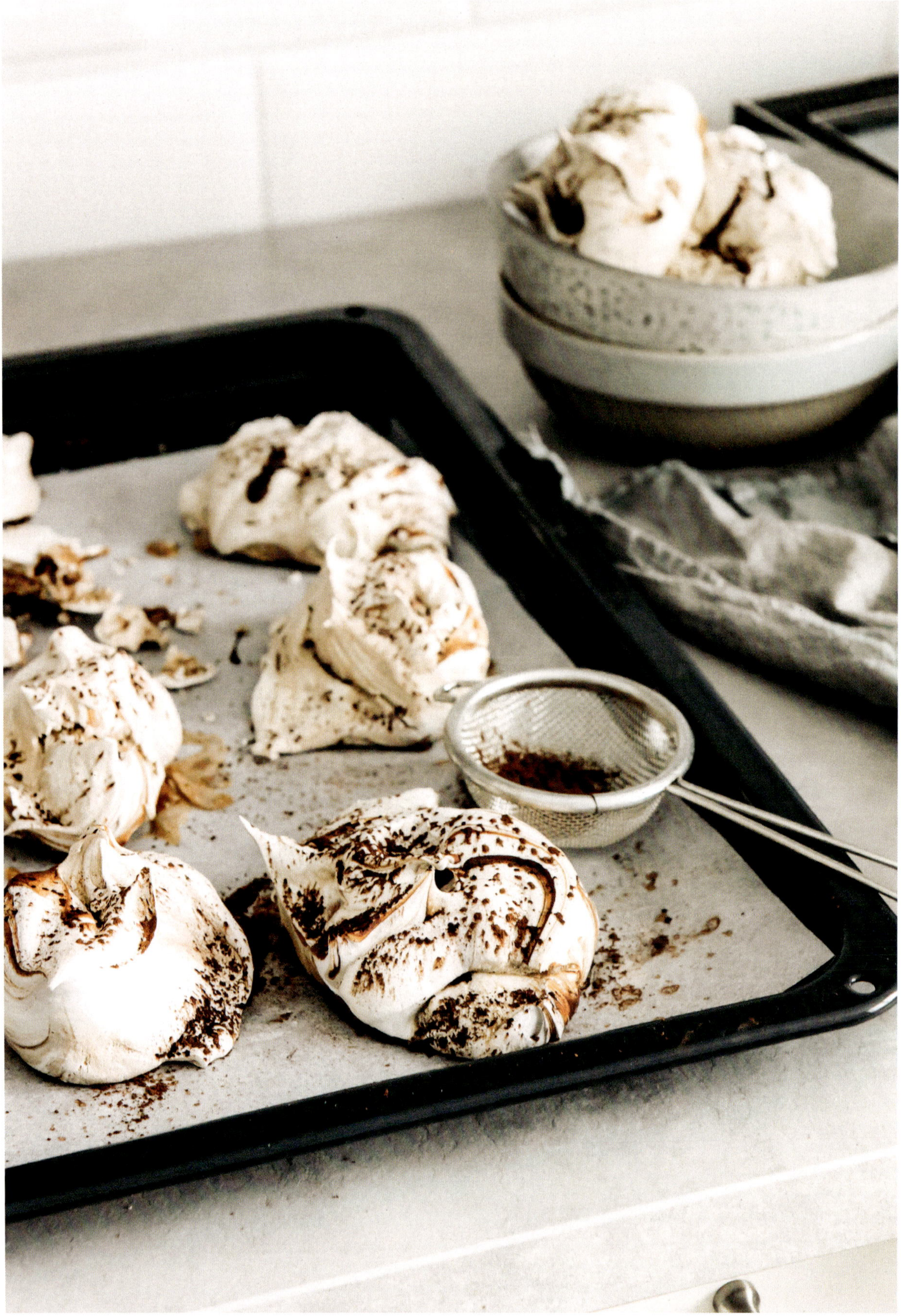

The Best Ever

★★★★★

BAKING COOKBOOK

SWEET AND SAVOURY DELIGHTS FOR ULTIMATE GOODNESS

★ 175 ★

Winning Recipes

HERRON

Contents

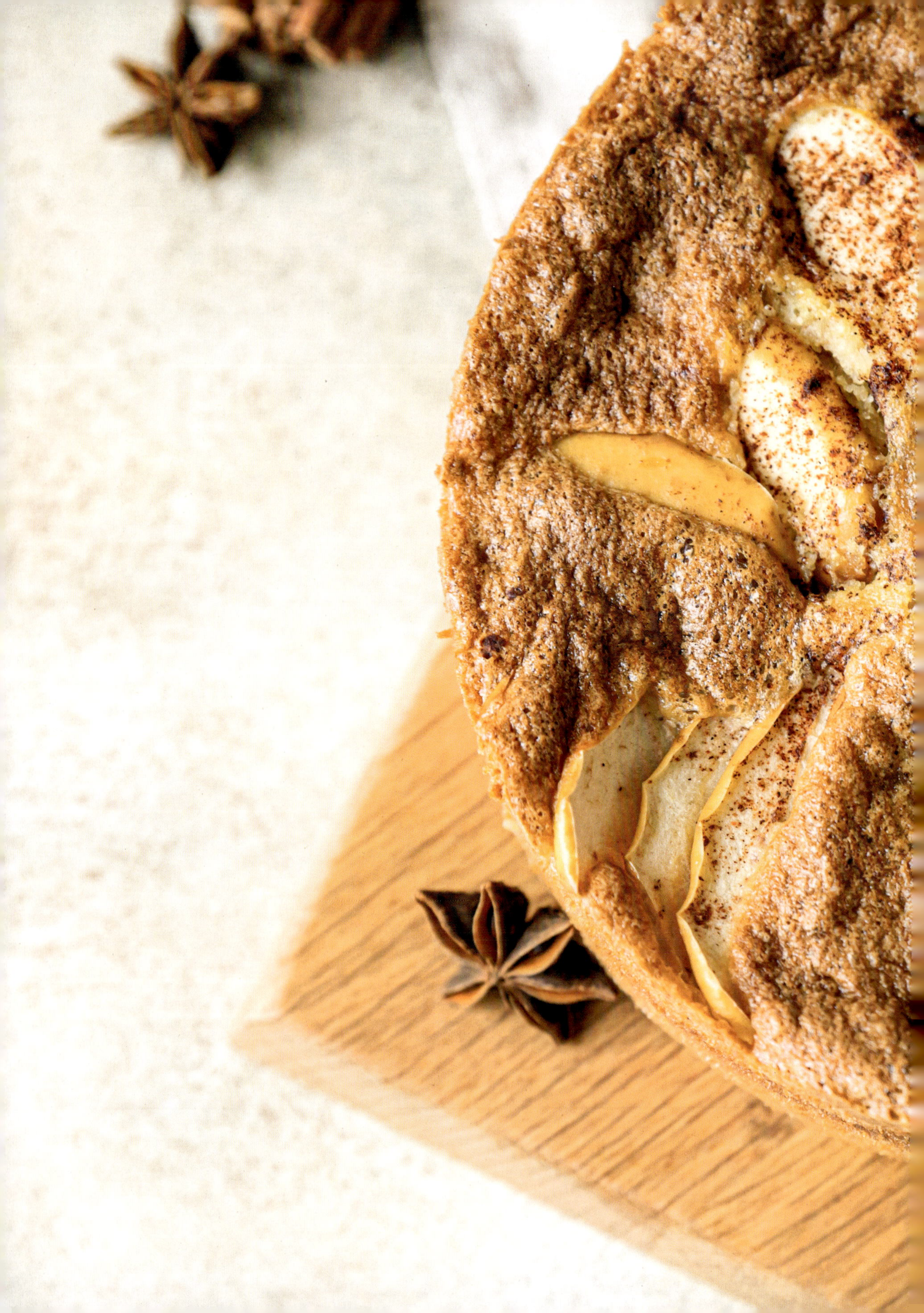

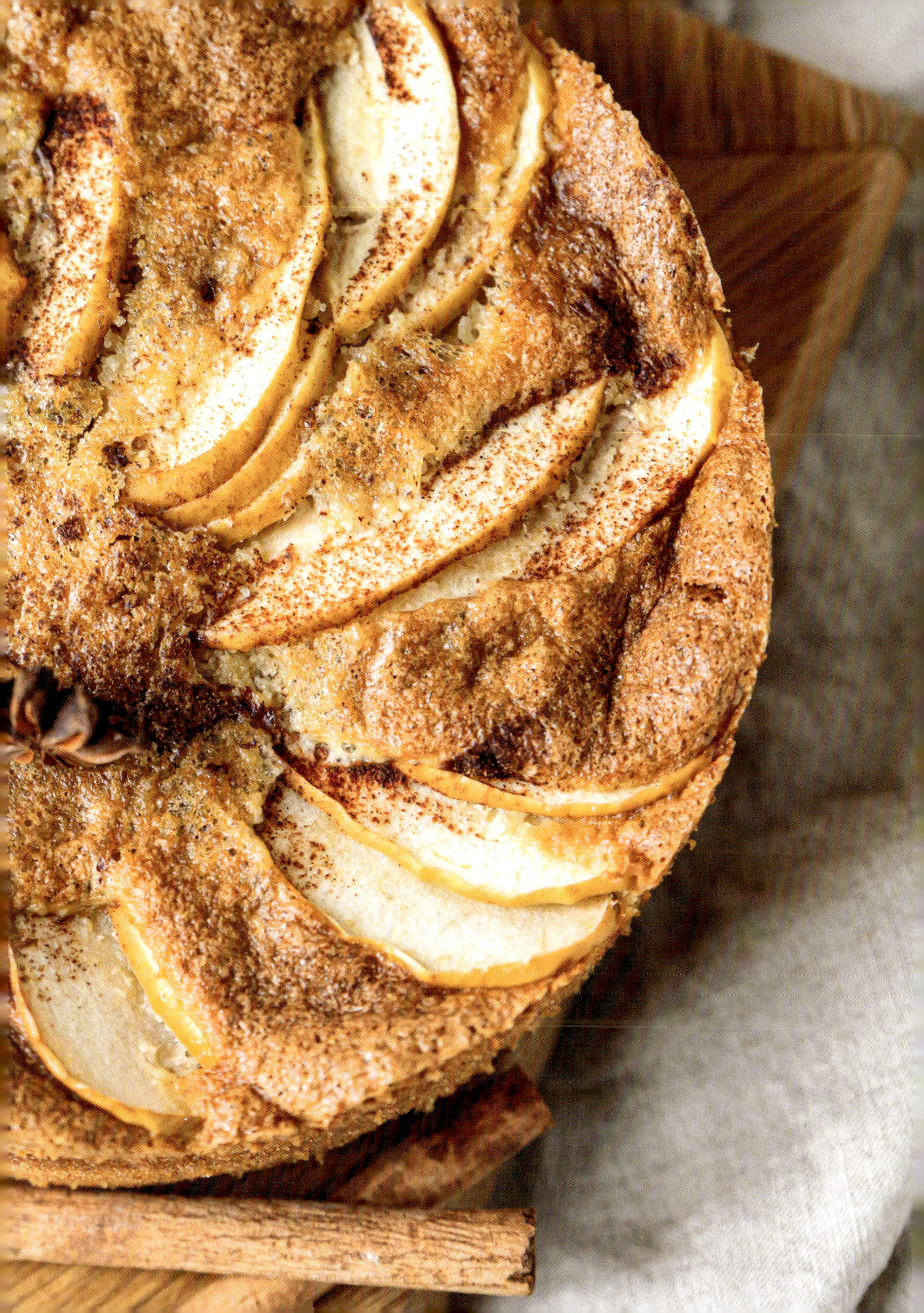

1

Easy

Puff Pastry

MAKES 1 QUANTITY
PREP + COOK TIME: 40 MINS + 2 HOURS CHILLING

2 cups (250g) plain flour
Pinch of salt
2/3 cup (150ml) iced water
225g butter

Put the flour and salt in a food processor. With the motor running slowly pour in iced water. When the dough comes together, cover with plastic wrap and chill for 20 minutes.

Transfer to a lightly floured surface and roll into a 25cm circle.

Place the butter in between two sheets of greaseproof paper and roll with a rolling pin to soften. Cut the butter in half and repeat the process until the butter is pliable but still cold. Reshape to a rough 15cm square.

Put the butter in the centre of the pastry and fold over the right and left sides of the circle, overlapping in the middle. Roll with a rolling pin to a slightly longer rectangle, then fold up the bottom third up to cover the middle third, then fold down the top third like an envelope. Seal the dough gently by pressing down on the edges with the rolling pin. Turn the dough a quarter turn.

Roll the dough out to a long rectangle (roughly 20 x 40cm). Fold up the thirds once again. Seal the edges and turn the dough a quarter turn. Repeat the rolling and folding one more time, then cover and chill for 20 minutes.

Repeat this step (rolling, folding, turning, rolling, folding) twice more, chilling each time.

Chill for 1 hour before using.

Shortcrust Pastry

MAKES 1 QUANTITY
PREP + COOK TIME: 15 MINS + 2 HOURS CHILLING

2 cups (250g) plain flour
125g chilled butter, diced
Pinch of salt
1 egg, chilled
1 tbsp chilled water

Process flour, butter and salt in a food processor until mixture resembles breadcrumbs.

Whisk egg and water together in a small bowl. With the motor running add to the food processor and continue to process until the mixture begins to form large clumps.

Turn pastry out on to a work surface and knead gently to bring together. Form into a disc. Wrap in plastic wrap or greaseproof paper and refrigerate for at least 2 hours before using.

To make shortcrust pastry without a food processor, rub the butter into the flour with your fingertips until the mixture resembles breadcrumbs. Pour the egg and water mixture all over the crumb mixture, then cut in with a butter knife. Use your hands to gently bring the mixture together, then knead, shape and refrigerate as above.

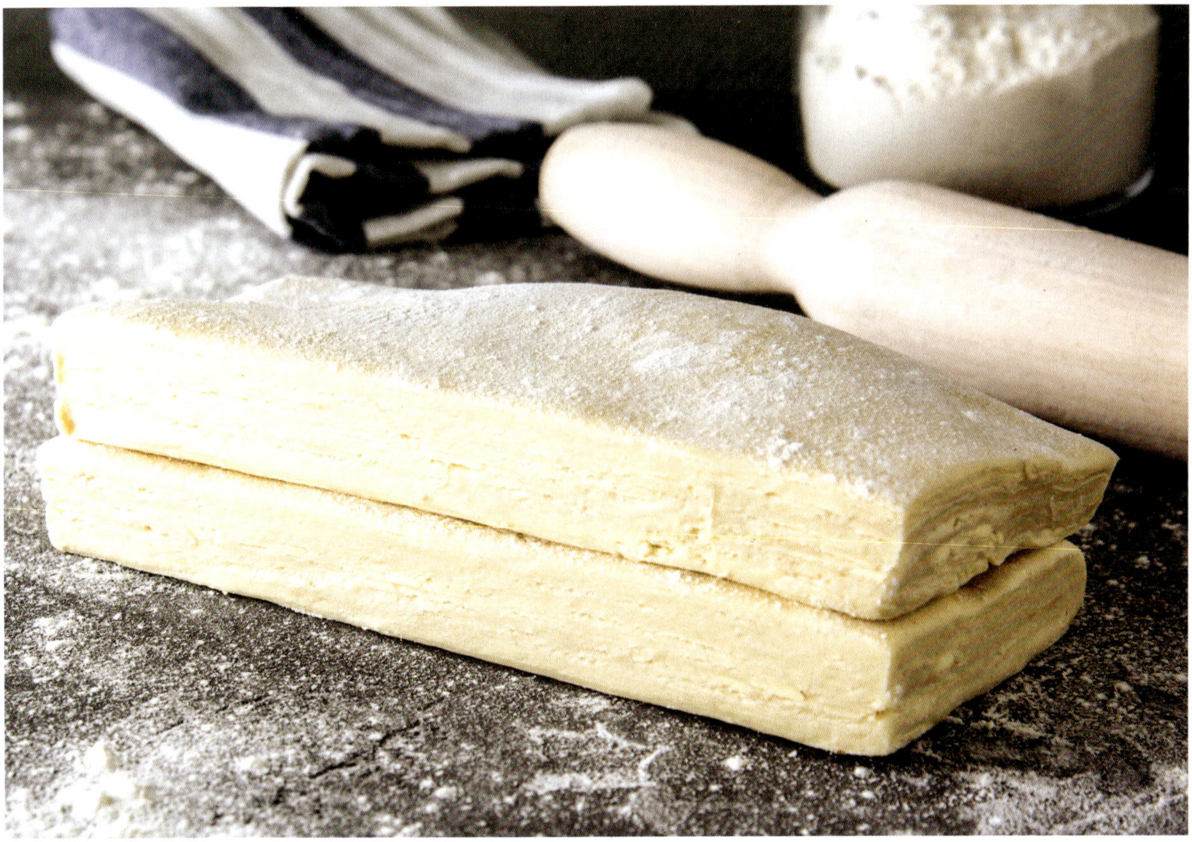

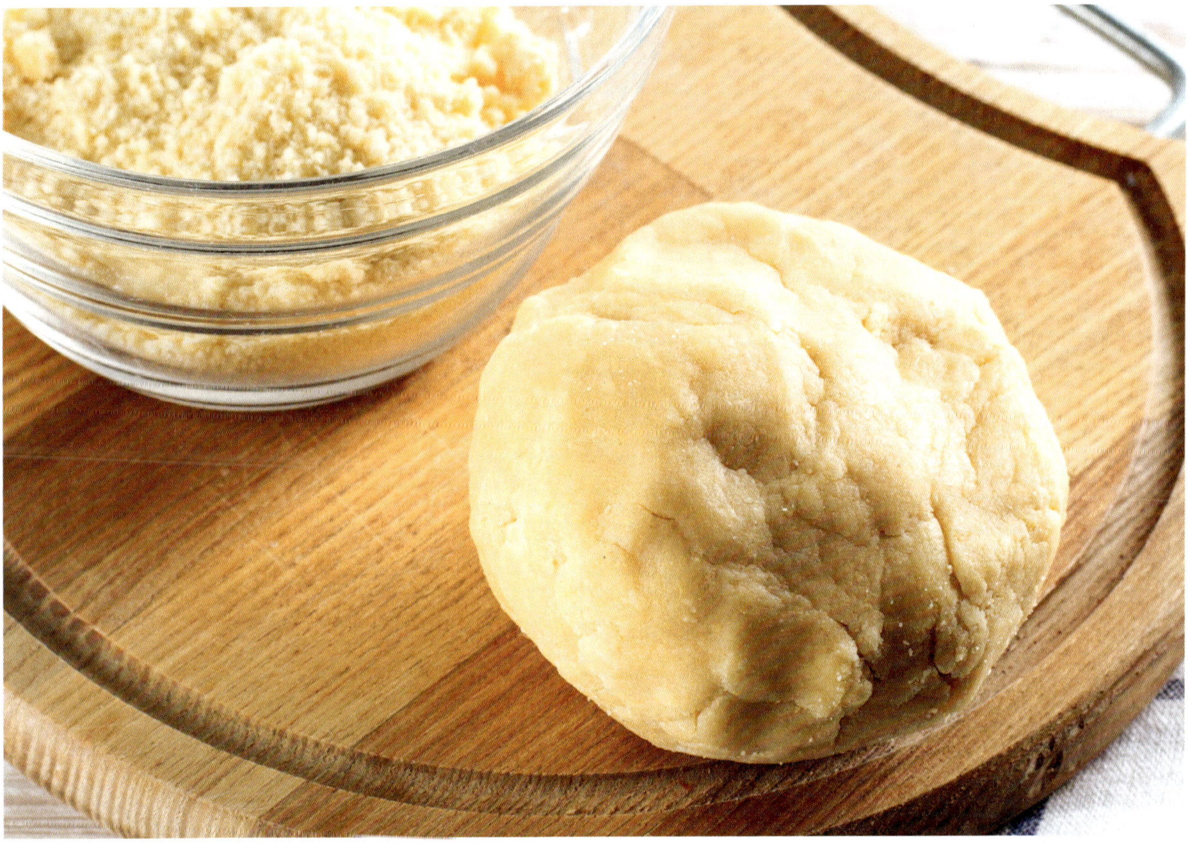

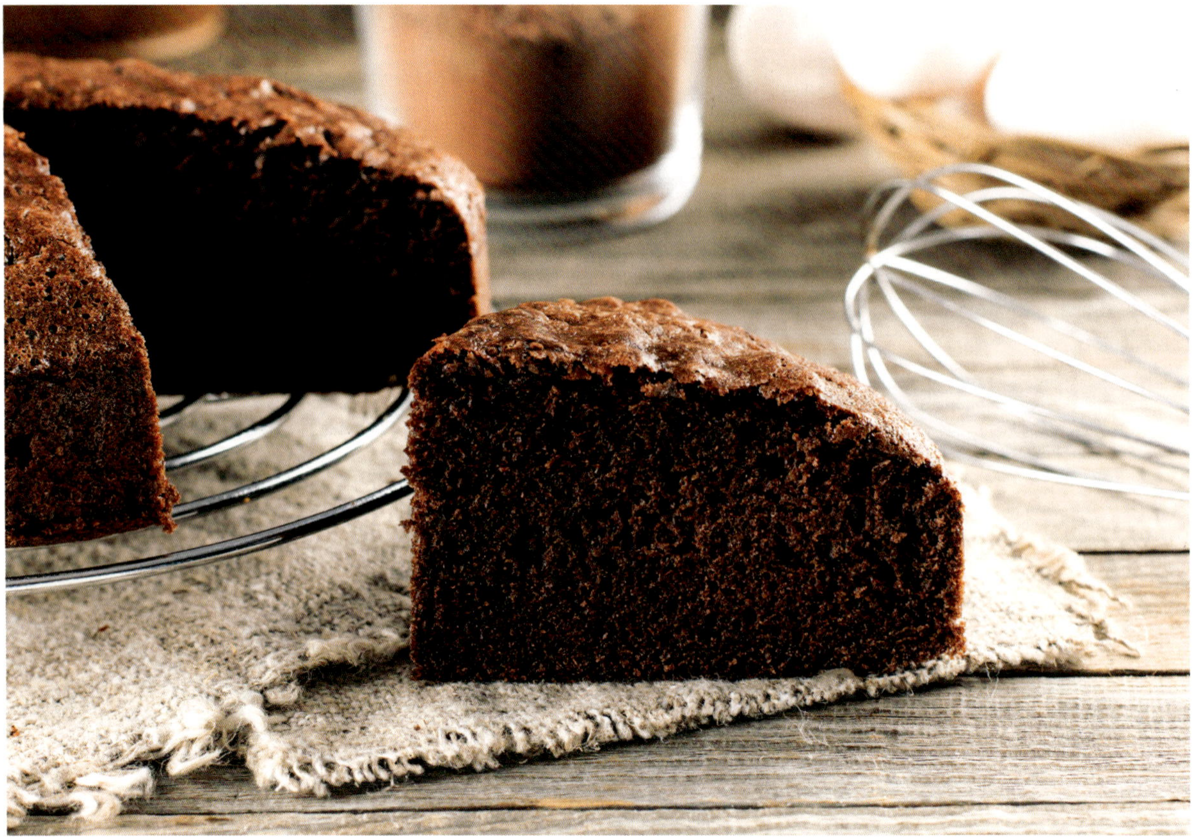

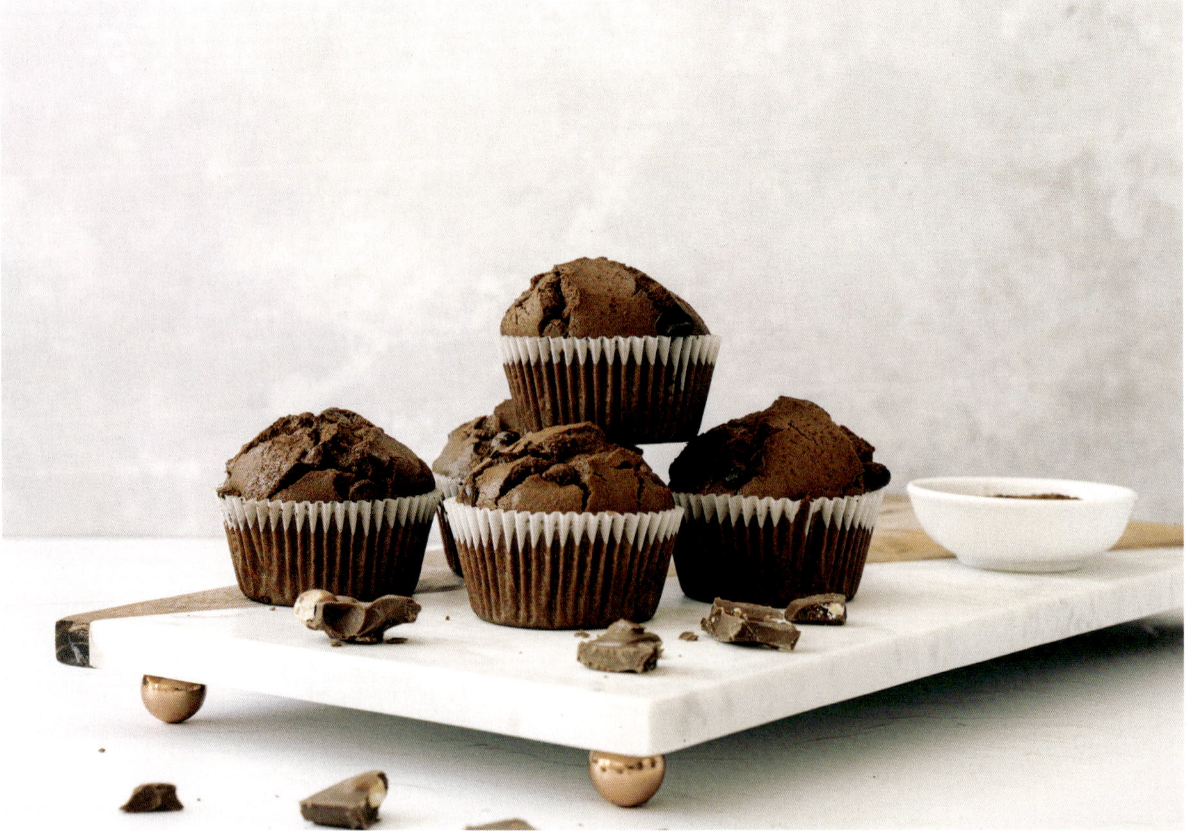

Chocolate Cake

SERVES 12
PREP + COOK TIME: 55 MINS

1 cup (200g) golden caster sugar
200g unsalted butter, softened
4 large eggs
1⅔ cups (200g) self-raising flour
2 tbsps cocoa powder
1 tsp baking powder
½ tsp vanilla extract
2 tbsps milk
Pinch of salt

Preheat oven to 170°C. Grease and line a 23cm springform cake tin with greaseproof paper.

In a large bowl, beat together sugar, butter, eggs, flour, cocoa powder, baking powder, vanilla, milk and salt. Pour the mixture into the prepared tin.

Bake for 20 minutes or until a skewer inserted into the centre comes out clean. Leave to cool in the tin for 10 minutes, before turning out onto a wire rack to cool completely.

Chocolate Muffins

MAKES 12
PREP + COOK TIME: 40 MINS

2½ cups (310g) self-raising flour, sifted
¾ cup (90g) cocoa powder, sifted
1 cup (220g) caster sugar
¾ cup (120g) dark chocolate chips
½ cup (125ml) vegetable oil
⅔ cup (160ml) milk
1 tsp vanilla extract
2 eggs

Preheat oven to 180°C. Line a 12-hole muffin tray with paper liners.

Combine flour, cocoa, sugar and chocolate chips in a large bowl. Make a well in centre. Whisk vegetable oil, milk, vanilla and eggs in a large jug. Pour oil mixture into well of dry ingredients. Using a metal spoon, stir gently until just combined. Spoon mixture into paper cases.

Place in the oven and bake for 25 minutes or until a skewer inserted into the centre comes out clean.

Stand in tray for 5 minutes. Transfer to a wire rack to cool.

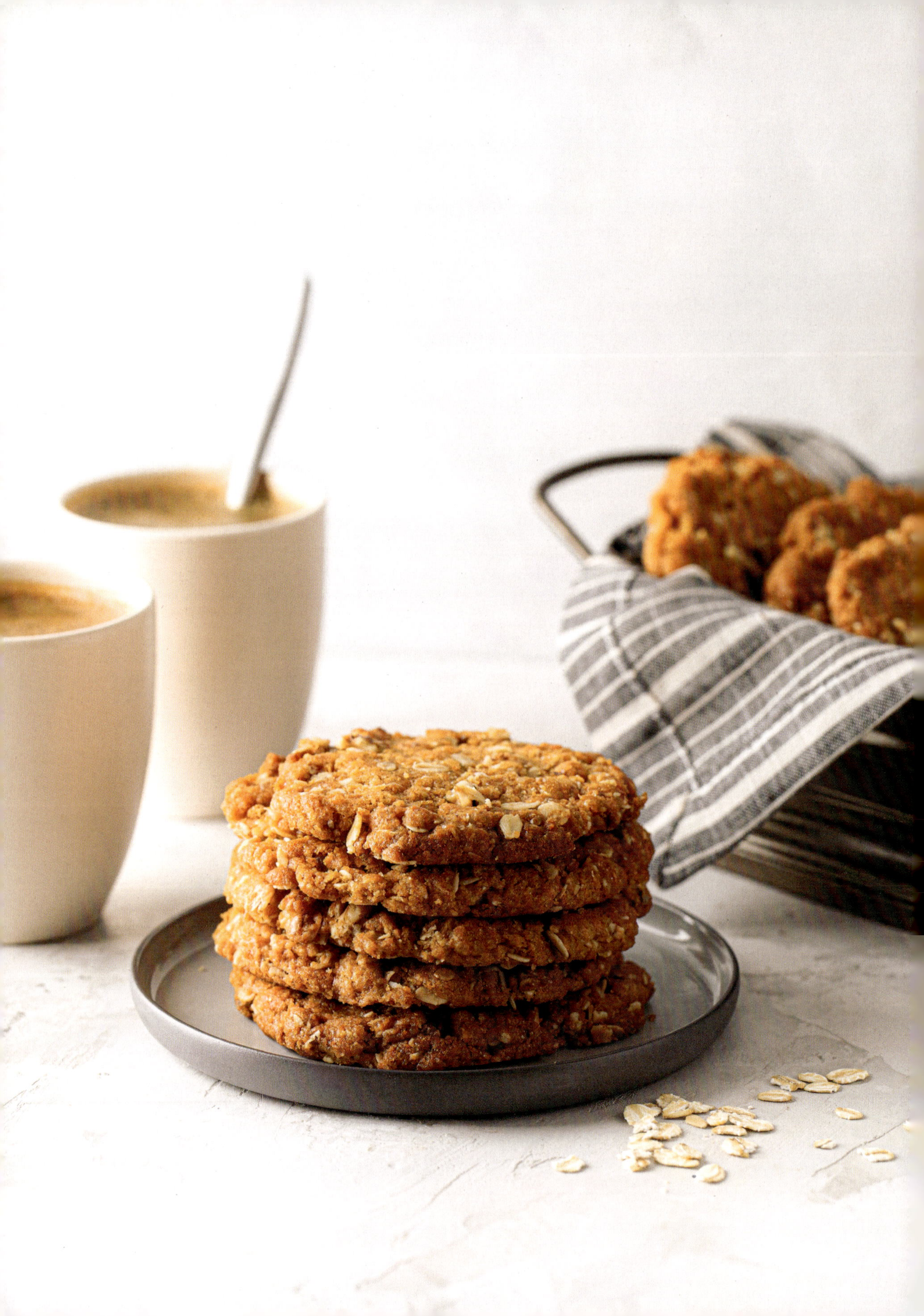

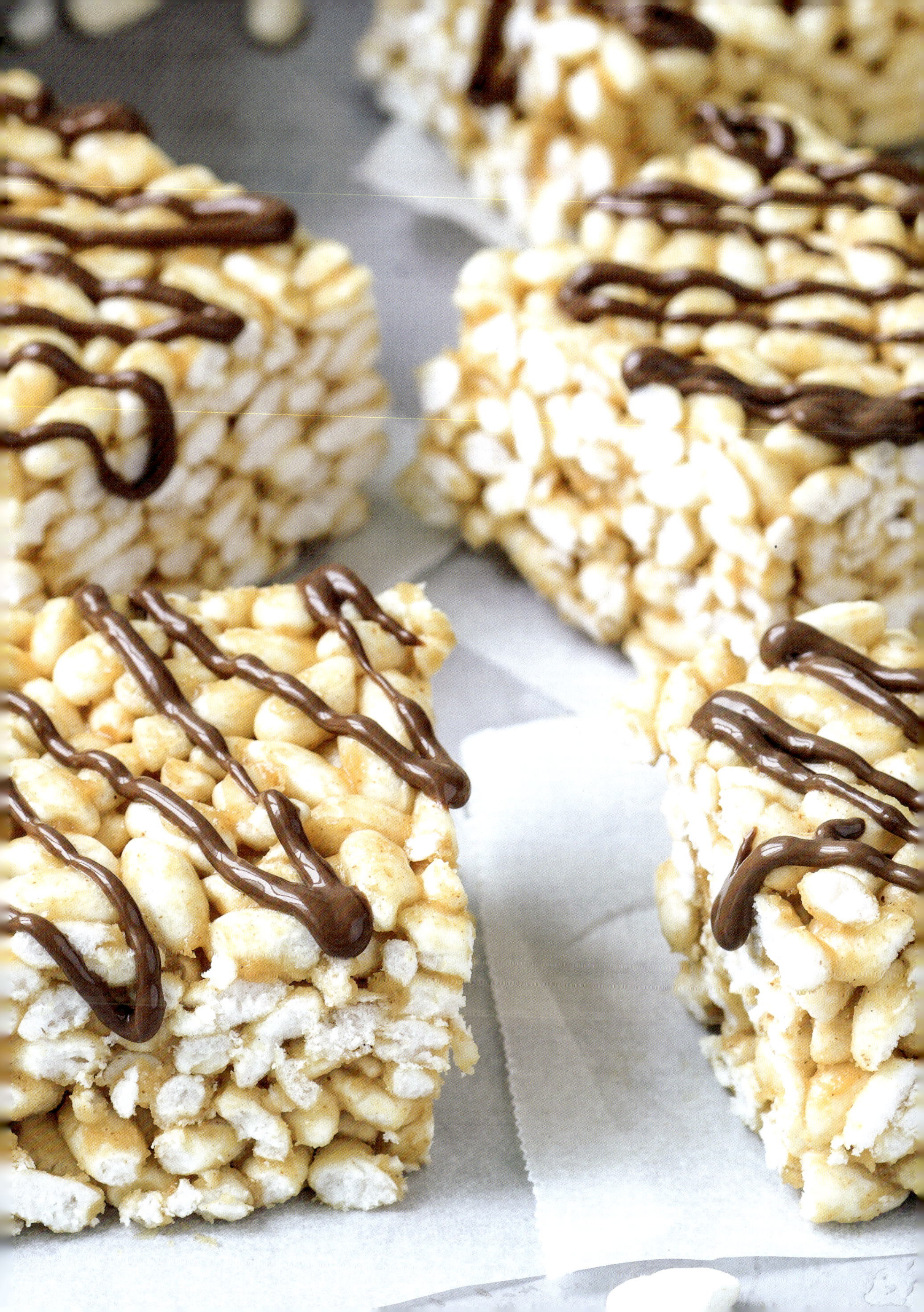

Anzac Biscuits

MAKES 26
PREP + COOK TIME: 35 MINS

1 cup (90g) rolled oats
1 cup (125g) plain flour, sifted
1 cup (220g) firmly packed brown sugar
½ cup (40g) desiccated coconut
125g butter, chopped
2 tbsps golden syrup
1½ tbsps water
½ tsp bicarbonate of soda

Preheat oven to 160°C. Grease and line a baking tray with greaseproof paper.

Combine oats, flour, sugar and coconut in a large bowl. Set aside.

Place butter, golden syrup and water in a small saucepan over low heat. Stir until smooth. Add the bicarb and stir again. Add the wet ingredients to the dry ingredients and mix well to combine.

Measure level tablespoons of mixture and roll into balls. Flatten slightly and then place evenly spaced on the prepared tray. Bake for 20 minutes or until golden. Cool on tray and then move to a wire rack.

Note: Anzac biscuits should be soft to touch. They will crisp on cooling. Increase/decrease the oven temperature and/or the baking time to produce crispier/softer biscuits.

Puffed Rice Slice

MAKES 16
PREP + COOK TIME: 1 HOUR
GLUTEN FREE

¾ cup + 1 tbsp (180g) sugar
180g butter
3 tbsps honey
½ tsp vanilla bean paste
6 cups (150g) puffed rice
90g dark chocolate, melted (optional)

Grease and line a 20cm square cake with greaseproof paper. Combine sugar, butter and honey in a pan over medium heat. Bring to a boil, stirring continuously, then reduce heat to medium-low and cook for a further 2 minutes. Stir in vanilla, then add to a large bowl along with the puffed rice. Stir well to combine. Pour mixture into the prepared tin and smooth with a spatula. Transfer to the fridge for 30-45 minutes to firm up, then slice into squares. Drizzle melted chocolate over the squares, if desired.

Shortbread Cookies

SERVES 24
PREP + COOK TIME: 1 HOUR

225g unsalted butter, softened
½ cup (110g) sugar
2 cups (250g) plain flour

Preheat oven to 180°C and line a baking tray. Cream together butter and sugar until light and fluffy. Add flour and mix until dough comes together. Scrape dough onto a piece of plastic wrap and shape into a disk. Seal the dough and chill until firm, about 30 minutes. Roll dough out on a floured surface and cut out cookies using a cutter. Place cookies on the baking tray and bake for around 20 minutes or until golden.

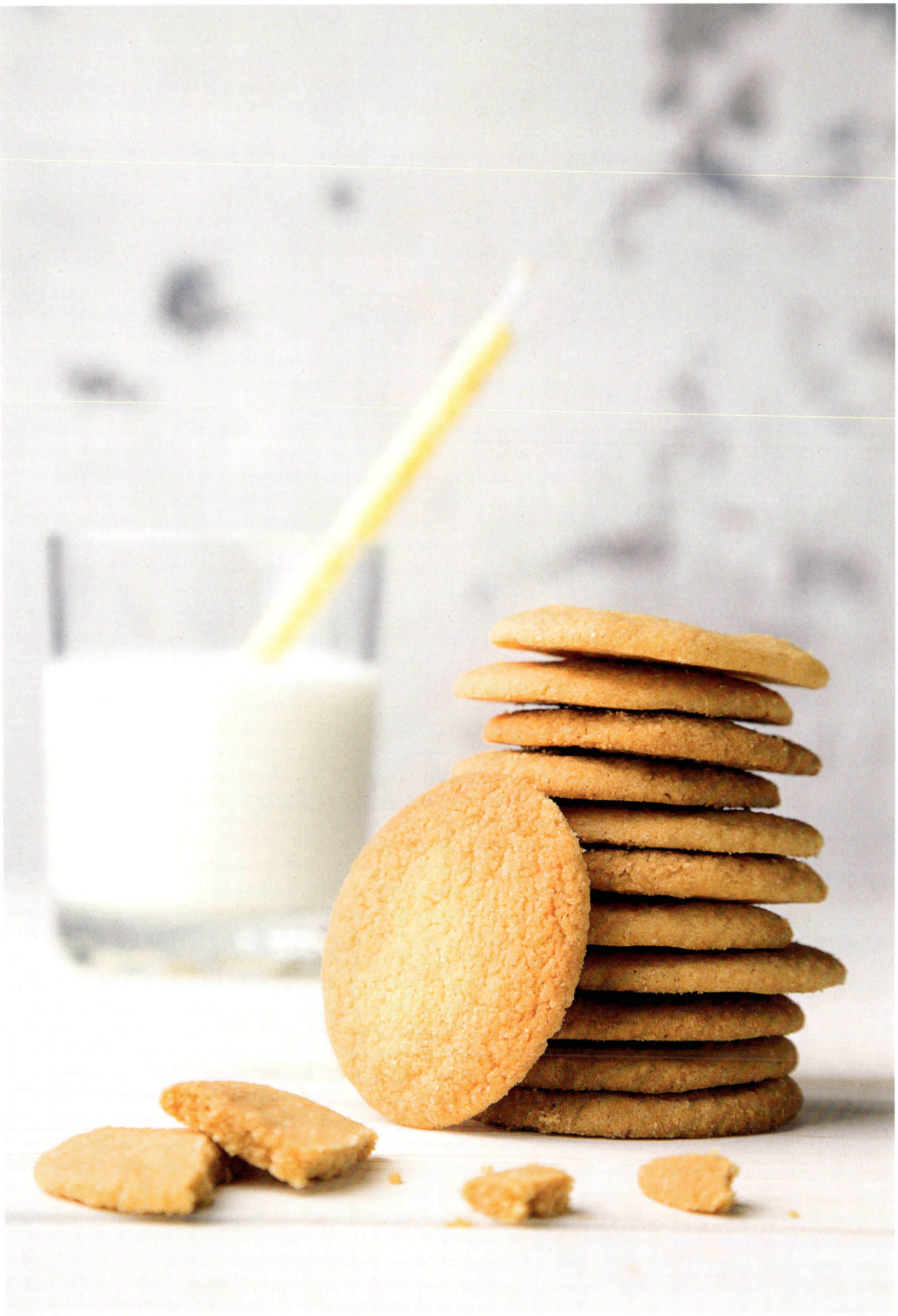

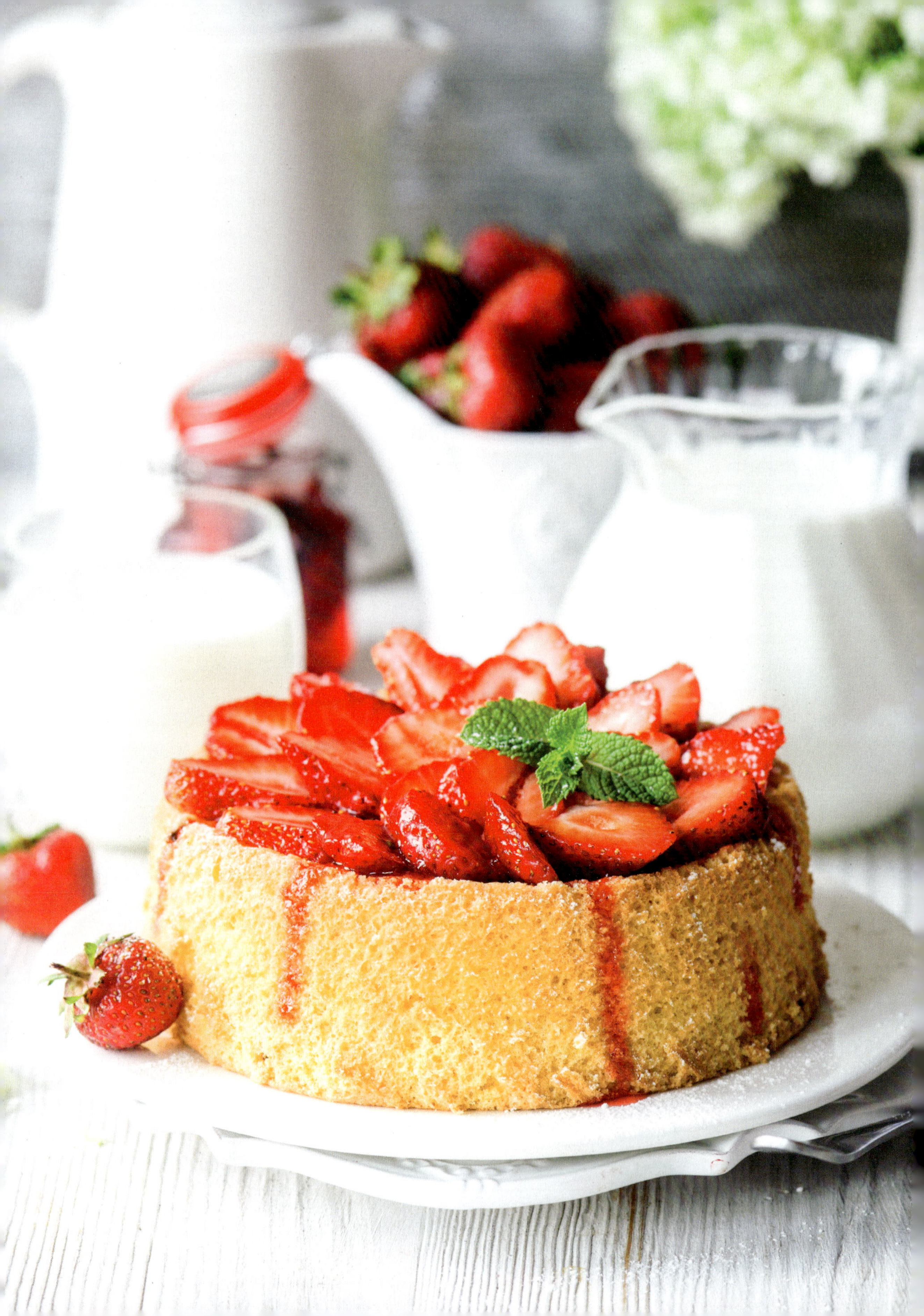

Vanilla Sponge

SERVES 12
PREP + COOK TIME: 1 HOUR 10 MINS

VANILLA SPONGE
¼ cup (30g) flour
9 eggs, separated
¾ cup (165g) sugar
1 cup (120g) almond meal
½ cup (60g) chopped almonds
2 tsps vanilla extract
3 tbsps milk
Glazed strawberries (see next recipe)
Cream to serve

Preheat oven to 180°C. Butter a 23cm springform pan, line the bottom with greaseproof paper and flour the sides.

Whisk together egg whites until soft peaks form using an electric hand mixer. Add ½ cup of sugar and continue whipping until stiff and glossy, about 30 seconds more.

In another bowl, whisk egg yolks with remaining ¼ cup of sugar until light and fluffy. Fold in egg whites, followed by almond meal, chopped almonds, flour, vanilla and milk.

Pour batter into the prepared tin and bake until slightly spongy in the centre, about 35-40 minutes. Let cool for 15 minutes in the tin, then remove the sides of the pan and let cool completely on a wire rack. The cake will fall slightly in the centre. Remove the bottom of the tin and the greaseproof paper before transferring to a serving platter.

Pour glazed strawberries into the sunken centre of the cake and gently spread into a circle on the surface, leaving a border all around. Let cool until set, about 30 minutes.

Serve with cream.

Glazed Strawberries

SERVES 12
PREP + COOK TIME: 10 MINS
GLUTEN FREE • DAIRY FREE

1 cup (325g) strawberry jam
1½ tbsps water
3 cups (600g) strawberries, hulled and halved

In a medium saucepan, bring jam and water to a boil and stir to remove any lumps. Add strawberries all at once and fold together with a spatula until evenly coated. Serve with vanilla sponge.

Vanilla Cupcakes

MAKES 24
PREP + COOK TIME: 40 MINS

CUPCAKES

150g butter, room temperature

1½ cups (330g) caster sugar

2 eggs

2½ cups (310g) self-raising flour

1¼ cups (310ml) milk

2 tsps vanilla essence

ICING

100g butter, room temperature

1½ cups (235g) icing sugar

2 drops vanilla essence

2 tbsps milk

Preheat oven to 190°C. Line two 12-hole muffin tins with paper cases.

Using an electric mixer, cream together butter and sugar until light and fluffy. Add eggs and beat to combine. Add the sifted flour, milk and vanilla and stir until a smooth batter forms. Spoon mixture into the cases to about two-thirds full.

Bake for 20 minutes until golden and springy to touch. Turn out onto a wire rack to cool while you prepare the icing.

In an electric mixer, beat butter until it is pale and fluffy. Sift over the icing sugar and add the vanilla essence and milk. Beat until the mixture has a light, fluffy texture. Add extra milk for a softer consistency. Spread or pipe icing over cupcakes and top with decorations as desired.

Cheat's Mini Chocolate Croissants

MAKES 32
PREP + COOK TIME: 45 MINS

2 sheets frozen puff or shortcrust pastry, thawed

⅔ cup (100g) chocolate chips

1 egg, beaten

Icing sugar for dusting

Preheat oven to 175°C. Line two baking trays with greaseproof paper.

Place the pastry sheets on a lightly floured work surface. Cut each pastry sheet in half, then cut each half into four even rectangles. Now, cut each rectangle diagonally into two triangles.

Place about 1 teaspoon of chocolate chips down the centre of each triangle. Then, starting at the wider end, roll up each triangle. Place each croissant seam-side down so that the tip of the triangle is tucked under the rolled croissant. Bend the edges slightly to create a crescent shape and place on the prepared baking trays.

Lightly brush tops of croissants with beaten egg.

Bake for 20-25 minutes or until golden brown.

Dust with icing sugar to serve.

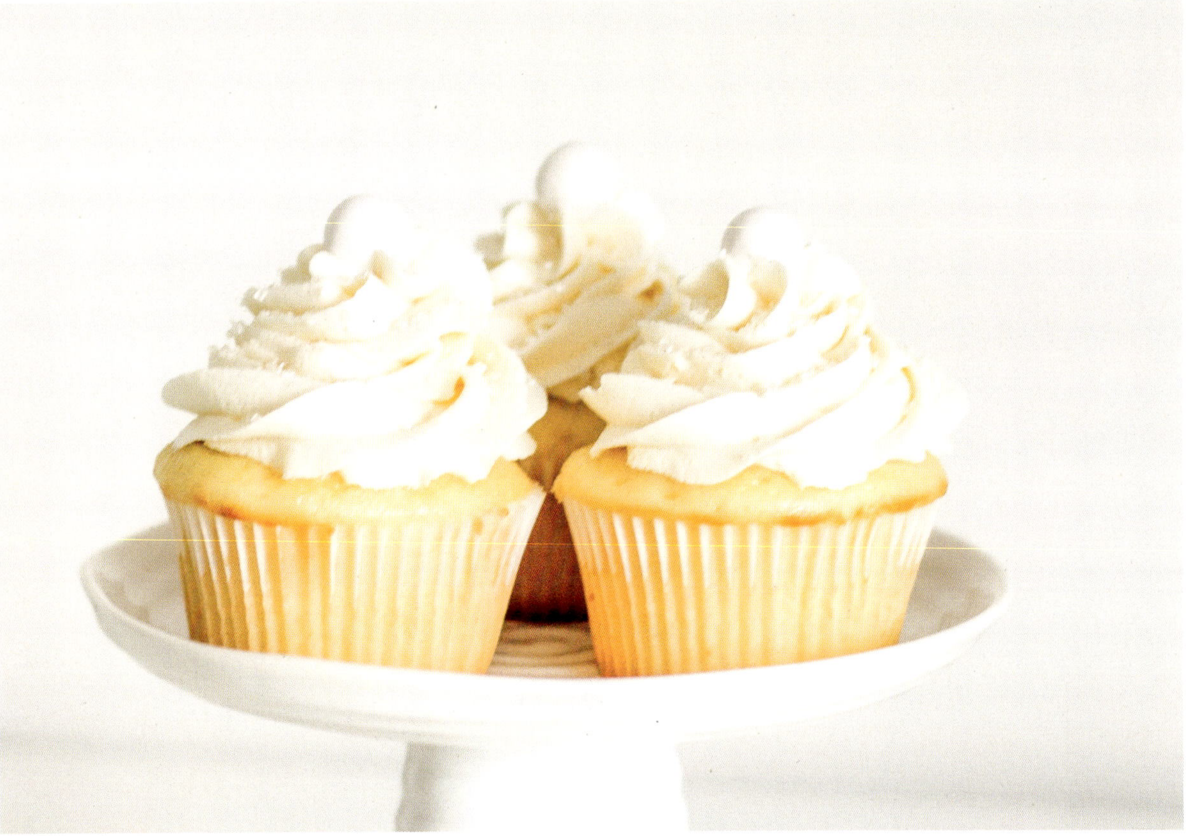

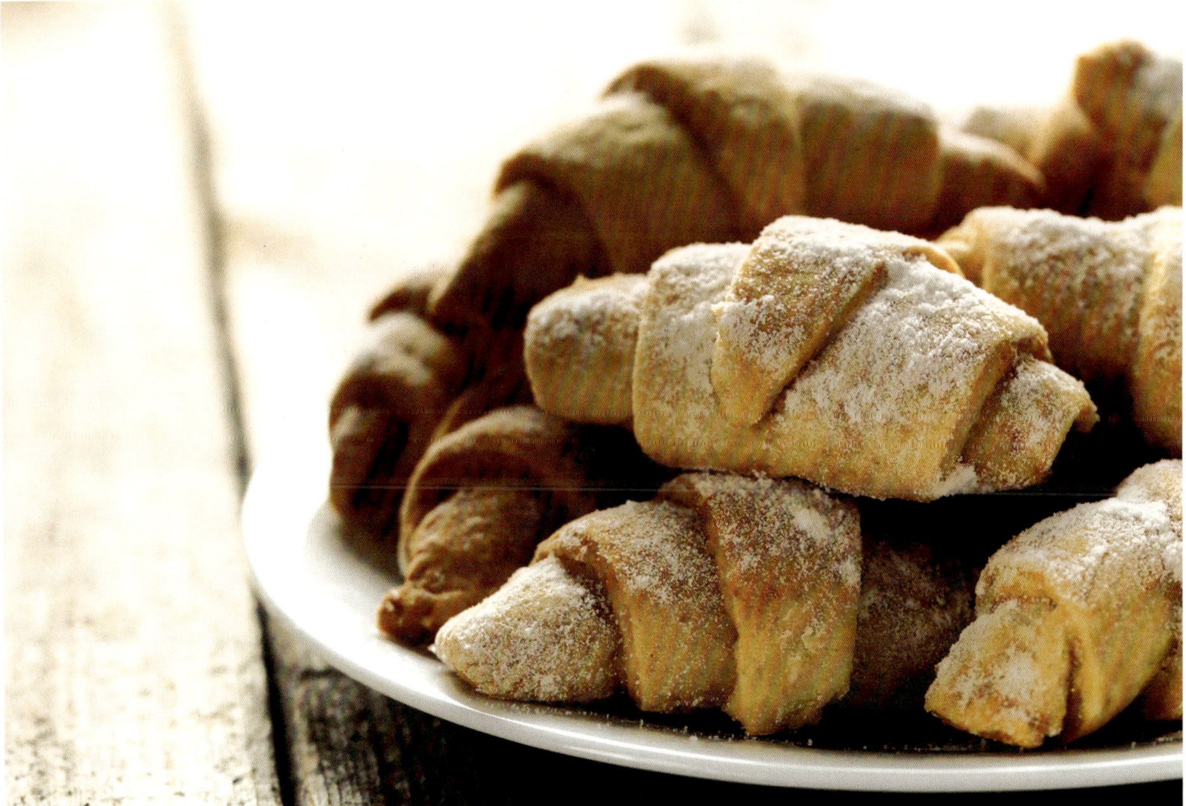

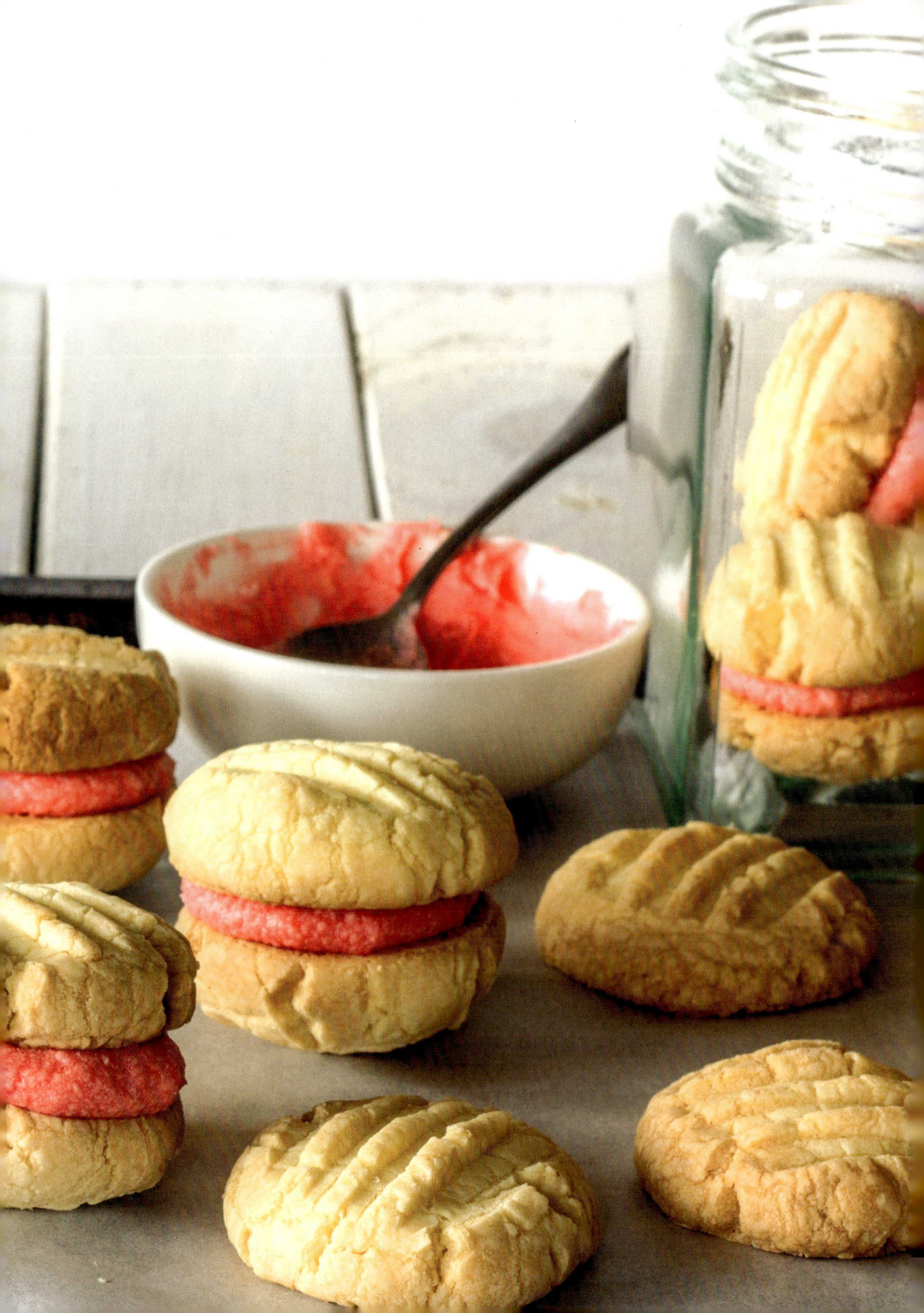

Raspberry Melting Moments

MAKES 25
PREP + COOK TIME: 50 MINS

BISCUITS

125g butter, room temperature
1 cup (125g) plain flour
⅓ cup (50g) icing sugar
⅓ cup (50g) custard powder

RASPBERRY FILLING

60g butter, room temperature
1 cup (155g) icing sugar
6 frozen raspberries, thawed
1 tbsp lemon juice

Preheat oven to 160°C. Line two baking trays with greaseproof paper.

Using an electric mixer, beat butter until pale and creamy. Add the flour, icing sugar and custard powder and stir to combine with a metal spoon.

Roll teaspoonfuls of dough mixture into balls. Place 3cm apart on the lined trays. Gently flatten with a fork dusted in icing sugar. Depress tines of fork in centre to create a marking on the biscuit.

Bake for 15 minutes or until just cooked through. Remove and set aside to cool for 30 minutes.

Using an electric mixer, beat butter and icing sugar until light and fluffy. Add raspberries and lemon juice and beat until combined. Spread the butter mixture over the flat side of half the biscuits and sandwich together with remaining biscuits.

Passionfruit Filling

MAKES ENOUGH FOR 25 BISCUITS
PREP + COOK TIME: 10 MINS
GLUTEN FREE

60g butter, room temperature
1 cup (155g) icing sugar
1 large passionfruit
1 tbsp lemon juice

Using an electric mixer, beat butter and icing sugar until light and fluffy. Add passionfruit pulp and lemon juice and stir to combine.

Lemon Filling

MAKES ENOUGH FOR 25 BISCUITS
PREP + COOK TIME: 10 MINS
GLUTEN FREE

60g butter, room temperature
1 cup (155g) icing sugar
Zest of 1 lemon
1 tbsp lemon juice

Using an electric mixer, beat butter and icing sugar until light and fluffy. Add lemon zest and juice and stir to combine.

Chocolate Filling

MAKES ENOUGH FOR 25 BISCUITS
PREP + COOK TIME: 10 MINS
GLUTEN FREE

60g butter, room temperature
150g dark chocolate

Melt the butter and chocolate in a heatproof bowl over a pan of simmering water. Take off the heat and stir to combine. Allow to cool before using.

Linzer Cookies

MAKES 20

PREP + COOK TIME: 1 HOUR 20 MINS + COOLING

340g butter, softened
¾ cup (165g) sugar
1 tsp vanilla extract
3 cups (375g) plain flour + more as needed
2 tbsps water
½ tsp salt
¾ cup (245g) raspberry jam
Icing sugar for dusting

Preheat the oven to 175°C. Line two baking trays with greaseproof paper.

Cream together butter and sugar with an electric hand mixer until light and fluffy. Add vanilla, flour, water and salt and mix on low speed until the dough comes together. Transfer the dough to a lightly floured work surface and shape into a flat disk. Wrap in greaseproof paper or plastic wrap and place in the fridge for 30 minutes.

Roll out the chilled dough to a ½cm thickness. Using a 5-7cm round cookie cutter, cut out as many cookies as possible. Rework any leftover dough and repeat until no dough remains, adding a few tablespoons of flour if it's too sticky. Using a smaller round cutter, make holes in the middle of half of your rounds. Place cookies on prepared baking trays and chill for an additional 15 minutes.

Bake the cookies for 15-20 minutes, until the edges begin to brown. Allow the cookies to cool to room temperature.

Dust the cut out cookies with icing sugar and spread raspberry jam on each solid cookie. Sandwich your cookies together and serve.

Cheat's Raspberry Tiramisu

SERVES 2

PREP + COOK TIME: 30 MINS

3⅔ cups (450g) frozen raspberries
⅓ cup (100ml) rosé wine
4 tbsps caster sugar
2¼ cups (500g) mascarpone
2 oranges, zested
2½ cups (600ml) double cream
18 pink savoiardi or sponge fingers
Cocoa powder for dusting
2 cups (250g) fresh raspberries
Icing sugar for dusting

Place the frozen raspberries into a saucepan with the rosé and 2 tablespoons caster sugar, and heat over medium-low heat for 3-4 minutes until the raspberries are defrosted and the sugar is dissolved. Push half of the mixture through a sieve into a bowl to make a raspberry puree. Set both the bowl and the pan aside.

Whisk the mascarpone with the orange zest and remaining 2 tablespoon of caster sugar. Whisk the double cream until soft peaks form then fold into the mascarpone.

Dip the sponge fingers into the pureed raspberries, then arrange three sponge fingers each on two small plates.

Dollop some of the cream mixture over the top of the fingers, then top with cooked raspberry mixture from the pan.

Repeat two more layers of sponge fingers, mascarpone cream and raspberries, placing each layer of sponge fingers perpendicular to the one below. Dust with cocoa powder, decorate with fresh raspberries, then dust with icing sugar to serve.

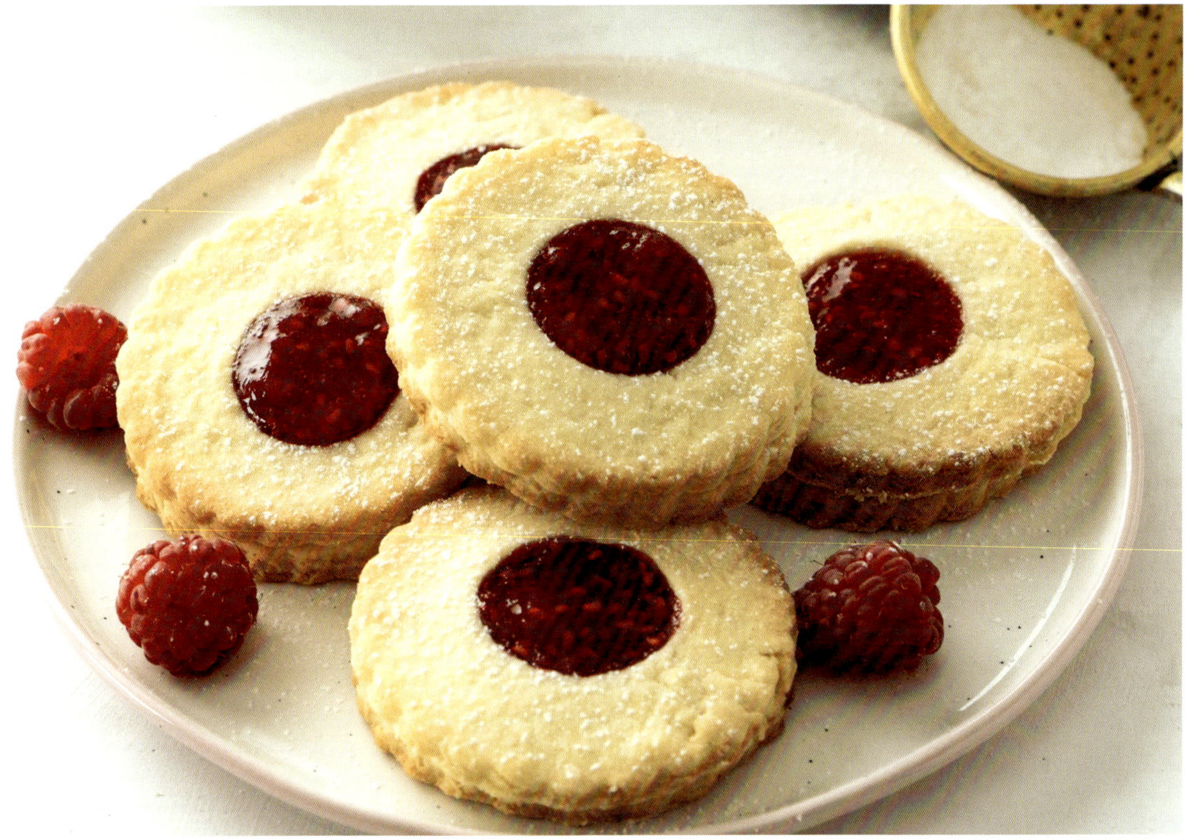

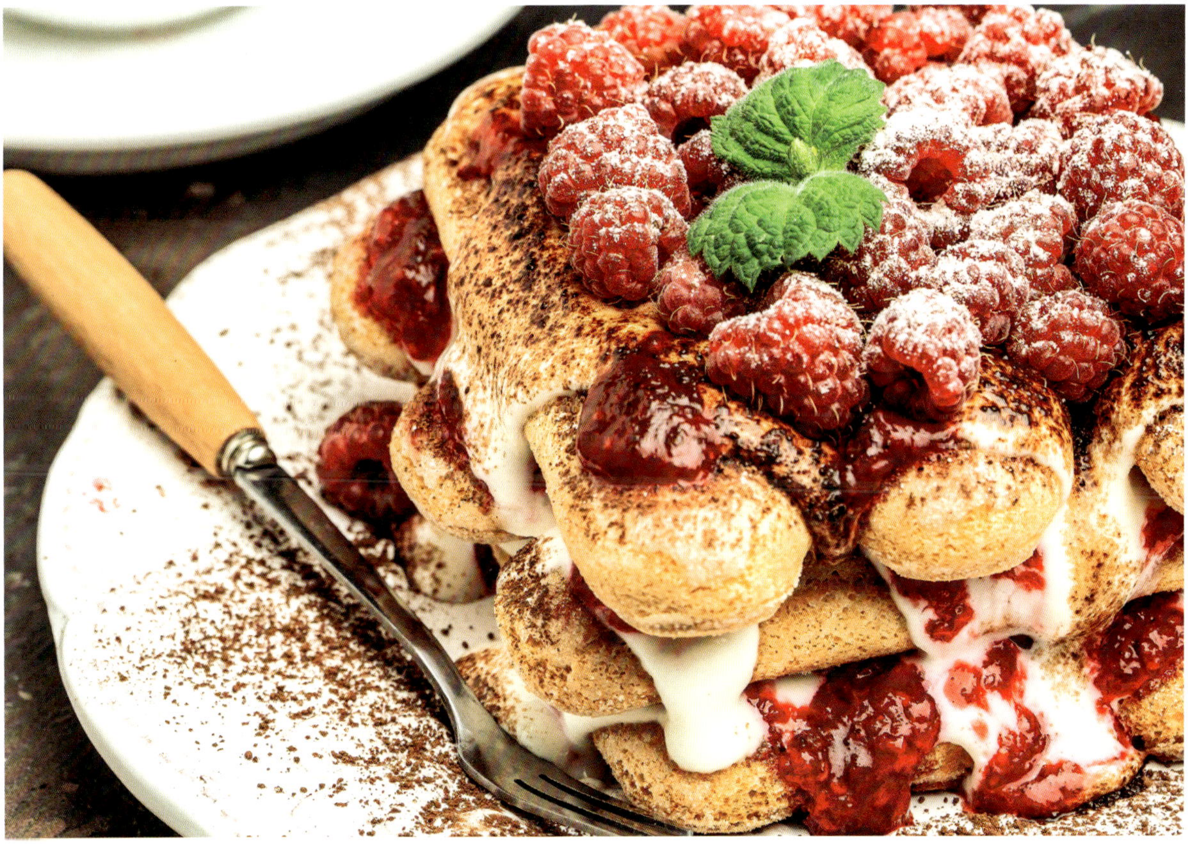

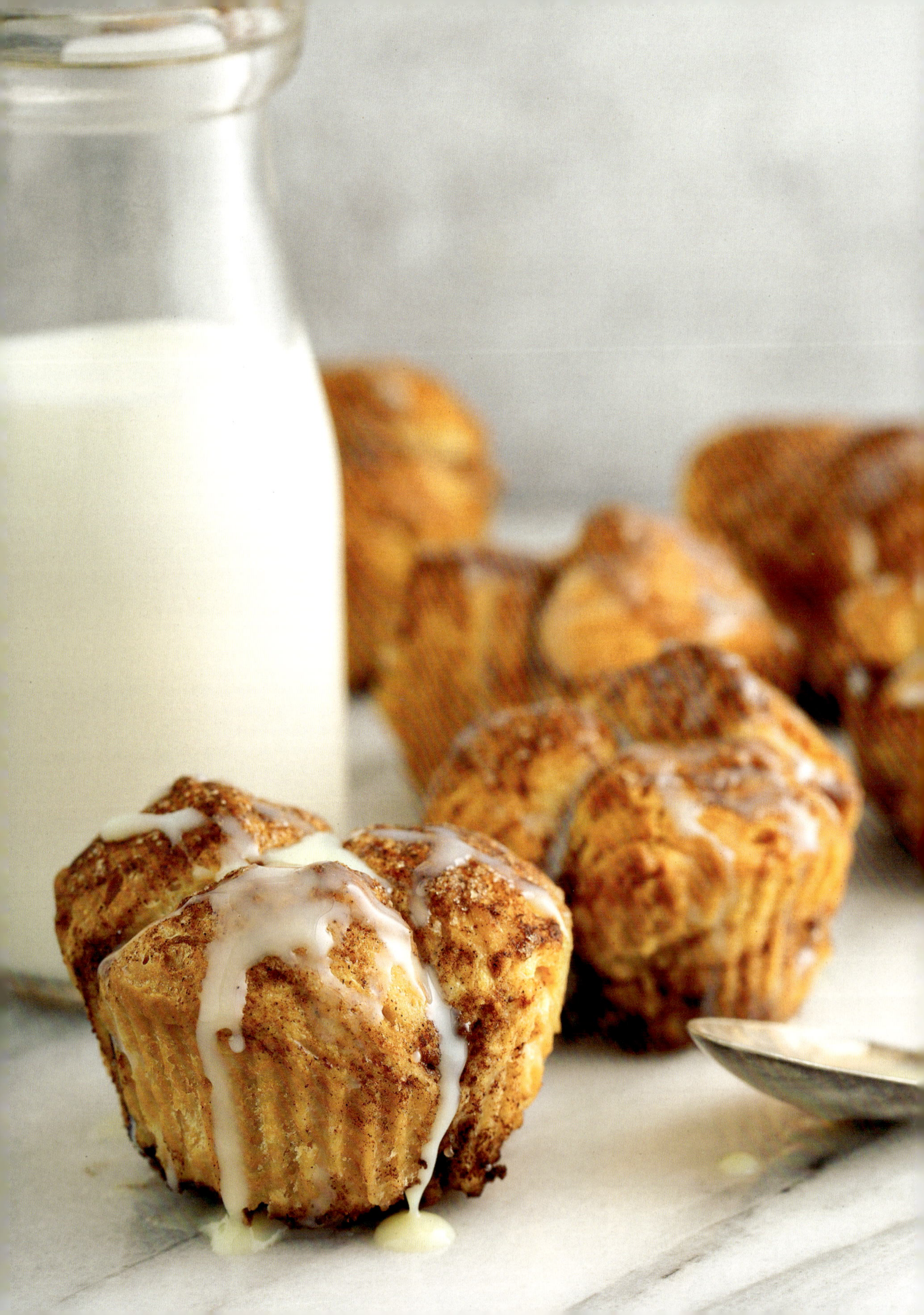

Monkey Bread Muffins

MAKES 12
PREP + COOK TIME:

2 cups (250g) + 2 tbsps flour
½ cup (110g) + 3 tbsps sugar
1 tbsp baking powder
½ tsp salt
⅓ cup (80ml) milk
½ cup (125ml) buttermilk
⅓ cup (85g) + 6 tbsps butter, melted
¾ cup (150g) firmly packed brown sugar
2 tsps cinnamon
Simple glaze (see next recipe)

Preheat oven to 175°C. Grease a 12-hole muffin tin.

Add all the flour, 3 tablespoons of sugar, baking powder and salt to a medium bowl. Stir to combine. Add the milk, buttermilk and ⅓ cup melted butter. Stir with a fork until just combined.

Add the remaining ½ cup of sugar to another bowl. Drop the dough 1 teaspoon at a time into the sugar. When you have about 12 dough balls shake to roll and coat the dough in the sugar. Place a dough balls into each muffin cup. Repeat with the remaining dough, filling the muffin cups with dough balls.

In a small bowl mix together the 6 tablespoons melted butter, brown sugar and cinnamon. Spoon 1 tablespoon of the mixture over each of the muffins.

Bake for 18-22 minutes until golden brown. Remove from the oven and wait for 5 minutes before removing the muffins from the pan with a fork.

Drizzle the glaze over the top with a small spoon.

Serve while still warm.

Simple Glaze

MAKES ENOUGH FOR 12 MUFFINS
PREP + COOK TIME: 5 MINS
GLUTEN FREE

½ cup (80g) icing sugar
1 tsp milk

Place icing sugar and milk in a small bowl. Mix well until smooth and pourable.

Drizzle over muffins to serve.

Chocolate Chip Cookies

MAKES 15
PREP + COOK TIME: 35 MINS

150g butter, room temperature
½ cup (100g) caster sugar
½ cup (110g) packed brown sugar
1 tsp vanilla extract
1 egg
1¾ cups (215g) plain flour
½ cup (85g) dark chocolate chips
½ cup (85g) milk chocolate chips

Preheat oven to 180°C. Line two baking trays with greaseproof paper.

Cream together butter, sugars and vanilla with an electric hand mixer for 1-2 minutes until light and fluffy. Add egg and beat to combine. Add the flour in two batches, beating after each addition. Add the dark and milk choc chips and mix thoroughly.

Measure level tablespoons of the dough. Roll into balls and place evenly spaced on prepared trays. Press down slightly on each ball.

Bake for 15 minutes or until golden. Remove from the oven and transfer to a wire rack to cool.

Highlander Shortbread

MAKES 18
PREP + COOK TIME: 1 HOUR

⅓ cup (75g) caster sugar
150g salted butter, room temperature
1⅔ cups (200g) plain flour
2 tbsps cornflour
100g demerara sugar

Preheat oven to 160°C. Grease two baking trays with butter.

In a large bowl, cream together the caster sugar and butter with an electric hand mixer until light and fluffy. Sift in the flour and cornflour and mix with a wooden spoon to form a stiff dough. Tip the dough onto a lightly floured work surface and gently knead until smooth.

Roll your dough into a ball then shape into a long sausage about 5cm in diameter. Wrap in plastic wrap and transfer to the fridge for 30 minutes to firm up.

Sprinkle the demerara sugar onto an ungreased baking tray. Roll the sausage-shaped dough in the sugar, ensuring it is completely coated all over.

Cut the sugar-coated dough into circles around 1cm thick and transfer to your pre-greased baking trays.

Bake for around 10-15 minutes until the tops are lightly golden.

Remove from the oven and leave to cool on the tray for around 10 minutes, before transferring to a wire rack to cool completely.

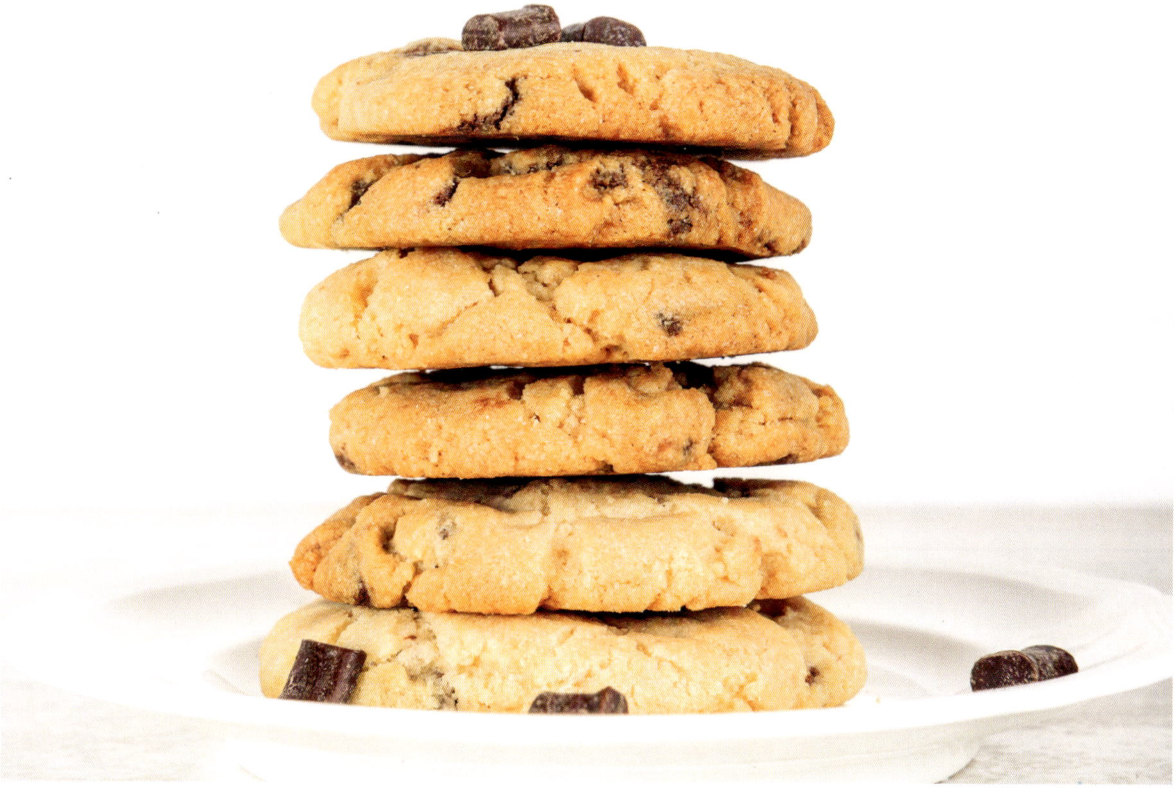

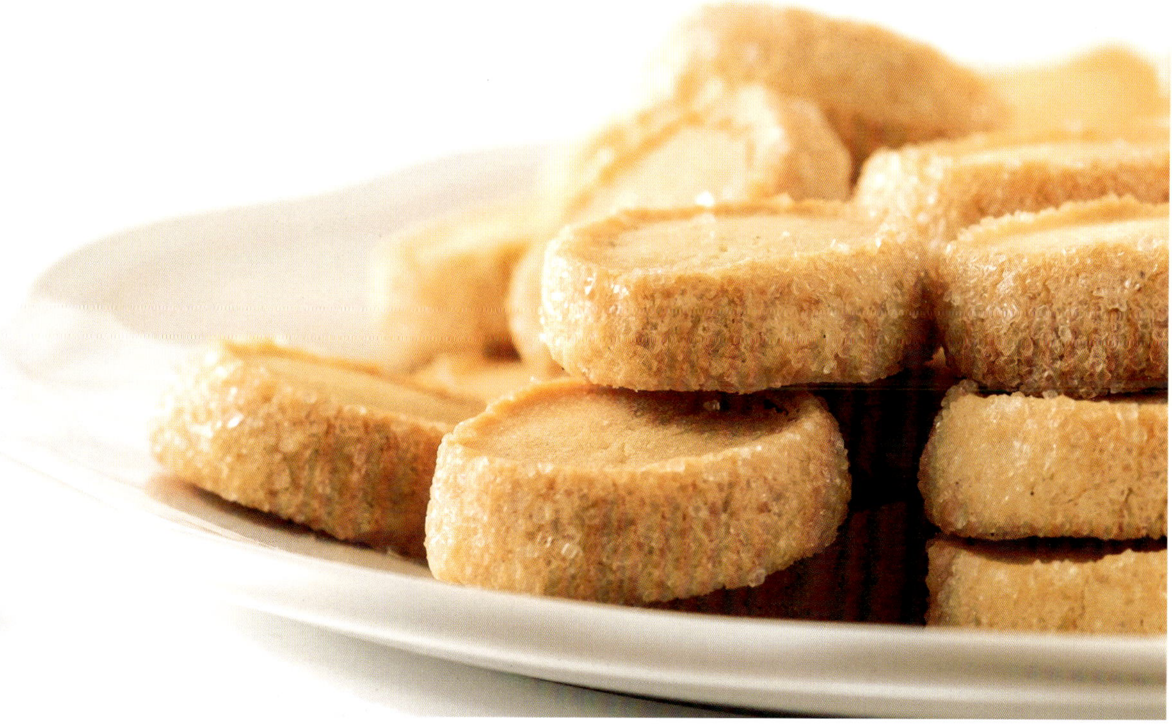

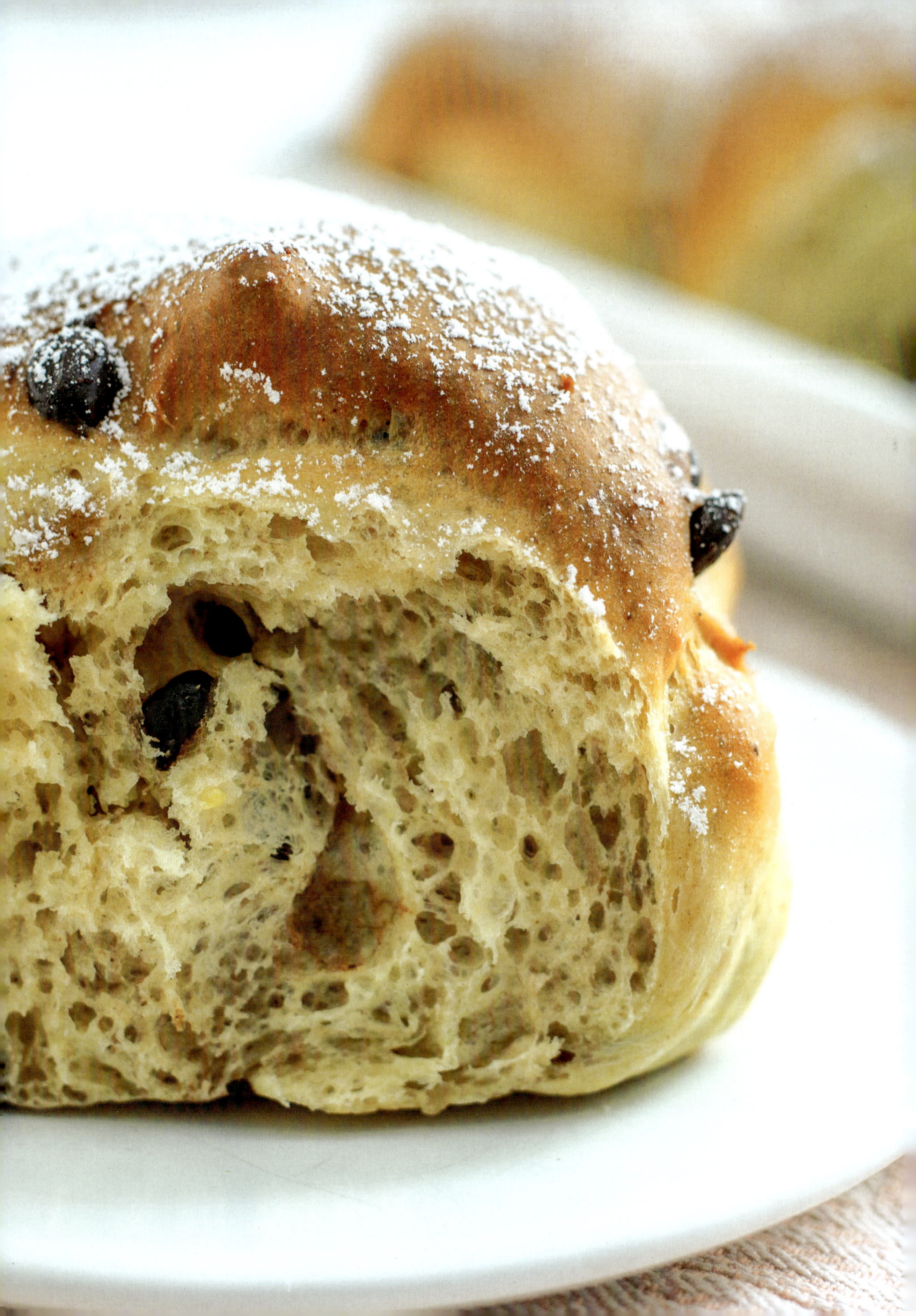

Chocolate Chip Buchteln

MAKES 15
PREP + COOK TIME: 2 HOURS 50 MINS

1 cup (250ml) milk
4 cups (500g) plain flour
¼ cup (50g) sugar
10g instant yeast
60g butter, softened
1 egg + 1 egg yolk
1 tsp vanilla extract
1¼ cups (200g) dark chocolate chips
Icing sugar for dusting

Heat the milk until it is just lukewarm.

Add flour and sugar to a large bowl and whisk together. Make a well in the centre and pour in the yeast and then the milk. Stir the yeast and milk together, then cover the bowl and set aside somewhere warm for 10 minutes.

After 10 minutes stir to combine the milk mixture with the flour and sugar.

Add the butter, egg, egg yolk and vanilla extract. Mix in an electric mixer with a dough hook on low speed for 10 minutes or until the dough is a smooth.

Transfer to a greased bowl and cover with a tea towel. Set aside somewhere warm to rest for 30 minutes.

After 30 minutes, add in the chocolate chips and knead by hand until the chocolate chips are dispersed throughout the dough.

Preheat oven to 175°C. Grease a 23 x 33cm rectangular baking tin.

Divide the dough into 15 equal pieces. Shape each piece of dough into a ball. Place each ball into the greased tin. Cover the tin with a tea towel and place somewhere warm for another 30 minutes.

After the 30 minutes bake the buns for 20-25 minutes until deep golden brown. Dust with icing sugar and serve warm.

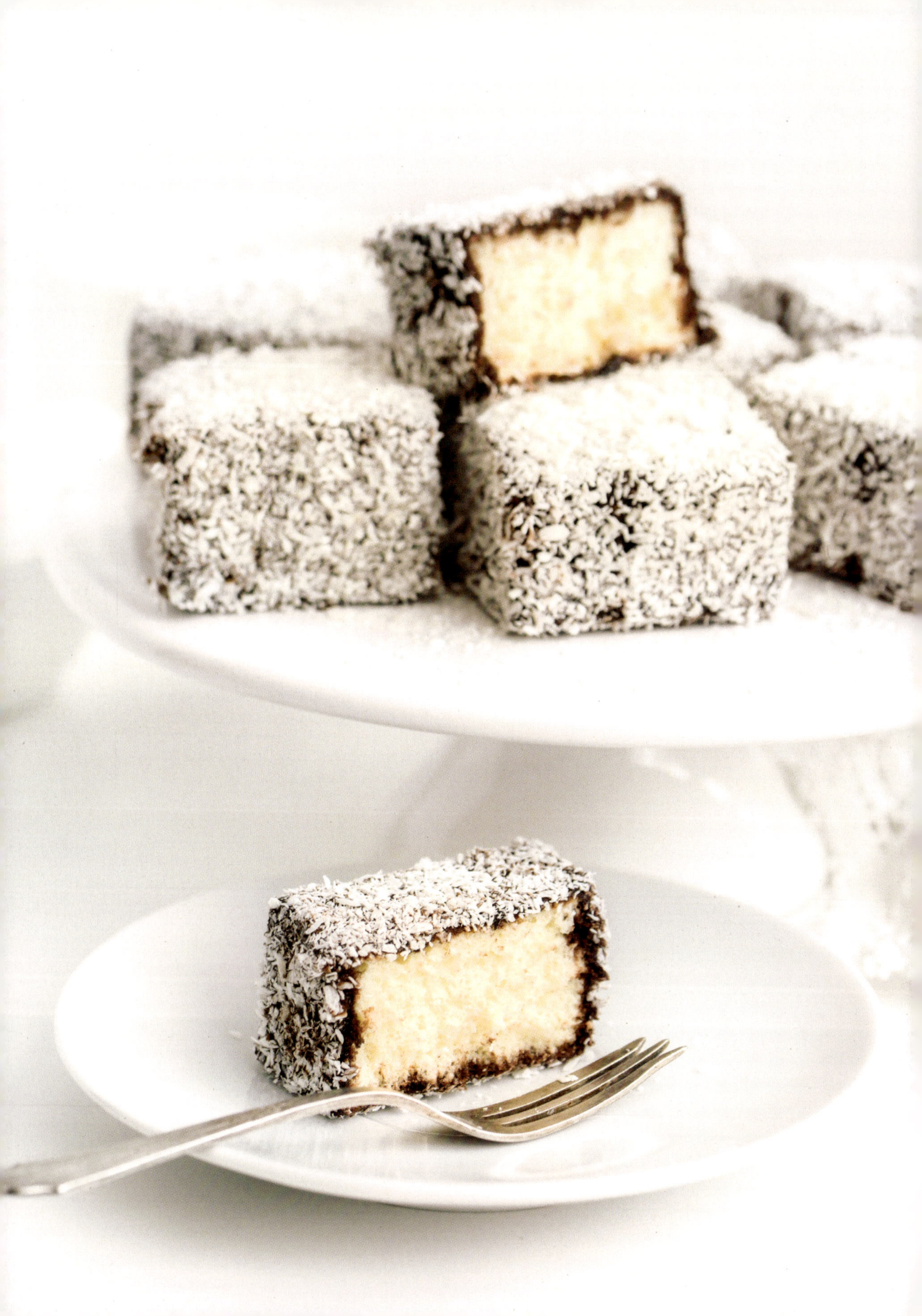

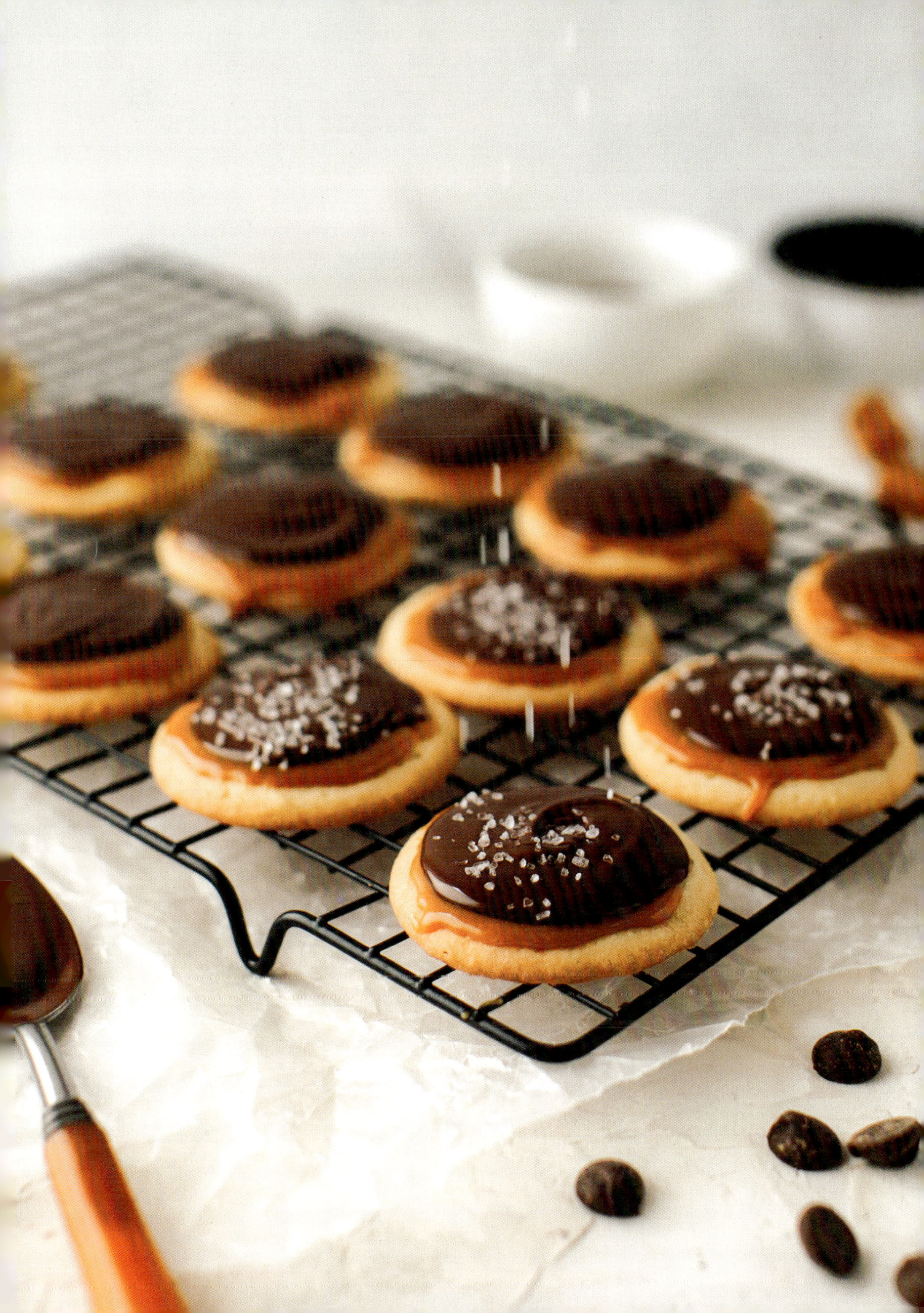

Lamingtons

MAKES 25
PREP + COOK TIME: 1 HOUR 10 MINS + COOLING

CAKE
1½ cups (185g) plain flour
2 tsps baking powder
¼ cup (40g) cornflour
200g butter, softened
1 cup (230g) caster sugar
2 tsps vanilla extract
3 eggs
½ cup (125ml) milk

ICING
1 tbsp unsalted butter
200g dark chocolate (70% cocoa content)
3¼ cups (500g) icing sugar, sifted
½ cup (125ml) milk
3⅔ cups (325g) desiccated coconut

Preheat the oven to 180°C. Grease and line an 18 x 30cm cake tin with greaseproof paper.

Sift the flour, baking powder and cornflour into a large bowl. Add the butter, sugar, vanilla, eggs and milk. Beat with an electric hand mixer on low until all of the ingredients are incorporated. Beat on high until the mixture is thick and pale. Pour into the prepared baking tin and bake for 30-35 minutes, or until a skewer inserted into the centre comes out clean.

Leave the cake in the tin for 5 minutes before turning out onto a wire rack to cool completely. Cut the sponge into about 25 squares.

Melt the butter and chocolate in a heatproof bowl over a pan of simmering water. Add the icing sugar and milk and whisk to combine.

Place coconut in a shallow dish.

Using two forks dip each square of sponge in the chocolate icing, then roll in the coconut. Transfer to a wire rack to set for 1 hour before serving.

Sugar Biscuits

SERVES 40
PREP + COOK TIME: 35 MINS

225g unsalted butter, softened
1 cup (220g) caster sugar
1½ tsps vanilla extract
1 large egg
3 cups (450g) plain flour
¾ tsp baking powder
¾ tsp salt + more to serve
Caramel sauce to serve (see recipe on page 80)
Melted chocolate to serve

Preheat oven to 160°C. Line two baking trays.

Cream together butter and sugar. Add vanilla, egg, flour, baking powder and salt. Mix well. Turn out onto a floured surface and roll out to 3mm thickness. Cut out circles with a cookie cutter. Place on trays and bake for 10 minutes. When cool spread with caramel sauce and melted chocolate and sprinkle with salt.

Meringues

MAKES 18
PREP + COOK TIME: 2 HOURS 30 MINS
GLUTEN FREE • DAIRY FREE

4 egg whites
1 cup (225g) caster sugar
1 tsp vanilla extract
Grated dark chocolate to serve

Preheat oven to 120°C. Line two baking trays with greaseproof paper.

Whisk egg whites until stiff peaks form. Pour in half the sugar and vanilla at a time, whisking between each addition. Using two teaspoons, spoon meringue onto lined trays. Reduce the oven to 90°C. Bake for 1 hour 30 minutes. Turn oven off and leave meringues in the oven to cool completely. Top with grated chocolate to serve.

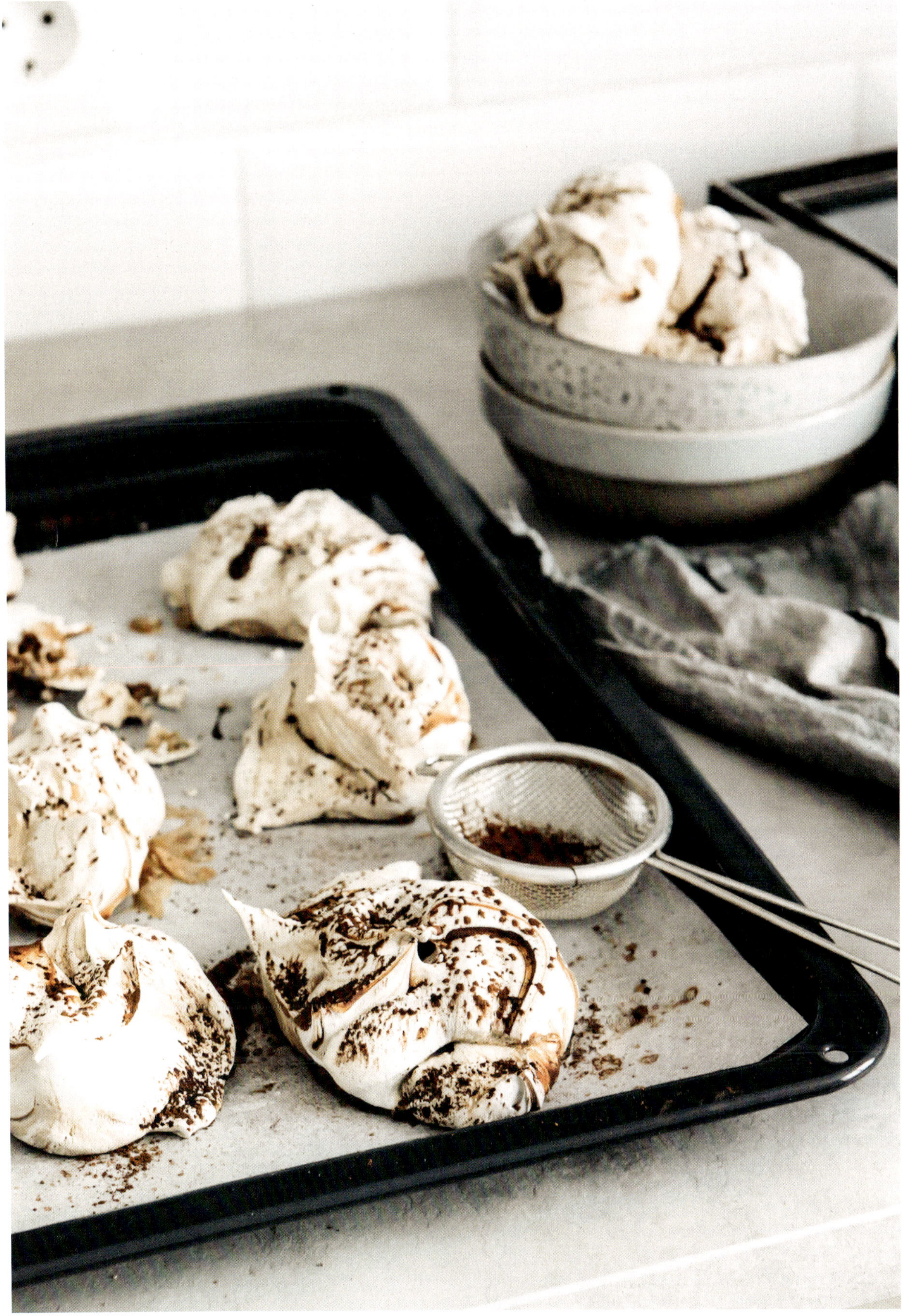

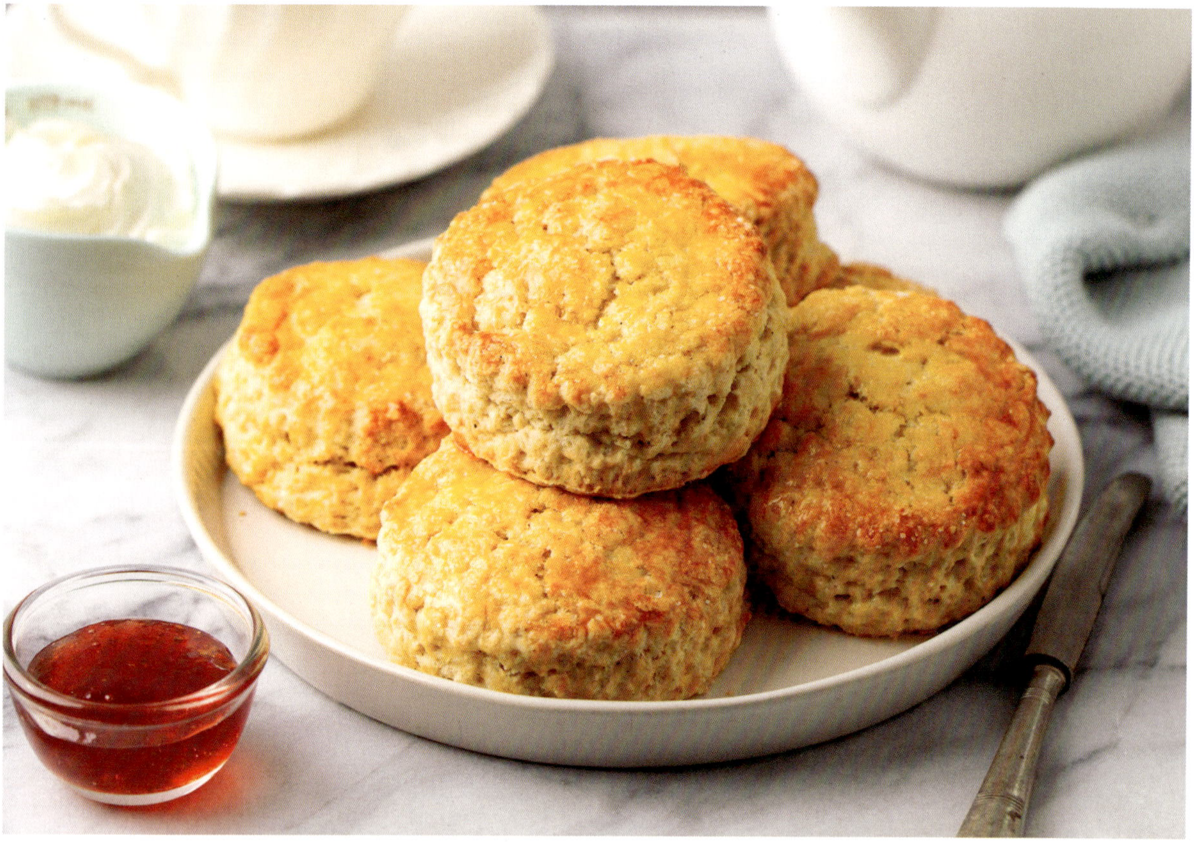

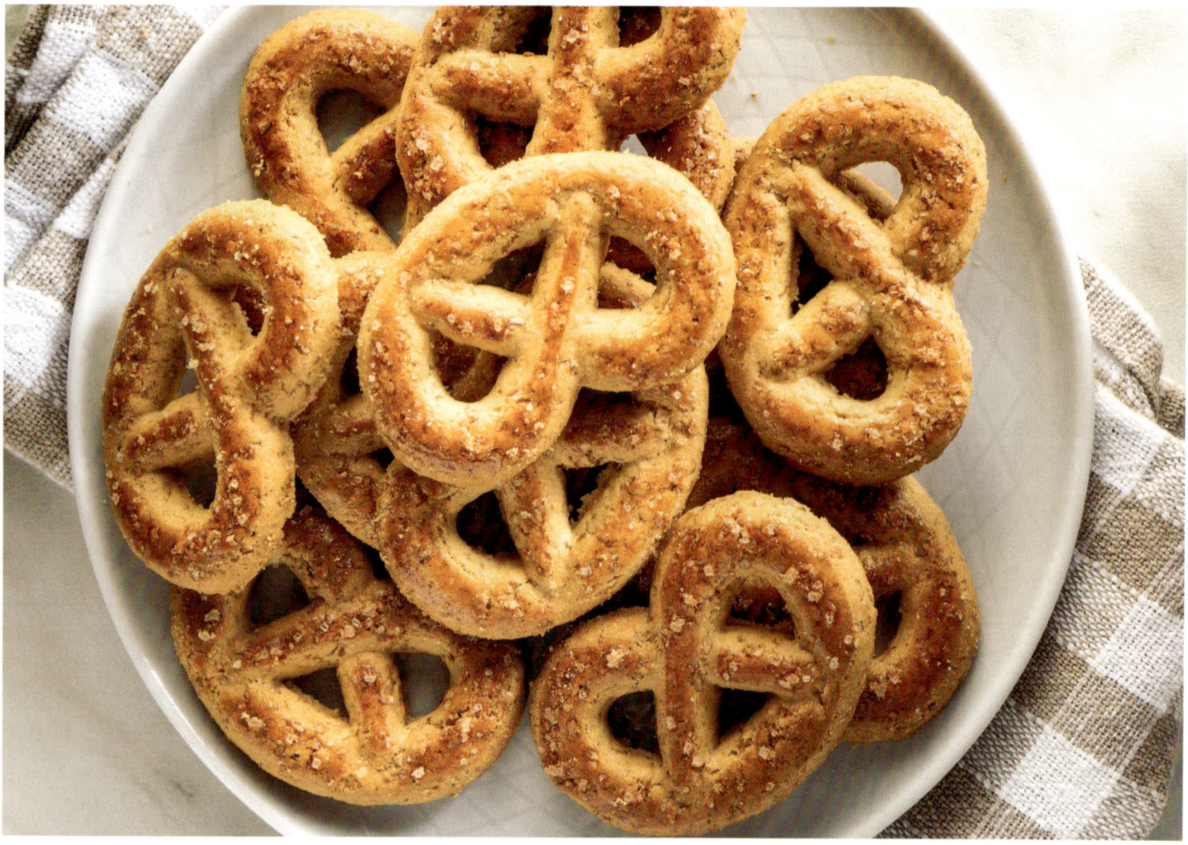

Scones

MAKES 16
PREP + COOK TIME: 35 MINS

3½ cups (435g) self-raising flour
Pinch of salt
60g butter, chilled, chopped
1¼ cups (310ml) milk, chilled
Jam and cream to serve

Preheat oven to 220°C. Dust a baking tray with flour.

Combine flour and salt in a bowl. Rub butter into flour using fingertips, until resembling fine breadcrumbs. Make a well in the centre and pour in 1 cup of milk. Stir with a metal spoon and add more milk as required to form a loose dough. Use hands to gently bring the dough together.

Turn dough onto a floured surface. Knead gently for 30 seconds or until just smooth. Roll dough to 2cm thickness. Cut out circles with a cutter, rerolling and cutting scraps. Place scones close together on the prepared tray. Brush with milk.

Bake for 20 minutes until risen and golden. Transfer to a wire rack to cool. Slice and serve with jam and cream.

Vanilla Pretzel Cookies

MAKES 60
PREP + COOK TIME: 1 HOUR

150g unsalted butter, room temperature
⅓ cup (70g) caster sugar
¼ tsp salt
1 tbsp vanilla bean paste
1 egg yolk
1½ cups (185g) plain flour
1 large egg white, lightly beaten with 1 tsp cold water
¼ cup (55g) sugar

Cream together the butter and caster sugar with an electric mixer until light and fluffy. Add salt, vanilla and egg yolk and beat to combine. Add the flour and mix to incorporate.

Divide the dough in half and roll each piece into a 15cm-long log. Wrap each log in greaseproof paper and twist the ends to seal. Chill the dough for 30 minutes.

Preheat oven to 175°C. Line two baking trays with greaseproof paper.

Using a large knife, slice the dough into 12cm-thick discs. Roll each disc of dough into a 15cm-long rope. Form each rope into the pretzel shape and place 5cm apart on the prepared baking tray. Using a pastry brush, gently brush the egg white mixture over the tops of each cookie, then sprinkle with the sugar.

Bake for 15 minutes until golden brown. Cool the cookies on the baking tray for 5 minutes before transferring to a wire rack to cool completely.

2

Chocolate

Brownie Biscuit Slice

MAKES 16
PREP + COOK TIME: 1 HOUR

BISCUIT BASE

1¼ cups (155g) plain flour
½ cup (110g) firmly packed brown sugar,
125g butter, melted

BROWNIE

150g dark chocolate, chopped
150g butter, chopped
1 cup (220g) caster sugar
2 eggs, lightly beaten
⅓ cup (40g) plain flour
2 tbsps self-raising flour
¼ cup (30g) cocoa powder
⅓ cup (40g) chopped pecans
⅓ cup (100g) caramel sauce to serve (see recipe on page 80)

Preheat oven to 160°C. Grease and line a 20 x 30cm baking tin with greaseproof paper, extending paper 2cm above edges.

To make the base, combine flour and sugar in a medium bowl. Stir in butter. Press evenly over base of pan.

Bake for 10-12 minutes, or until golden. Set aside to cool.

To make brownie, place chocolate and butter in a large, heatproof bowl over a pan of simmering water. Stir until melted and smooth.

Remove bowl from the heat. Stir in sugar, then eggs until fully combined. Sift in flours and cocoa. Stir until combined. Fold in chopped pecans. Pour mixture over cooked base.

Bake for 30-35 minutes, or until just firm to touch. Cool in pan.

Lift slice from the pan, cut into squares and drizzle with caramel sauce.

Chocolate Meringue Cookies

MAKES 18-20
PREP + COOK TIME: 30 MINS
GLUTEN FREE

170g dark chocolate
2 large egg whites, at room temperature
⅛ tsp cream of tartar
½ tsp vanilla extract
Pinch of salt
¼ cup (55g) sugar
½ cup (80g) milk chocolate chips

Set two oven racks in the middle positions and preheat the oven to 175°C. Line two baking trays with greaseproof paper.

Break the chocolate into small pieces and place in a heatproof bowl over a pan of simmering water. Heat gently, stirring, until the chocolate is melted. Remove from heat and set aside.

In a large bowl, using an electric hand mixer, beat the egg whites with the cream of tartar, vanilla and salt until soft peaks form. Gradually add the sugar, continuing to beat until stiff peaks form. Pour the warm chocolate and chocolate chips into the bowl and fold with a spatula until just combined.

Drop heaping tablespoons of the batter about 3cm apart on the prepared baking trays. Bake for 8-10 minutes, or until the cookies look dry on the surface but are still very gooey inside when pressed. Allow to cool for 5 minutes on the baking trays before transferring to a wire rack to cool completely.

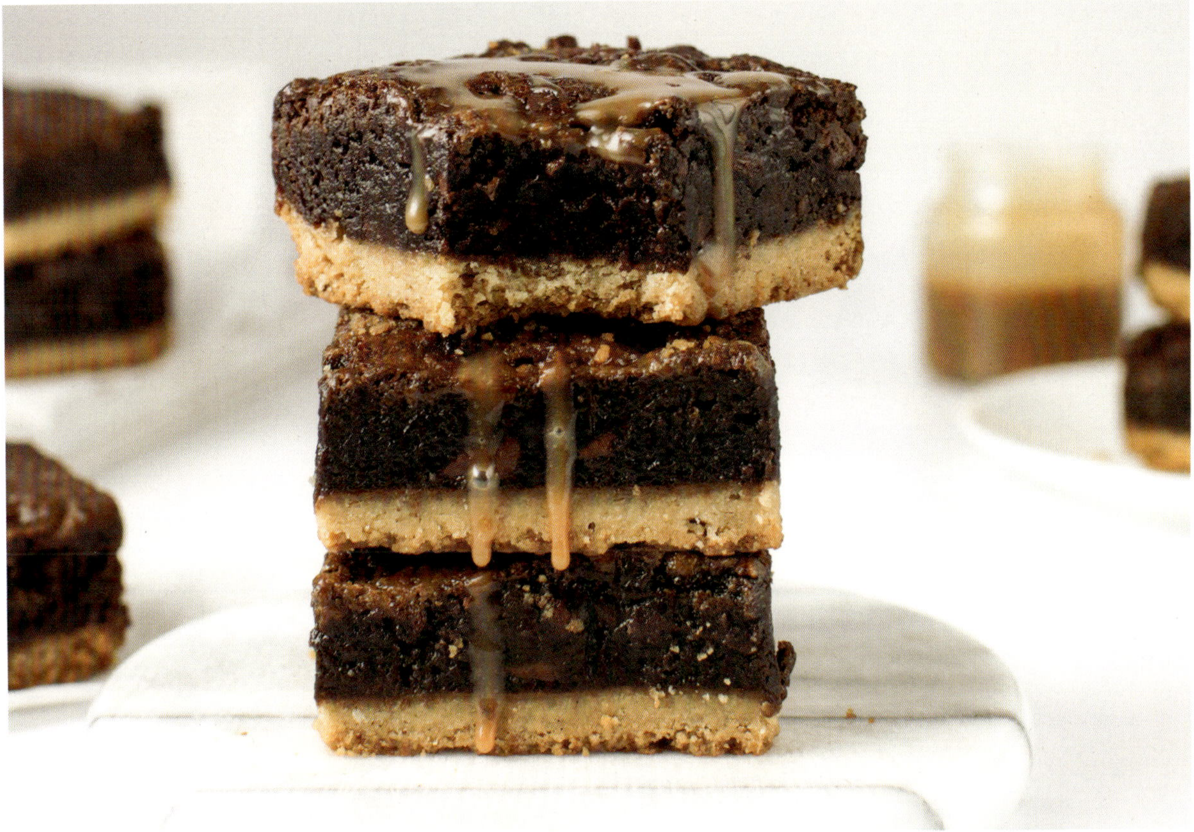

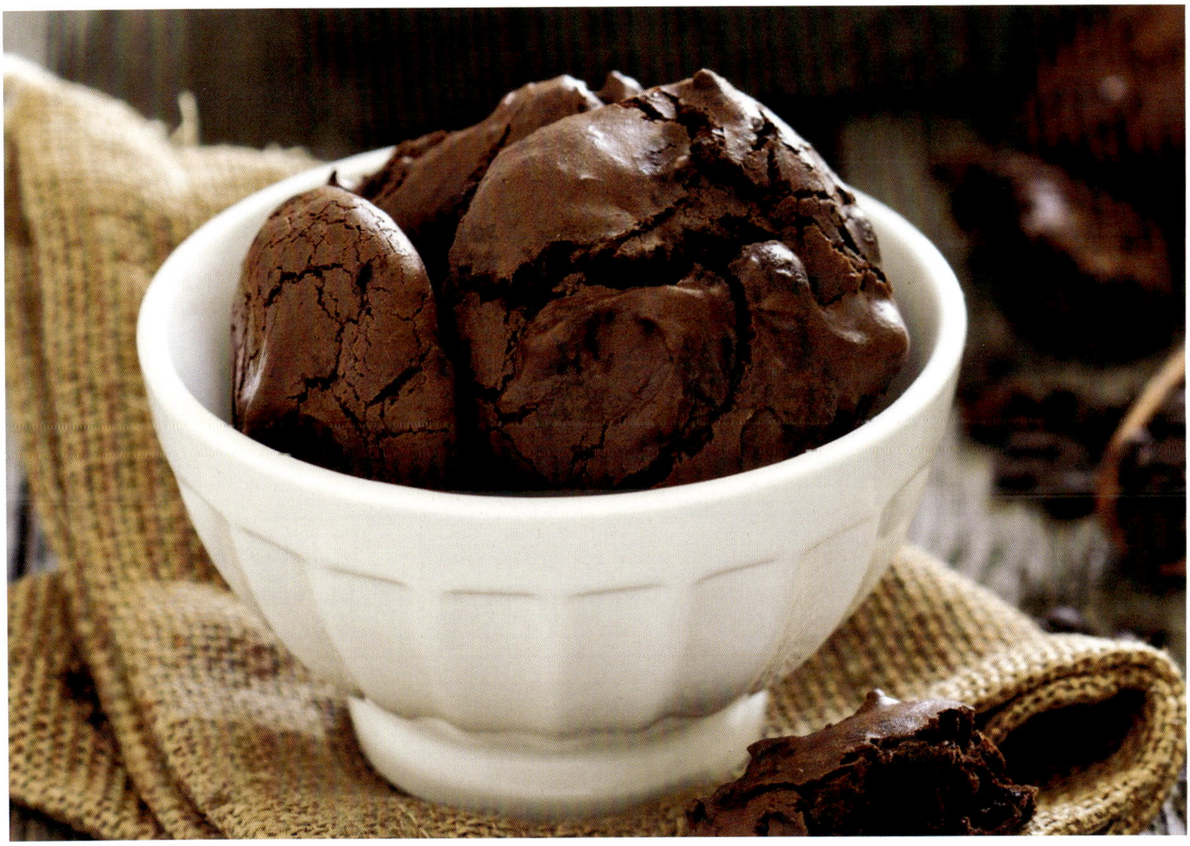

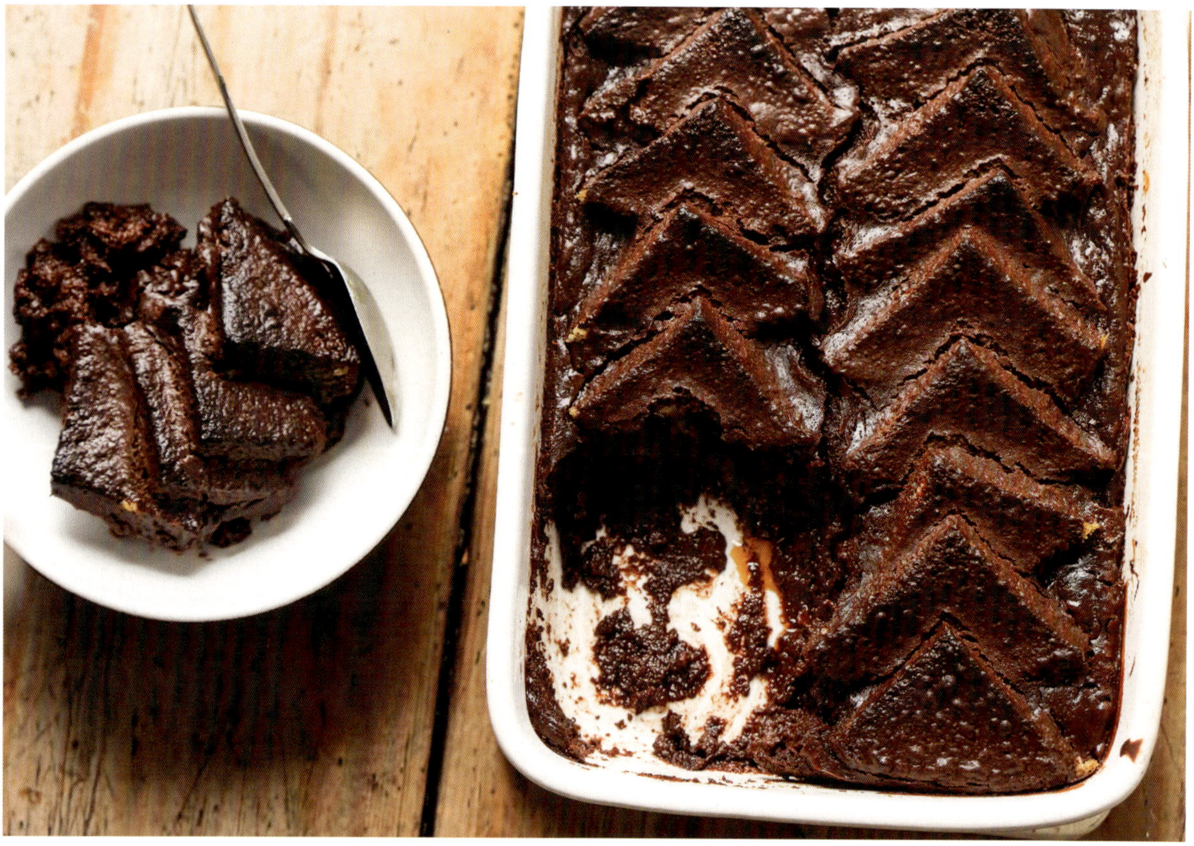

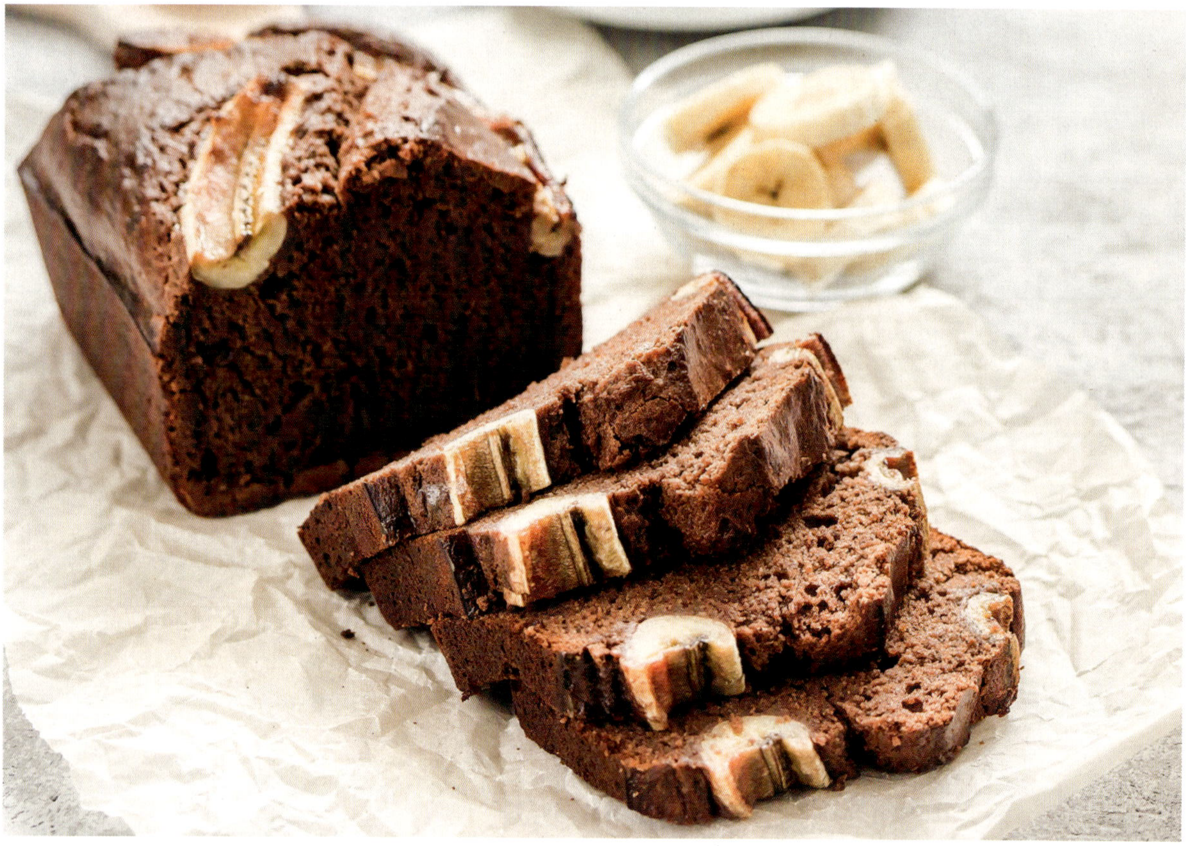

Chocolate Bread & Butter Pudding

SERVES 6
PREP + COOK TIME: 1 HOUR

1 large loaf bread, cut into 5mm-thick slices
150g dark chocolate, chopped
1⅔ cups (425ml) thickened cream
4 tbsps dark rum
½ cup (110g) caster sugar
75g butter
Pinch of cinnamon
1 tsp vanilla extract
3 large eggs

Preheat oven to 180°C.

Remove crusts from the bread and cut each slice into four triangles.

Place the chocolate, cream, rum, sugar, butter, cinnamon and vanilla in a heatproof bowl set over a pan of gently simmering water. Stir until the chocolate and butter are melted. Remove from the heat.

In a separate bowl, whisk the eggs, then pour in chocolate mixture. Whisk to combine.

Spoon a thin layer of the chocolate mixture into the base of a rectangular baking dish, then arrange the bread triangles over the chocolate in two layers of overlapping rows. Pour the remaining chocolate mixture all over the bread. Allow to stand for 15 minutes then transfer to the oven.

Bake for 30-35 minutes until crunchy on top and soft inside.

Chocolate Banana Bread

SERVES 10
PREP + COOK TIME: 1 HOUR 15 MINS

1 cup (125g) plain flour
½ cup (60g) cocoa powder
1 tsp bicarbonate of soda
½ tsp salt
4 large, very ripe bananas
60g unsalted butter, melted and slightly cooled
¼ cup (60ml) light olive oil or melted coconut oil
¾ cup (165g) packed light brown sugar
1 large egg, room temperature
1 tsp vanilla extract
½ cup (80g) chocolate chips

Preheat oven to 175°C. Grease a 23cm loaf tin.

In a medium bowl, whisk together the flour, cocoa powder, bicarb and salt. Set aside.

In a large bowl, mash three of the bananas with a fork. Add the melted butter and oil and stir to combine. Mix in the brown sugar, egg and vanilla extract. Stir the dry ingredients into the wet ingredients until just combined. Fold in the chocolate chips. Pour batter into prepared pan. Slice the remaining banana lengthwise and place on top of the bread.

Bake for 50-65 minutes, or until a skewer inserted into the centre comes out mostly clean.

Allow to cool in the tin for 15 minutes before turning out onto a wire rack to cool completely. Cut into slices and serve.

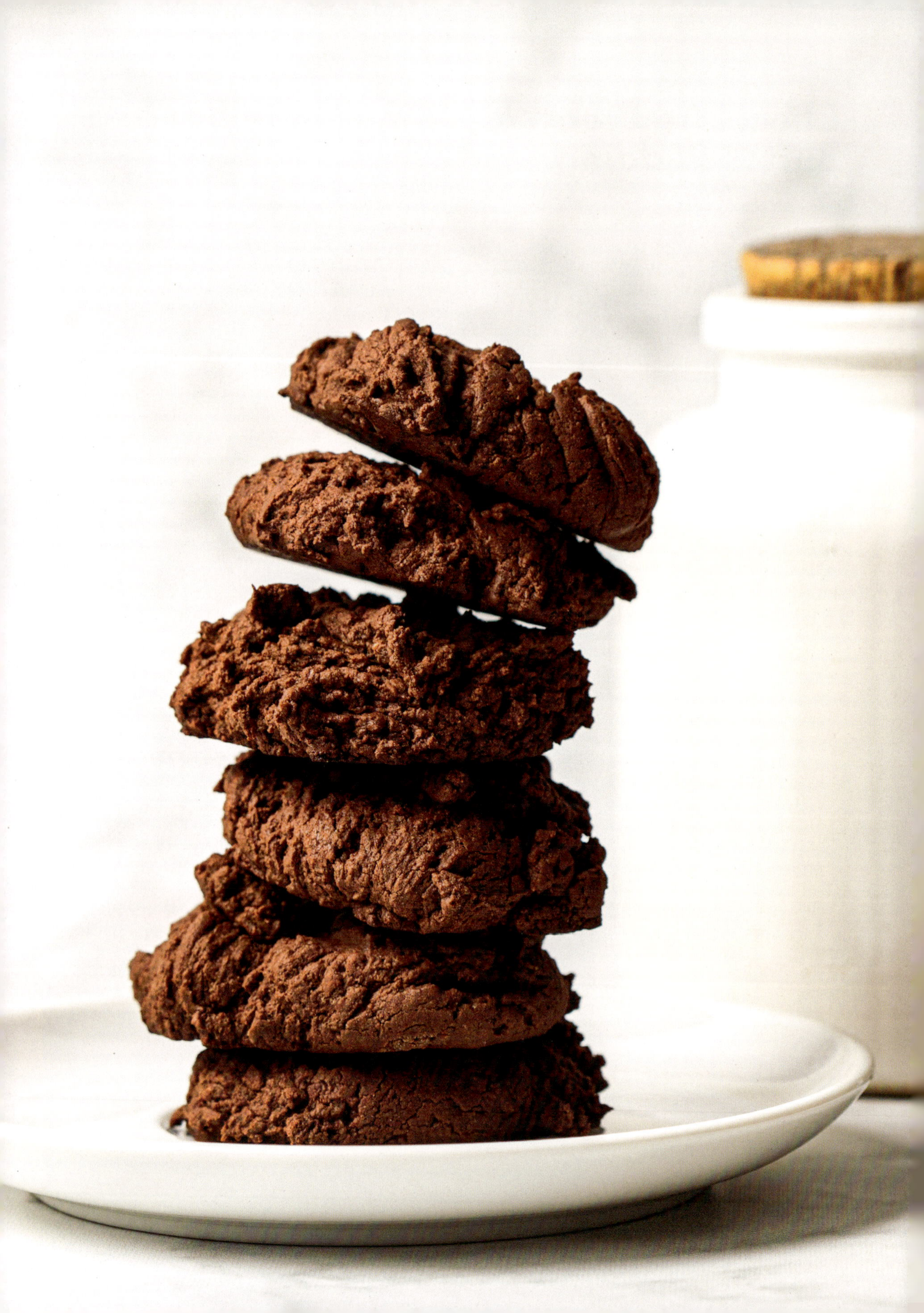

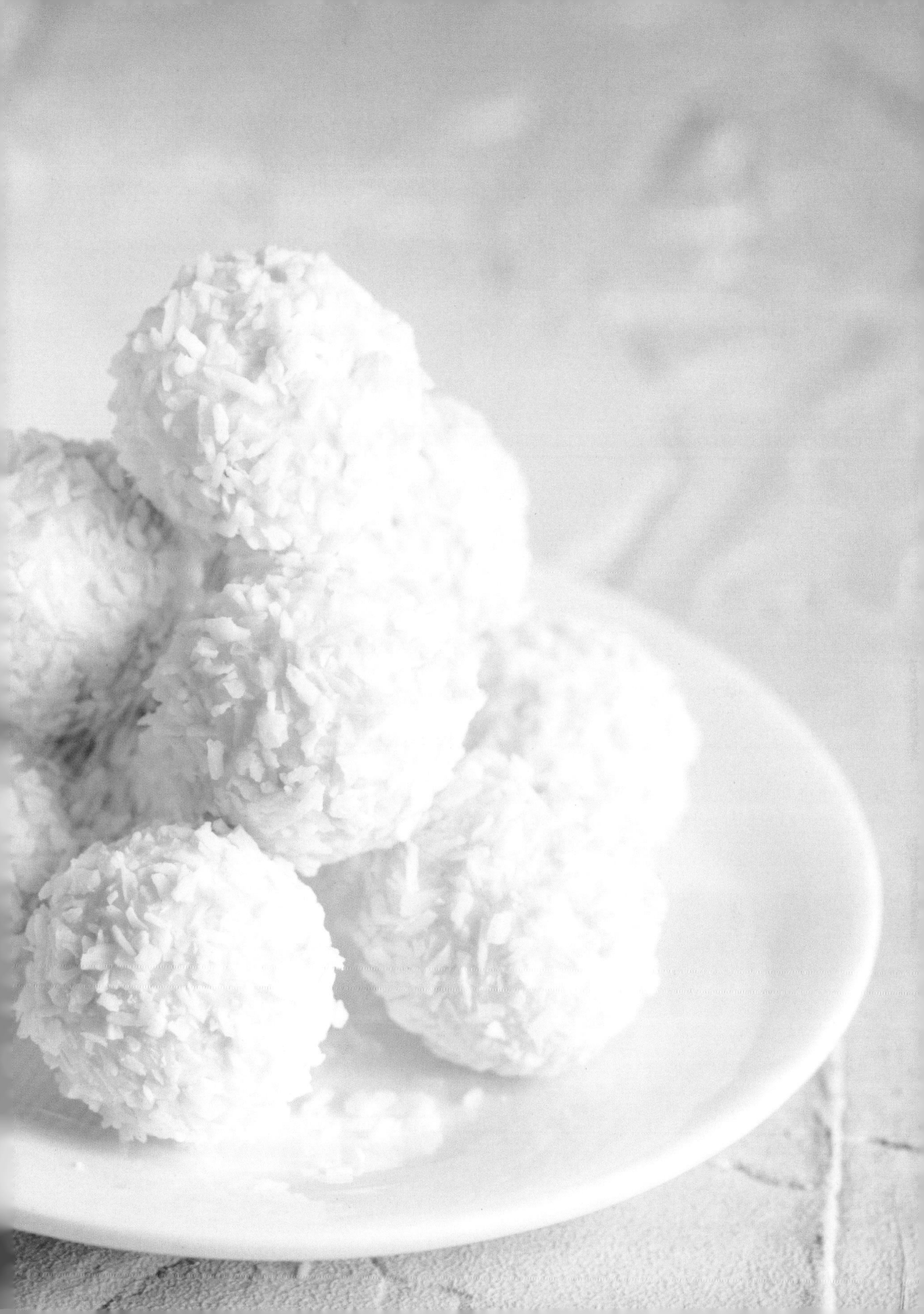

Double Choc Chip Cookies

MAKES 12
PREP + COOK TIME: 35 MINS

125g butter, room temperature
½ cup (100g) caster sugar
½ cup (80g) brown sugar
1 egg
1 tsp vanilla extract
1½ cups (185g) self-raising flour
½ cup (60g) cocoa powder
¾ cup (130g) dark chocolate chips

Preheat oven to 160°C and line two baking trays with greaseproof paper.

Cream together butter and sugars with an electric hand mixer until light and fluffy. Add egg and vanilla and whisk to combine. Stir in flour and cocoa then fold through chocolate chips.

Measure level tablespoons, rolling into balls and placing on prepared trays approximately 3cm apart. Press down slightly on each ball.

Bake for 15 minutes or until golden brown. When cooked, remove from the oven and transfer to a wire rack to cool.

Snowballs

MAKES 20
PREP + COOK TIME: 20 MINS + CHILLING
GLUTEN FREE

200g white chocolate, coarsely chopped
¼ cup (60ml) thickened cream
¼ cup (20g) + ⅓ cup (30g) shredded coconut
½ tsp vanilla extract

Place chocolate and cream in a medium, heatproof bowl set over a saucepan of simmering water. Stir until melted. Remove from heat and stir in ¼ cup shredded coconut and vanilla extract. Cover the bowl and refrigerate for 4 hours or until firm. Scoop mixture into balls. Roll in remaining coconut and refrigerate until firm.

Chocolate Caramel Popcorn

SERVES 8
PREP + COOK TIME: 40 MINS
GLUTEN FREE

16 cups (190g) plain popped popcorn
225g butter
1 cup (200g) light brown sugar
⅓ cup (115g) golden syrup
125g dark chocolate, melted

Preheat the oven to 150°C. Line a baking tray with greaseproof paper. Arrange popcorn on the tray.

In a small saucepan, melt butter and sugar together. Bring to a low boil and add the golden syrup. Boil for 4 minutes, stirring constantly. Pour caramel over popcorn. Bake in the oven for 30 minutes, stirring every 10 minutes. Pour melted chocolate over popcorn. Stir to coat then allow to harden before serving.

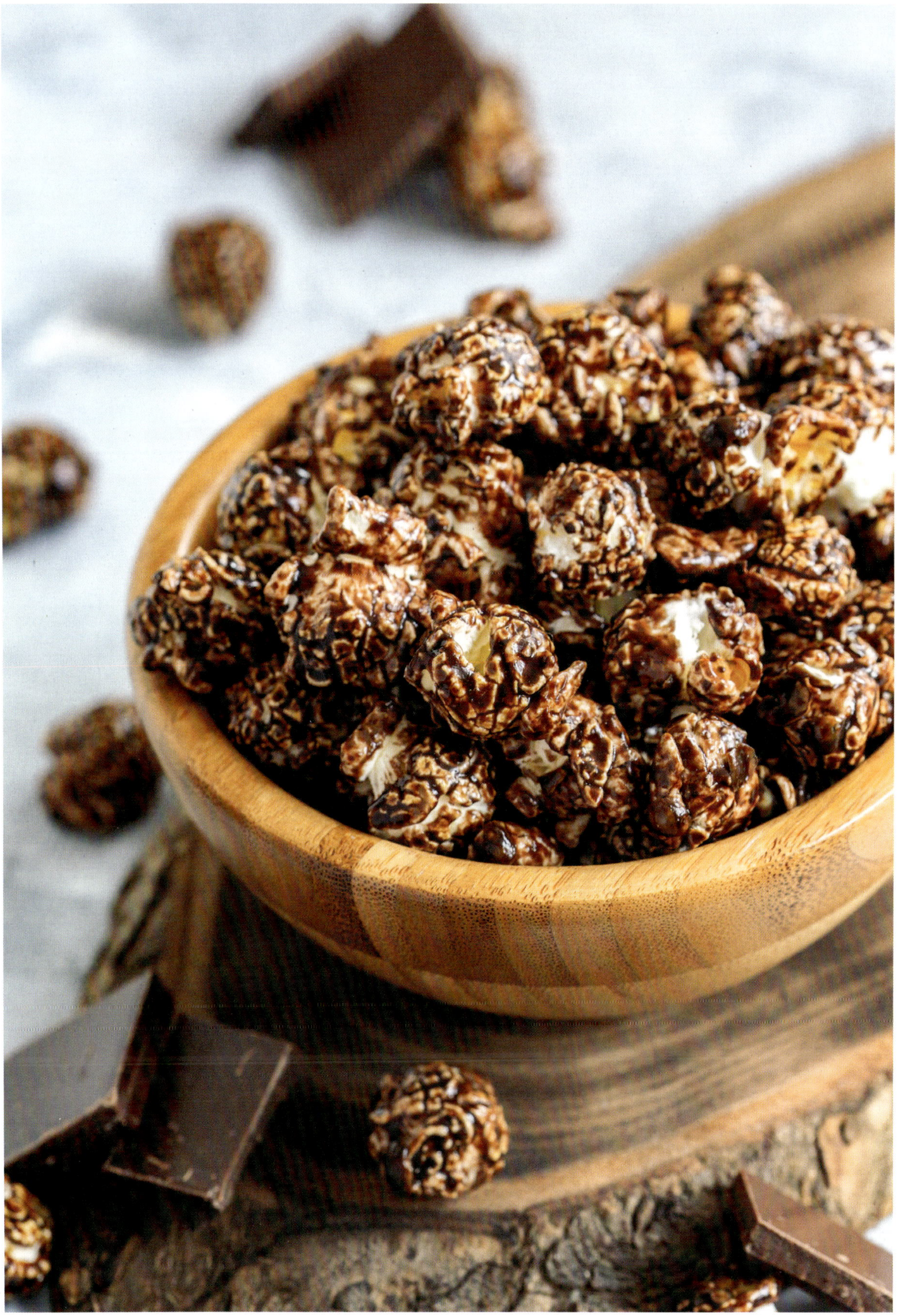

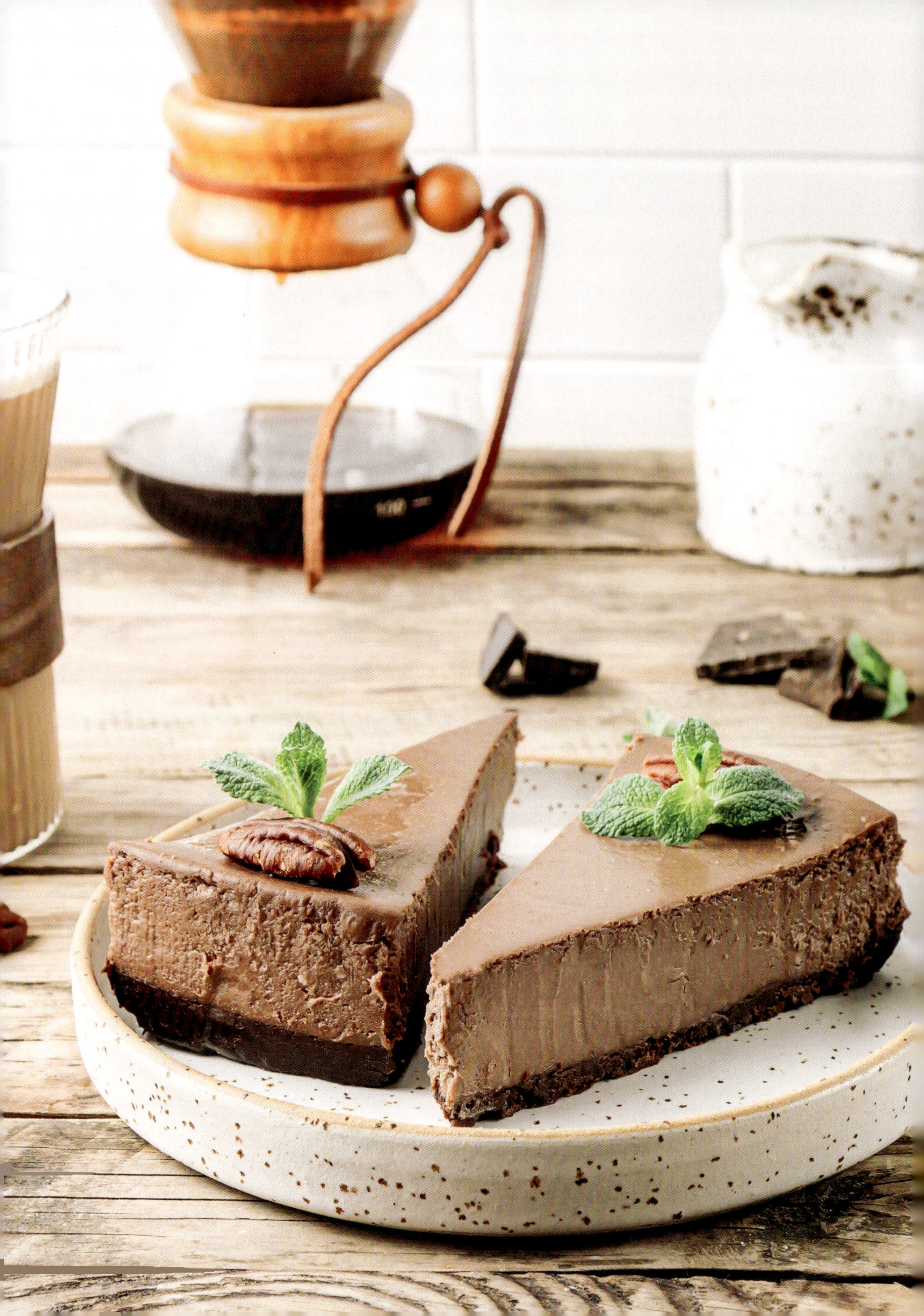

Chocolate Cheesecake

SERVES 12
PREP + COOK TIME: 1 HOUR 40 MINS + 4 HOURS COOLING AND CHILLING

BASE

160g butter

1 x 250g packet plain chocolate biscuits, roughly broken

½ tsp cinnamon

FILLING

270g dark chocolate, finely chopped

120g butter

¾ cup (165g) caster sugar

3 eggs

750g cream cheese, room temperature

2 tbsps cocoa powder

1 tsp vanilla extract

2½ cups (600ml) sour cream

12 pecan halves and mint sprigs to serve (optional)

Preheat oven to 160°C. Line a 23cm springform tin with greaseproof paper.

Melt the butter in a small pan over medium heat.

Place the biscuits, cinnamon and melted butter in the bowl of a food processor and process until well combined. Transfer to the prepared tin and press firmly with the back of a spoon. Cover with plastic wrap and put in the fridge to chill for 30 minutes.

Meanwhile, place the chocolate and butter in a heatproof bowl over a saucepan of simmering water and stir for 5 minutes or until just melted.

Using an electric beater, beat sugar and eggs in a large bowl until light and fluffy. Add the cream cheese and beat until well combined. Add chocolate mixture, cocoa powder and vanilla and gently fold the mixture together with a metal spoon. Add the sour cream and stir to combine.

Pour the mixture on top of the biscuit base and smooth the surface with a spatula. Bake for 1 hour or until just firm in the centre.

After 1 hour, turn off the oven but leave cake inside with door ajar, for 2 hours or until cooled completely.

Remove from the oven, cover with plastic wrap and place in fridge for 2 hours to chill.

Decorate with pecan halves and mint sprigs, if desired, before slicing and serving.

Sesame Chocolate Cookies

MAKES 24
PREP + COOK TIME: 20 MINS + 1 HOUR CHILLING
GLUTEN FREE • DAIRY FREE

1 egg
½ cup (115g) tahini
½ cup (155g) maple syrup
¾ cup (90g) almond meal
½ cup (60g) cocoa powder
¼ cup (40g) coconut sugar
½ tsp baking powder
½ tsp bicarbonate of soda
½ tsp salt
1 tsp vanilla extract
½ cup (80g) dark chocolate chips
¼ cup (40g) + 1 tbsp sesame seeds
1 tsp salt

In a large bowl, whisk together egg, tahini and maple syrup. Add almond meal, cocoa powder, coconut sugar, baking powder, bicarb, salt and vanilla extract. Stir until fully combined. Fold in chocolate chips and ¼ cup sesame seeds. Cover and refrigerate for at least 1 hour.

Preheat oven to 175°C. Line two baking trays with greaseproof paper.

Roll dough into 3cm balls. Place on baking trays 5cm apart. Flatten slightly, then sprinkle with salt and remaining sesame seeds. Bake for 10-12 minutes, until puffed and set on the bottoms.

Allow to cool on the tray for a few minutes before transferring to a wire rack to cool completely.

Chocolate Apricot Loaf Cake

SERVES 10
PREP + COOK TIME: 1 HOUR 15 MINS

1¼ cups (225g) dried apricots, chopped
⅓ cup (100ml) boiling water
¼ cup (60ml) Greek yoghurt
4 tbsps butter, melted
1 large egg
⅓ cup (60g) brown sugar
3 tbsps honey
1 cup (115g) plain flour
1 heaped tbsp cocoa powder
½ tsp baking powder
½ tsp bicarbonate of soda
Pinch of salt
150g dark chocolate, roughly chopped

Preheat the oven to 160°C. Lightly grease a 1kg loaf tin and line with greaseproof paper.

Place the apricots in a bowl of boiling water and set aside for 5 minutes.

Transfer half the soaked apricots along with all the soaking water to a food processor. Add the yoghurt and melted butter and blend into a smooth paste.

Transfer to a bowl and stir in the egg, sugar and honey. Whisk to combine. Add the remaining apricots and stir well.

In a separate bowl, sift together the flour, cocoa, baking powder, bicarb and salt. Fold the dry ingredients into the wet until just incorporated. Fold in the chopped chocolate.

Spoon the mixture in large dollops into the prepared tin and bake for 50-60 minutes, or until a skewer inserted in the middle comes out clean.

Remove from the oven and allow to cool in the tin for 5 minutes before transferring to a wire rack to cool completely.

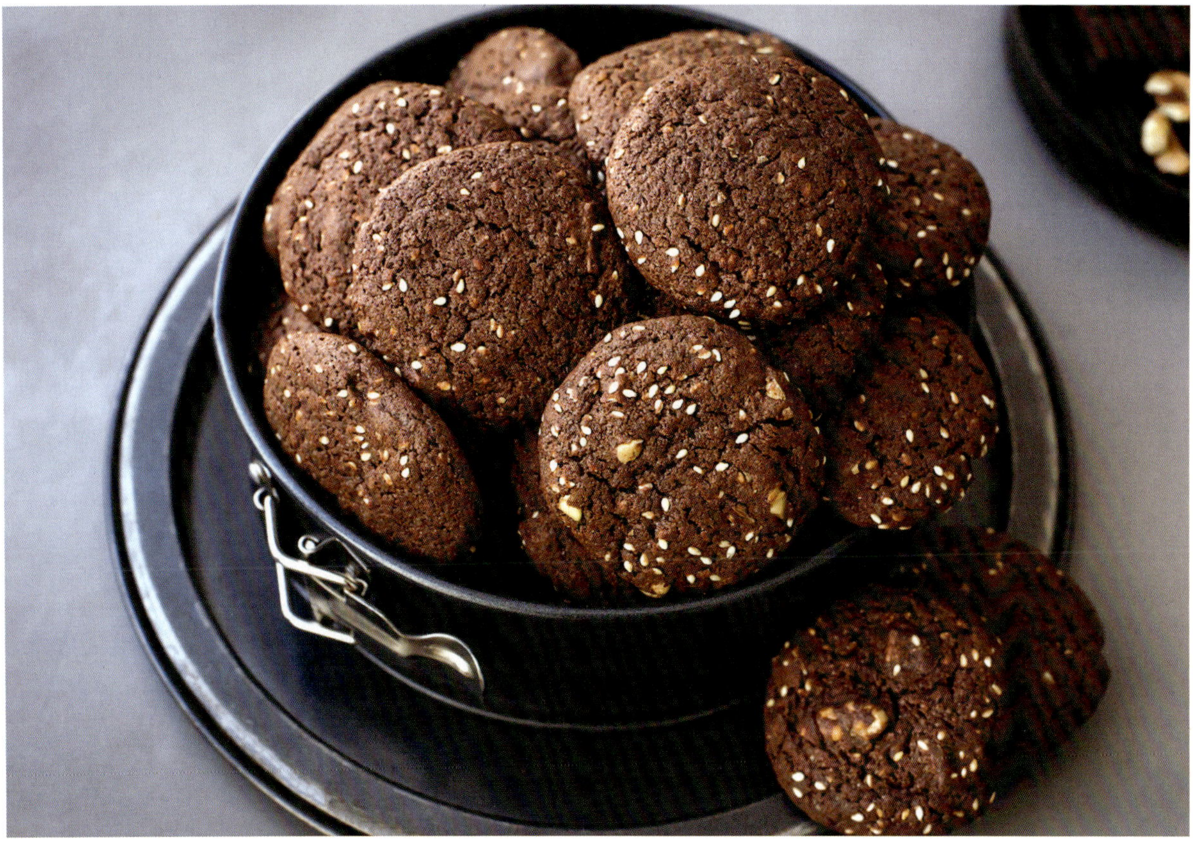

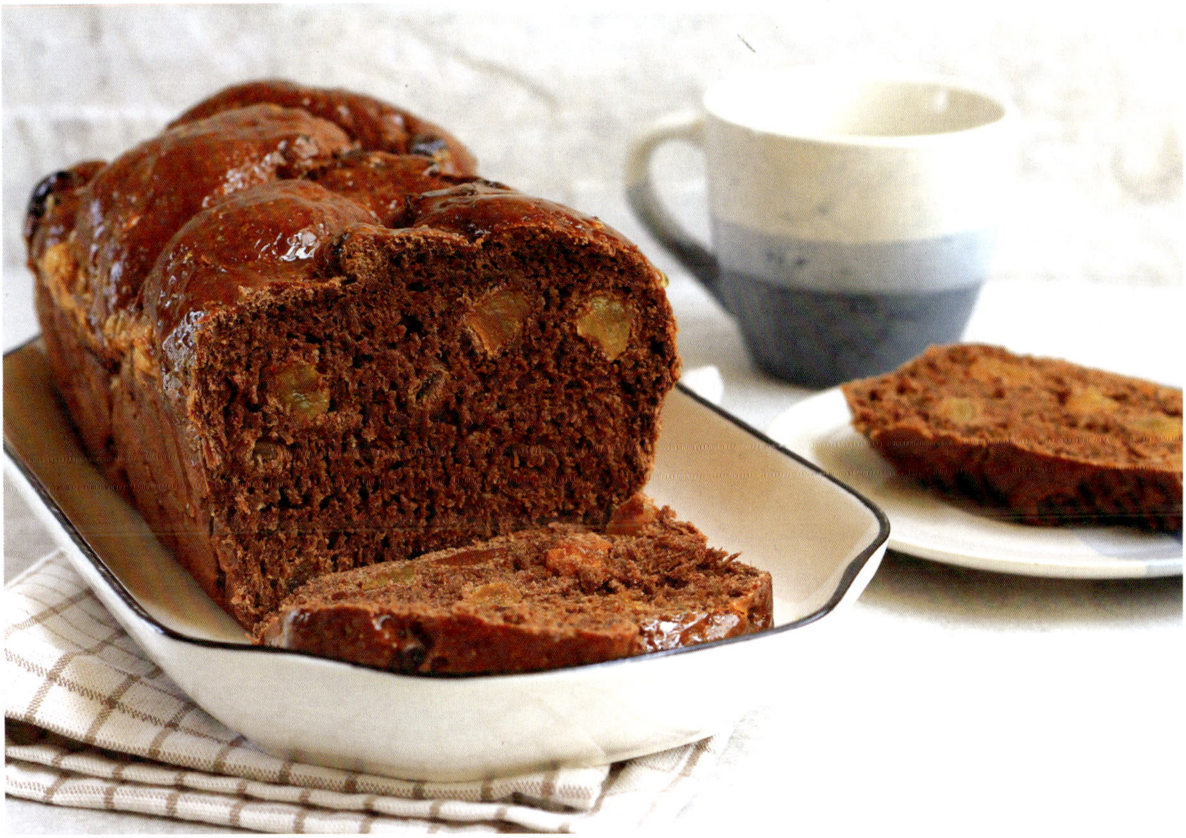

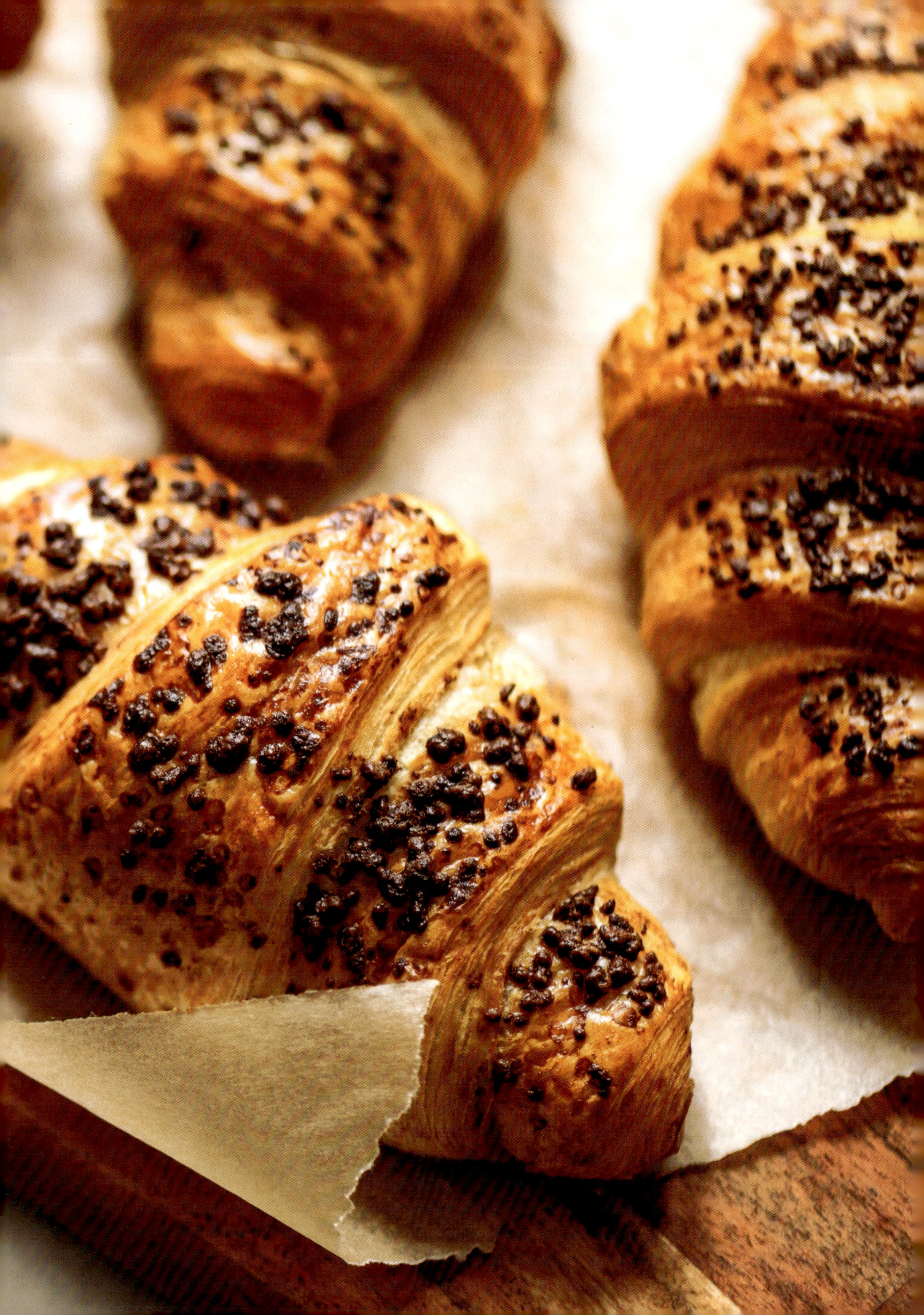

Chocolate Croissants

MAKES 16
PREP + COOK TIME: 1 HOUR, 30 MINS + CHILLING + RESTING DOUGH

DOUGH

60g unsalted butter, cubed and softened
4 cups (500g) plain flour
¼ cup (55g) sugar
2 tsps salt
1 tsp instant yeast
1½ cups (375ml) full-cream milk, chilled
113g dark chocolate, coarsely chopped + extra for decorating

BUTTER LAYER

340g unsalted butter, softened
2 tbsps plain flour

EGG WASH

1 large egg
2 tbsps full-cream milk

For the dough, place butter in the bowl of an electric stand mixer and add flour, sugar, salt and yeast. Turn the mixer on low-medium speed to gently combine the ingredients. With the mixer running, slowly pour in the milk. Once added, turn the mixer up to medium and beat the dough for at least 5 minutes. The dough will be soft and pull away from the sides of the bowl.

Remove the dough from the bowl and work into a ball. Place on a lightly floured or greaseproof-paper-lined baking tray. Flatten the dough out and cover with plastic wrap. Place the tray in the fridge and allow the dough to rest for 30 minutes.

Remove the dough from the fridge. Begin flattening out the dough on a floured surface or silicone mat. Roll it into a 35 x 25cm rectangle. Place the rolled-out dough back onto the lined baking tray. Cover the dough with plastic wrap, place the tray in the fridge and allow the dough to rest for 4 hours or overnight.

For the butter layer, beat the butter and flour together with a hand mixer until smooth. Transfer the mixture to a silicone mat or greaseproof-paper-lined baking tray and smooth into a 18 x 25cm rectangle.

Place the tray in the fridge for 30 minutes. Remove both the dough and butter from the fridge. Place the butter layer in the centre of the dough and fold each end of the dough over it. Seal the dough edges over the butter.

Roll the dough into a 25 x 50cm rectangle. Fold the dough lengthwise into thirds as if folding a letter. Turn the dough and roll out again into a 25 x 50cm rectangle, then fold lengthwise into thirds as if folding a letter.

Place the folded dough on the baking tray, cover with plastic wrap and chill for 30 minutes.

Roll the dough out once again into a 25 x 50cm rectangle. Fold the dough lengthwise into thirds as if folding a letter. Place the folded dough on the lined baking tray, cover with plastic wrap and chill for 4 hours or overnight.

Remove the dough from the fridge. On a lightly floured counter, roll the dough out into a 20 x 50cm rectangle. Using a sharp knife, slice the dough in half vertically. Each rectangle will be 10cm wide. Make three evenly spaced cuts horizontally, yielding 8 rectangles. Cut each rectangle in half lengthwise on the diagonal so you have 16 triangles.

Using your fingers or a rolling pin gently stretch each triangle to be about 20cm long. Place a few small pieces of chocolate in a single layer at one end and tightly roll the dough up in a crescent shape with the tip underneath. Repeat with remaining dough, placing the shaped croissants on two lined baking trays. Loosely cover with plastic wrap and allow to rest at room temperature for 1 hour, then place in the fridge to rest for 1 hour or up to 12 hours.

Preheat oven to 200°C. Whisk the egg wash ingredients together. Remove the croissants from the refrigerator. Brush each lightly with egg wash and sprinkle with pieces of chocolate.

Bake until croissants are golden brown, about 20 minutes. Remove chocolate croissants from the oven and place on a wire rack to cool for a few minutes before serving.

Cheesecake Brownies

MAKES 16
PREP + COOK TIME: 45 MINS

150g butter, chopped
300g dark chocolate, chopped
3 eggs
1 cup (220g) caster sugar
1½ cups (185g) plain flour
¼ cup (60ml) sour cream
250g cream cheese, room temperature

Preheat oven to 180°C. Grease a 20cm square cake tin with melted butter. Line with greaseproof paper, allowing the paper to overhang.

Combine the butter and chocolate in a large heatproof bowl over a pan of simmering water. Stir continuously until chocolate melts and mixture is smooth. Remove from heat. Set aside for 5 minutes to cool.

Whisk two of the eggs in a small bowl. Add to the chocolate mixture along with ⅔ cup sugar. Stir well to combine. Add flour and sour cream and stir to incorporate.

Use an electric hand mixer beat the cream cheese and remaining sugar in a bowl until smooth. Add the remaining egg and beat until just combined.

Spoon chocolate and cream cheese mixtures, alternately, over base of pan. Use a skewer to swirl, creating a marble effect. Bake in oven for 30 minutes or until a skewer inserted into the centre comes out clean.

Allow to cool for 1 hour before lifting out of the tin with the paper and slicing.

Chocolate Mint Slice

MAKES 16
PREP + COOK TIME: 1 HOUR 45 MINS + CHILLING

BASE
150g butter, softened
1 cup (200g) brown sugar
1 egg, room temperature
1 tsp vanilla extract
1 tsp peppermint extract
¾ cup (105g) plain flour
1 tsp baking powder
¼ cup (30g) cocoa powder
½ cup (40g) desiccated coconut

PEPPERMINT LAYER
2 cups (310g) icing sugar
30g butter
2-3 tbsps boiling water
2 tsps peppermint extract
1-2 drops green food colouring

CHOCOLATE TOPPING
200g dark chocolate, broken into small pieces
2 tbsps oil

Preheat oven to 160°C. Grease and line a 20 x 30cm slice tin with greaseproof paper.

Cream together butter and sugar until light and fluffy. Add egg, vanilla and peppermint extract and mix to combine. Sift in flour, baking powder and cocoa. Add the coconut, stir to combine. Spread mixture evenly into tray. Bake for 25-30 minutes or until just firm. Allow to cool slightly.

Beat together peppermint layer ingredients until smooth. Spread over warm base. Allow to cool.

Melt chocolate and oil in a heatproof bowl over a pan of gently simmering water. Pour the melted chocolate over the cooled peppermint filling and tilt the pan to cover the edges.

Transfer to the fridge for at least 2 hours until completely set. Slice and serve.

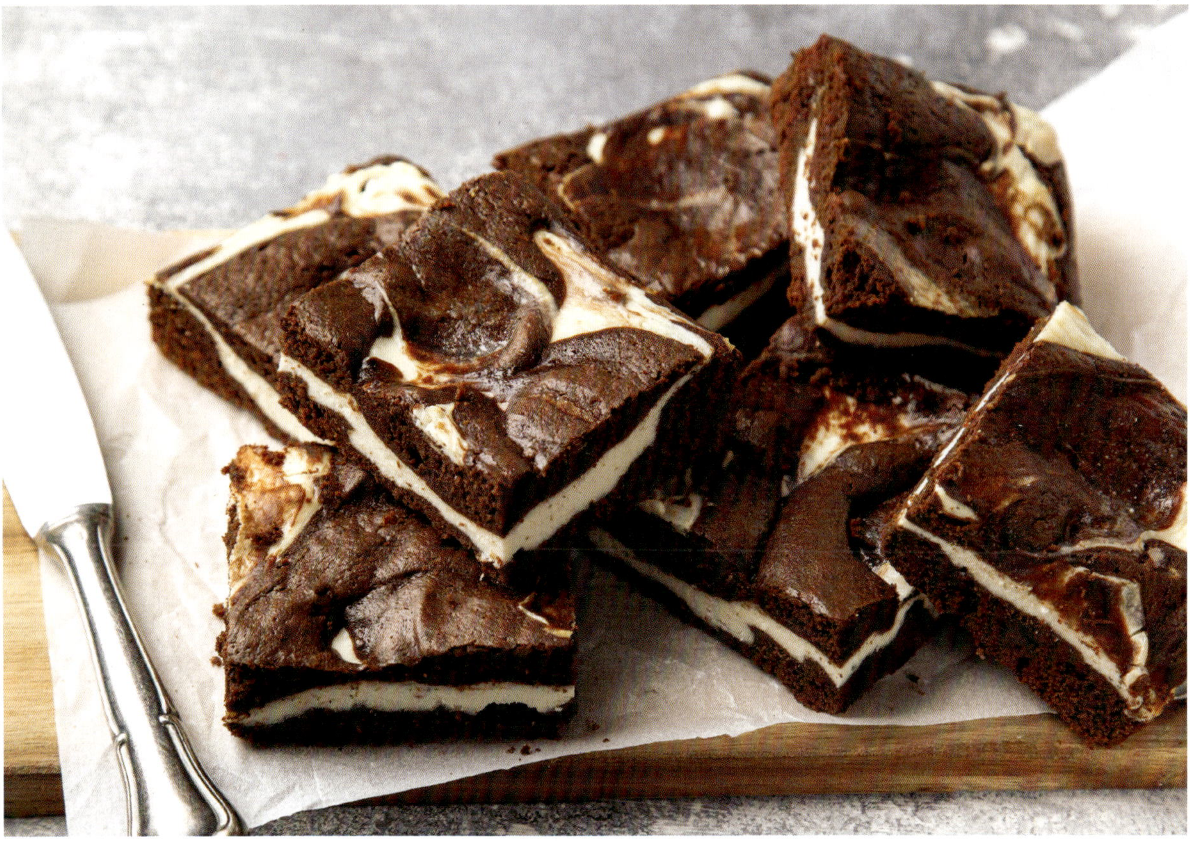

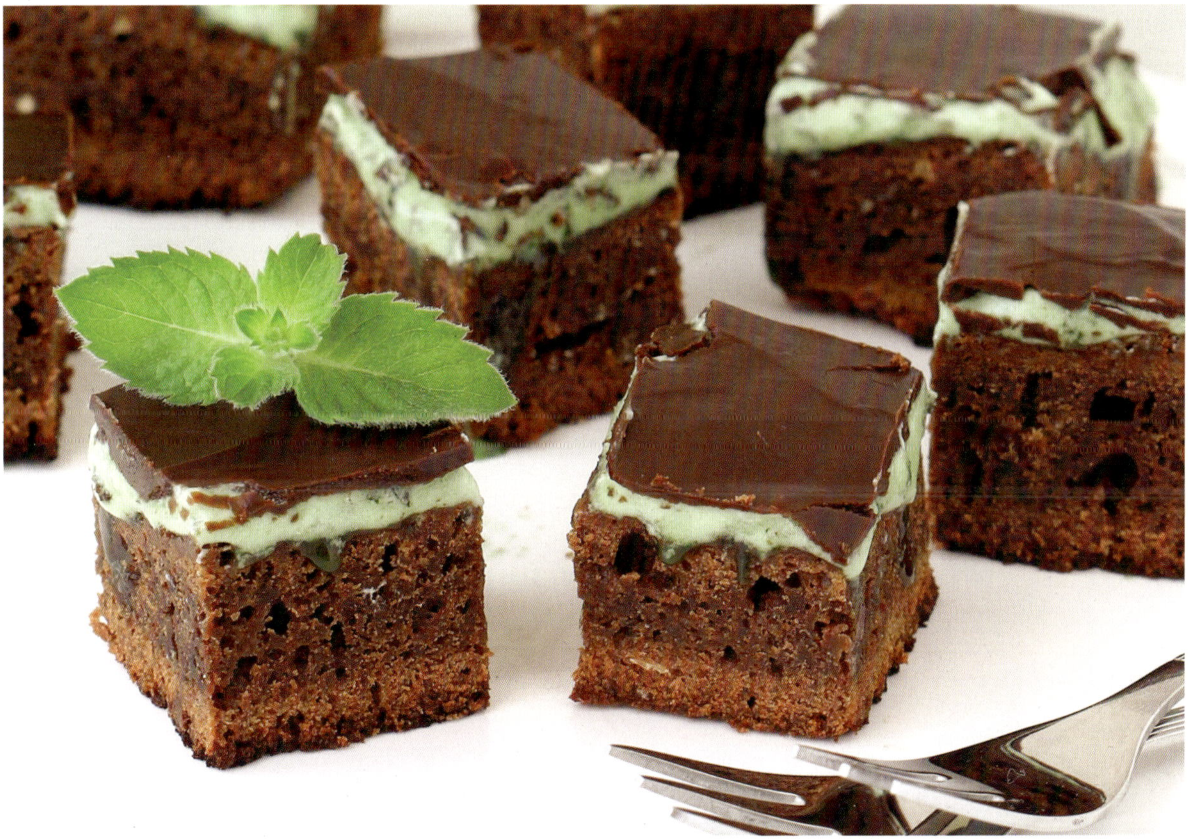

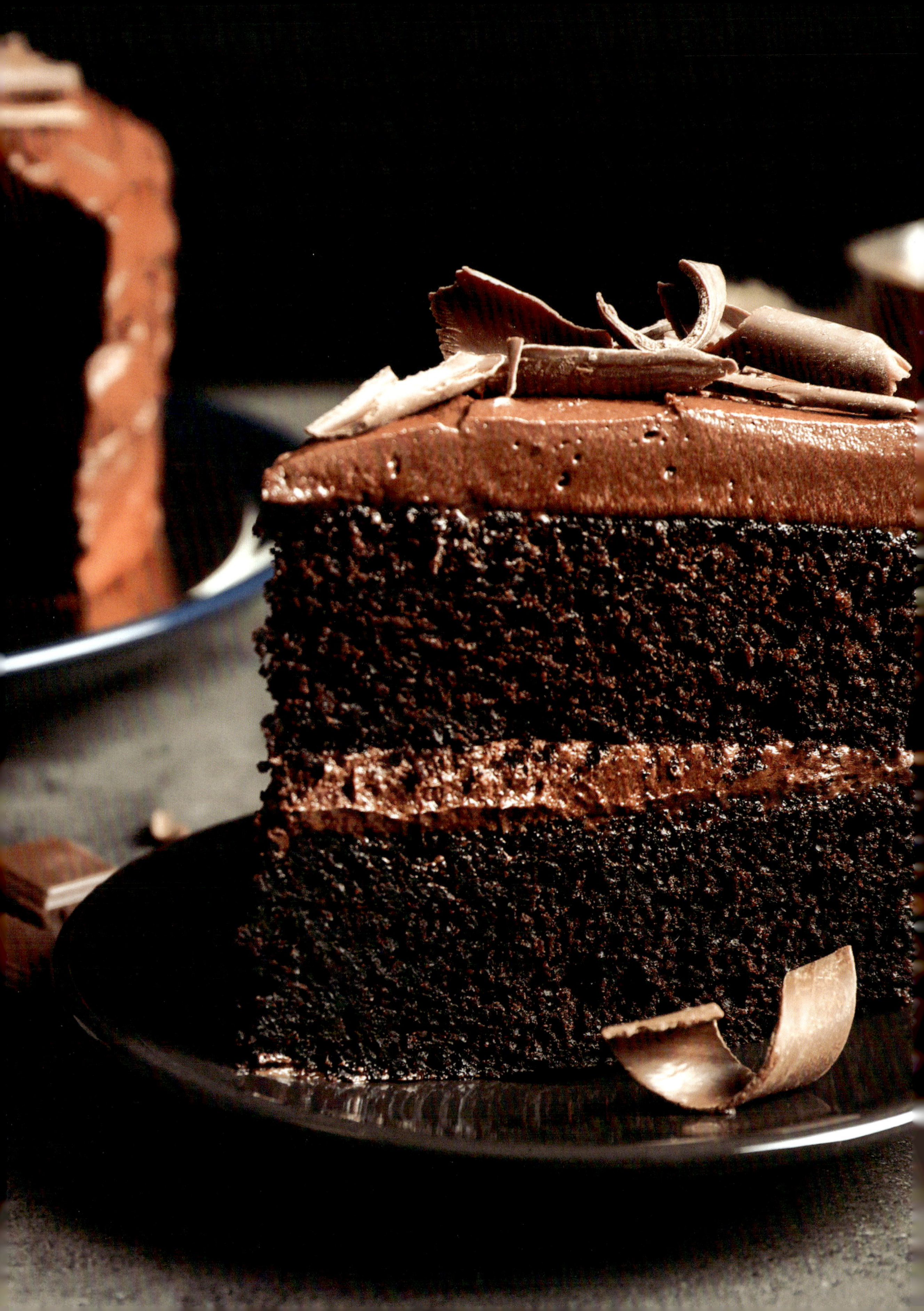

Chocolate Fudge Cake

SERVES 12-16
PREP + COOK TIME: 1 HOUR 10 MINS

1⅔ cups (250g) dark chocolate chips
200g unsalted butter
½ tsp salt
½ cup (125ml) vegetable or canola oil
2 tsps vanilla extract
2½ cups (550g) sugar
4 eggs
½ cup (60g) cocoa powder
2 tsps baking powder
2 cups (250g) plain flour
2 cups (500ml) boiling hot water
Chocolate buttercream icing
Chocolate shavings to decorate (optional)

Preheat oven to 150°C. Grease two 22cm spring-form cake tins and line with greaseproof paper.

Melt chocolate chips, butter and salt in a heatproof bowl in the microwave in 30-second bursts, mixing in between, until melted. Alternatively place chocolate and butter in a heatproof bowl set over a saucepan of simmering water and stir with a metal spoon until melted and glossy. Add oil, vanilla and sugar and mix to combine. Add eggs and mix until combined.

In a large mixing bowl sift the cocoa, baking powder and flour. Mix until smooth. Add hot water to dry ingredients and mix until incorporated. Pour the chocolate mixture into the bowl and stir to combine into a batter.

Pour batter evenly into the cake tins and bake for 50-60 minutes or until a skewer inserted into the centre of each cake comes out moist but clean.

Remove sides from the cake tins and transfer to a cooling rack to cool. Cool completely before carefully handling to remove bases.

Spread half the icing over the first cake to create a layer of filling. Top with the second cake and spread icing onto the top. Decorate with chocolate shavings, if desired, to serve.

Chocolate Buttercream Icing

MAKES 3 CUPS
PREP + COOK TIME: 10 MINS
GLUTEN FREE

1 cup (250g) unsalted butter, room temperature
3 cups (425g) icing sugar
½ cup (60g) cocoa powder
3 tbsp thickened cream (+ more as needed)
2 tsp vanilla extract
¼ tsp salt

Using a handheld mixer or stand mixer fitted with a whisk attachment, beat butter on high for 3 minutes until creamy and lighter in colour. Scrape down the bowl as needed.

Add the icing sugar, cocoa powder, cream, vanilla extract and salt to the bowl.

Beat on low speed until sugar is incorporated then beat for 3 minutes on medium-high until well blended. Add more cream if needed for a looser consistency.

Use immediately or store icing in the fridge until ready. Remove from the fridge and allow to come to room temperature before spreading.

Chickpea Chocolate Chips

MAKES 12
PREP + COOK TIME: 30 MINS
GLUTEN FREE • DAIRY FREE

- 1 x 400g can chickpeas, drained and rinsed
- ½ cup (125g) almond butter or cashew butter
- ⅓ cup (105g) maple syrup
- 2 tsps vanilla extract
- ½ tsp bicarbonate of soda
- ½ tsp baking powder
- ½ tsp salt
- ½ cup (80g) dark chocolate chips

Preheat oven to 175°C. Line a baking try with greaseproof paper.

Add the chickpeas and nut butter into a food processor and blend on high for 1 minute until smooth. Add the maple syrup and vanilla and continue to blend for 2-3 minutes, scraping down the sides as necessary. Add the bicarb, baking powder and salt, then blend for 30 seconds. Stir in the chocolate chips.

Drop rounded tablespoons of cookie dough onto the prepared baking tray, least 3cm between each cookie. Bake for 12-14 minutes until golden brown.

Vegan Brownies

MAKES 16
PREP + COOK TIME: 45 MINS
DAIRY FREE

- 1 cup (125g) plain flour
- ¼ cup (30g) cocoa powder, sifted
- 1 cup (200g) caster sugar
- 200g vegan dark chocolate, broken into pieces
- ⅓ cup (80ml) light olive oil
- 1 tsp vanilla extract
- 1 cup (250ml) almond milk
- ½ cup (60g) chopped walnuts

TO SERVE (OPTIONAL)

- 90g vegan dark chocolate, melted

Preheat oven to 160°C. Line a 20cm square cake tin with greaseproof paper.

In a large mixing bowl, add flour, cocoa powder and sugar and gently whisk to mix.

Place the chocolate in a heatproof bowl over a pan of simmering water. Stir for a few minutes until melted. Remove the bowl from the heat and add oil, vanilla and almond milk. Stir to combine then scrape the chocolate mixture into the flour mixture and stir to incorporate. Fold in the walnuts.

Transfer brownie batter to prepared tin and bake for 25-30 minutes or until a skewer inserted in the middle comes out with a few moist crumbs attached. Do not over-bake or brownies will be too dry. Transfer brownies to a wire rack to cool slightly before slicing into squares.

To serve, place the chocolate in a heatproof bowl over a pan of simmering water. Stir for a few minutes until melted, then drizzle over the brownie squares.

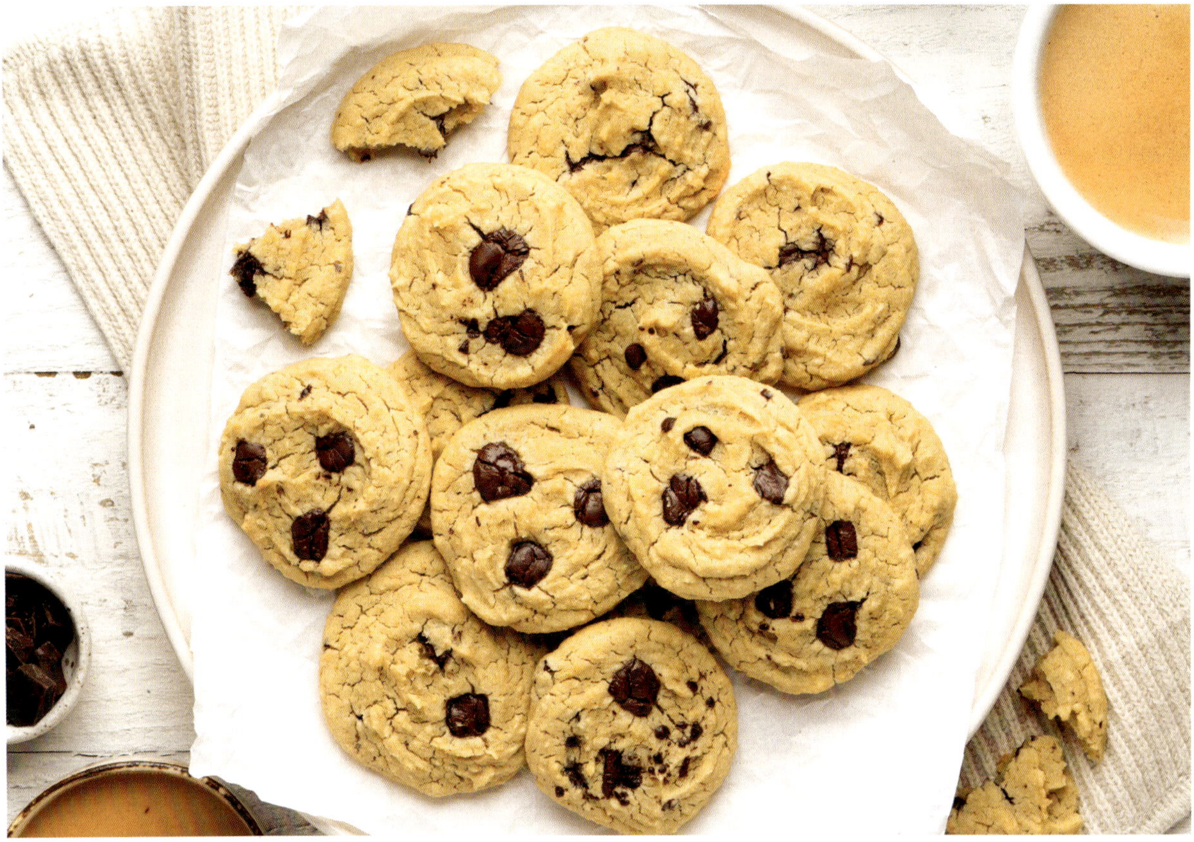

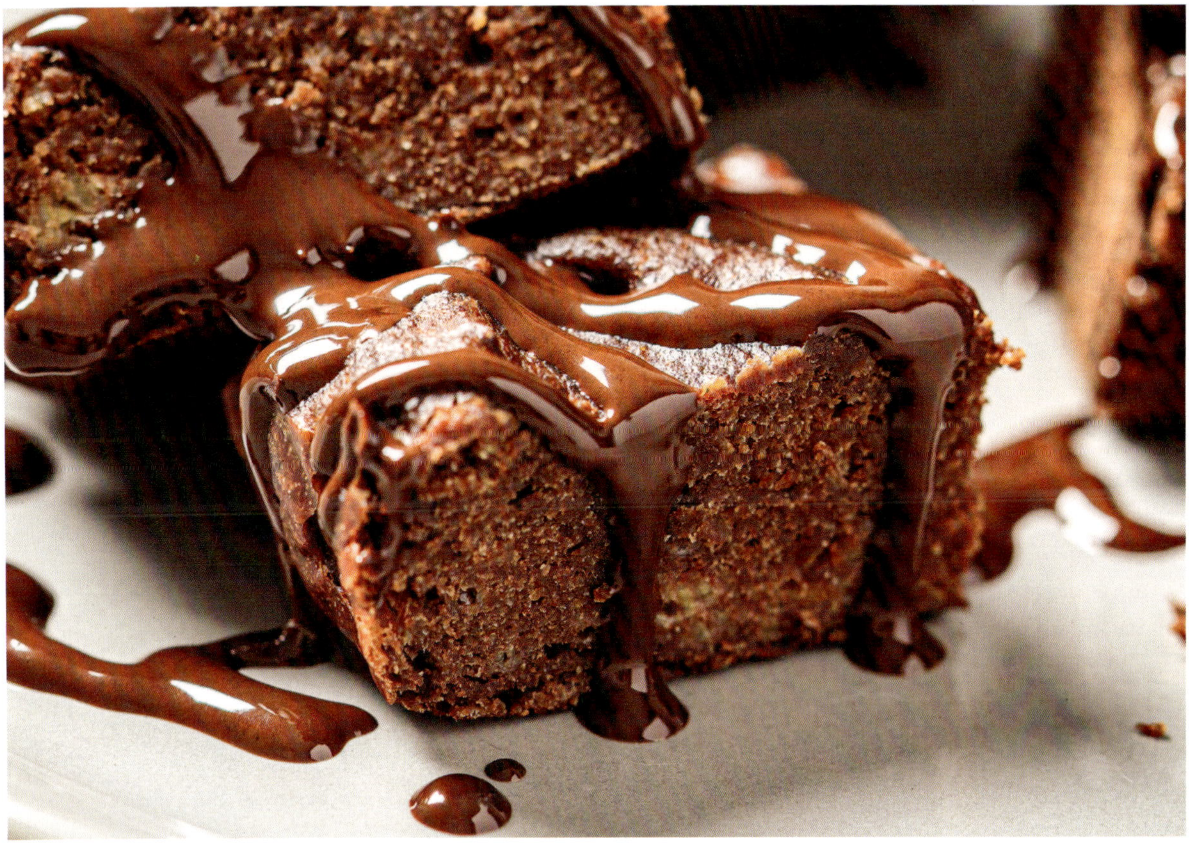

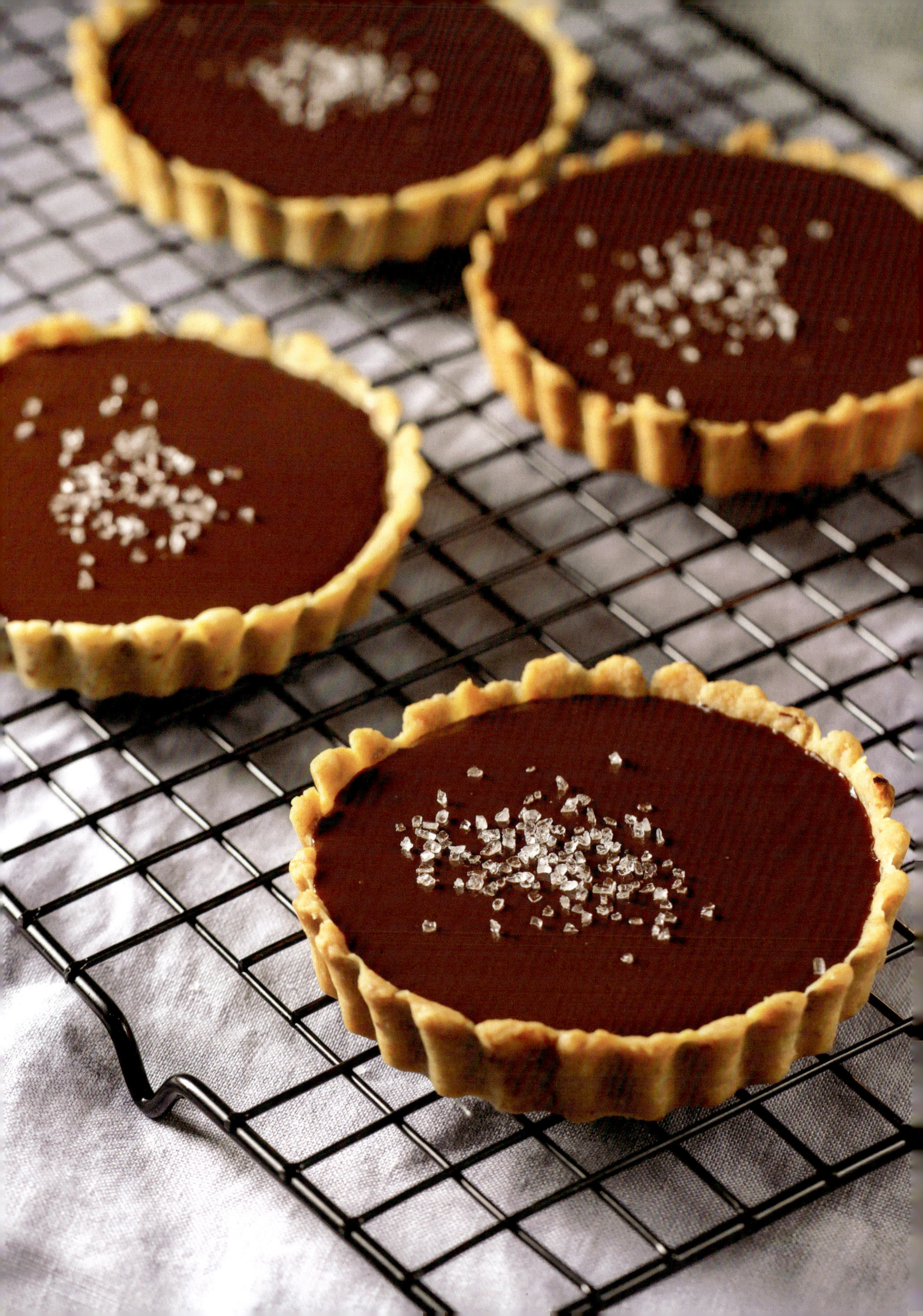

Salted Chocolate Tarts

MAKES 4
PREP + COOK TIME: 45 MINS + 1 HOUR 10 MINS CHILLING

PASTRY
1 cup (125g) plain flour
2 tbsps sugar
75g unsalted butter, softened
1 tsp vanilla extract
1 egg yolk

FILLING
120g dark chocolate, chopped
½ cup (125ml) double cream

TO SERVE
Salt flakes

Place the flour, sugar and butter into a food processor and process it until it resembles fine breadcrumbs. Add the vanilla and egg yolk and process until a smooth dough forms.

Turn the dough out onto a lightly floured surface. Shape into a disc. Wrap in greaseproof paper or plastic wrap and refrigerate for 30 minutes.

Divide the dough into four pieces. Press each piece evenly into a 12cm tart mould. Trim the excess with a sharp knife. Prick the base of each pastry case a few times with a fork. Place the tart cases on a baking tray and transfer to the freezer for 10 minutes.

Preheat the oven to 170°C.

Bake pastry cases for 20 minutes. Remove from the oven and leave to cool completely. Remove the cases from the moulds and set aside.

Place chocolate in a heatproof jug. Heat cream in a pan over medium-high heat until bubbles start appearing around the edges. Pour cream immediately over the chocolate and let it sit for 3 minutes. After 3 minutes whisk until smooth.

Pour the chocolate filling into the pastry cases.

Transfer to the fridge and chill for 30 minutes. Sprinkle each tart with a pinch of salt flakes to serve.

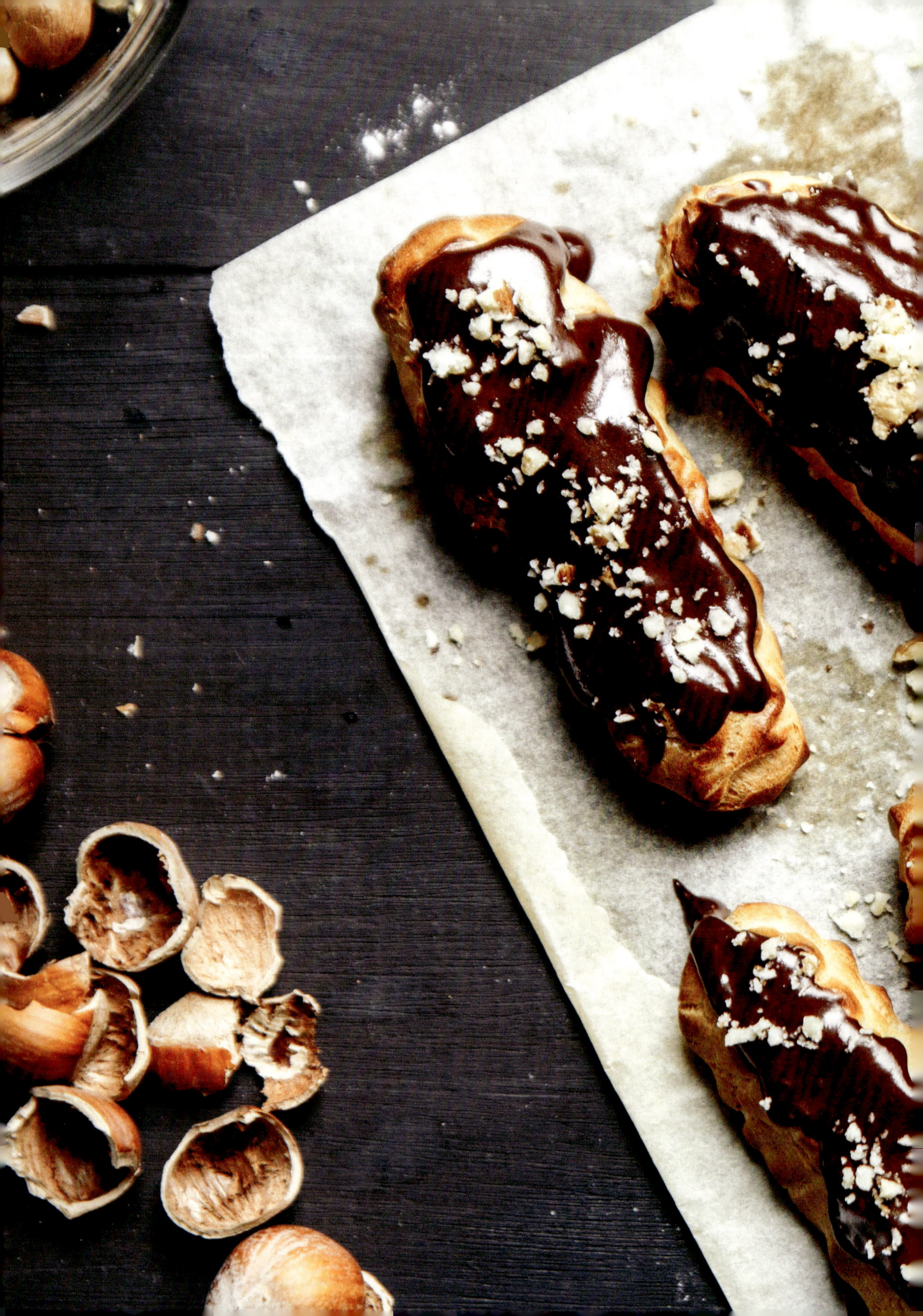

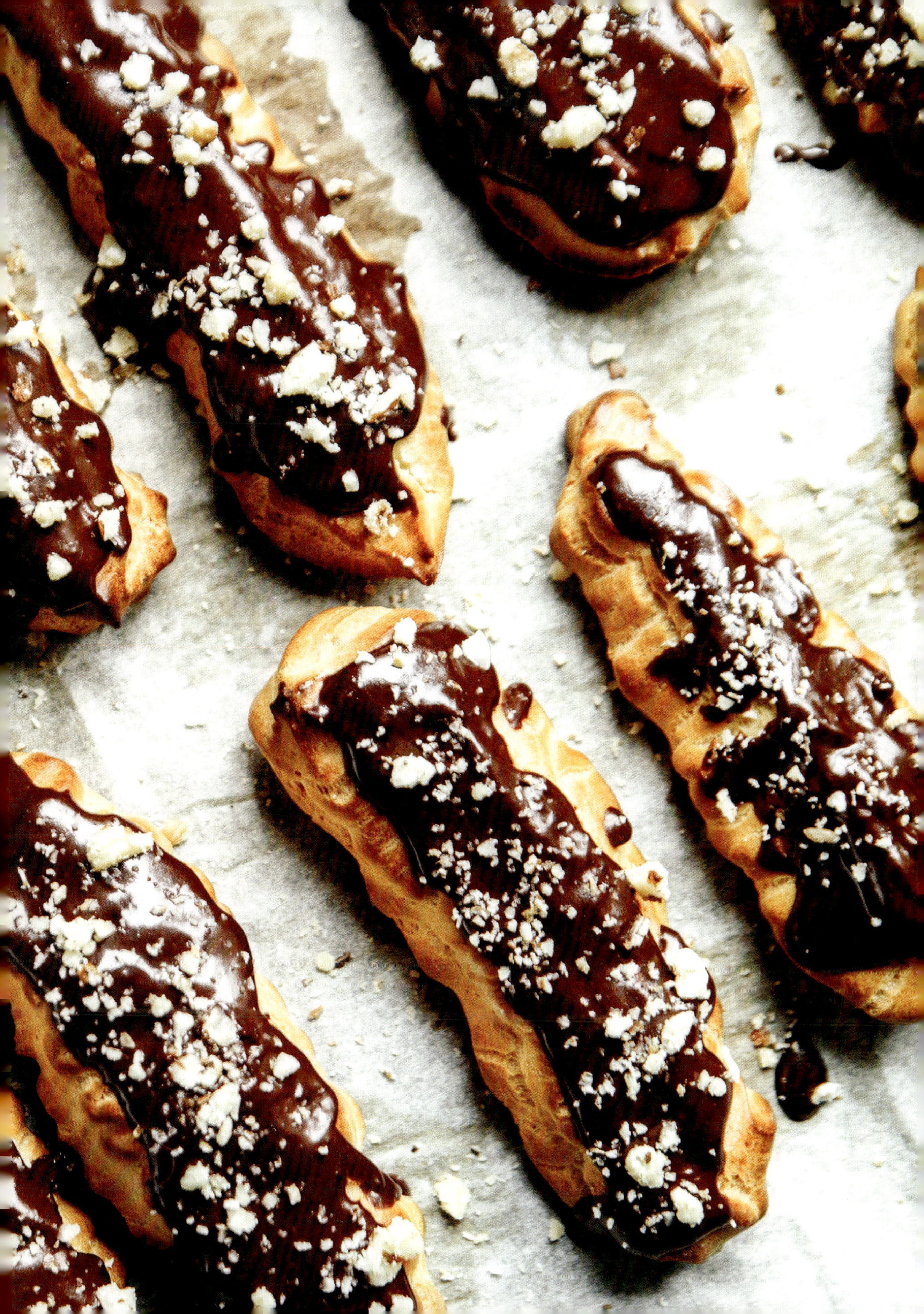

Chocolate Eclairs

MAKES 10
PREP + COOK TIME: 1 HOUR

135g butter
1 cup (240ml) water
2 tsps sugar
1 cup (120g) flour
½ tsp salt
4 large eggs, lightly beaten
2½ cups (600ml) thickened cream
2 tbsps icing sugar
1 vanilla bean, split and scraped
Chocolate ganache topping (see next recipe)
¼ cup (30g) chopped hazelnuts

Preheat the oven to 200°C. Line a baking tray with greaseproof paper.

Place butter, water and sugar into a large saucepan over a low heat. When butter is melted, increase heat and stir in flour and salt. Remove from heat and quickly beat the mixture until it forms a smooth paste. Transfer the mixture into a large bowl to cool for 10-15 minutes. Add the beaten eggs and stir vigorously until smooth and glossy. Transfer the dough into a pastry bag, fitted with a 1½cm round tip. Pipe out 10 lines 10cm long onto the baking tray.

Place in the oven and bake for 30-35 minutes, until golden brown. Prick with a skewer and set aside to cool.

Whip the cream, icing sugar and seeds scraped from the vanilla bean until soft peaks form.

Cut cooled eclairs in half. Fill with cream, drizzle with chocolate ganache topping and scatter with hazelnuts to serve.

Ganache Topping

SERVES 10
PREP + COOK TIME: 10 MINS
GLUTEN FREE

1½ cups (205g) dark chocolate chips
1 cup (240ml) thickened cream, warmed

Melt the chocolate and cream in a heatproof bowl over a pan of simmering water. Stir until smooth.

Chocolate Bundt

SERVES 10
PREP + COOK TIME: 1 HOUR 20 MINS

100g dark chocolate, roughly chopped
½ cup (55g) cocoa powder
1 tsp vanilla extract
⅔ cup (160ml) sour cream
⅓ cup (80ml) boiling water
200g unsalted butter, softened
2 cups (400g) caster sugar
3 eggs, room temperature
2½ cups (300g) plain flour
1 tsp baking powder
½ tsp bicarbonate of soda
½ tsp salt
Icing sugar for dusting

Preheat oven to 170°C. Grease a bundt tin.

Melt chocolate in a bowl over a pan of simmering water. Take off the heat and add cocoa, vanilla, sour cream and boiling water. Stir to a smooth paste. In another bowl cream butter and sugar until light and fluffy. Add eggs, one at a time, whisking after each addition. Stir in chocolate paste. Sift in flour, baking powder, bicarb and salt. Fold in with a metal spoon. Spoon mixture into the bundt tin. Bake for 45 minutes or until an inserted skewer comes out clean. Leave to cool for 15 minutes before turning out onto a wire rack. Dust with icing sugar to serve.

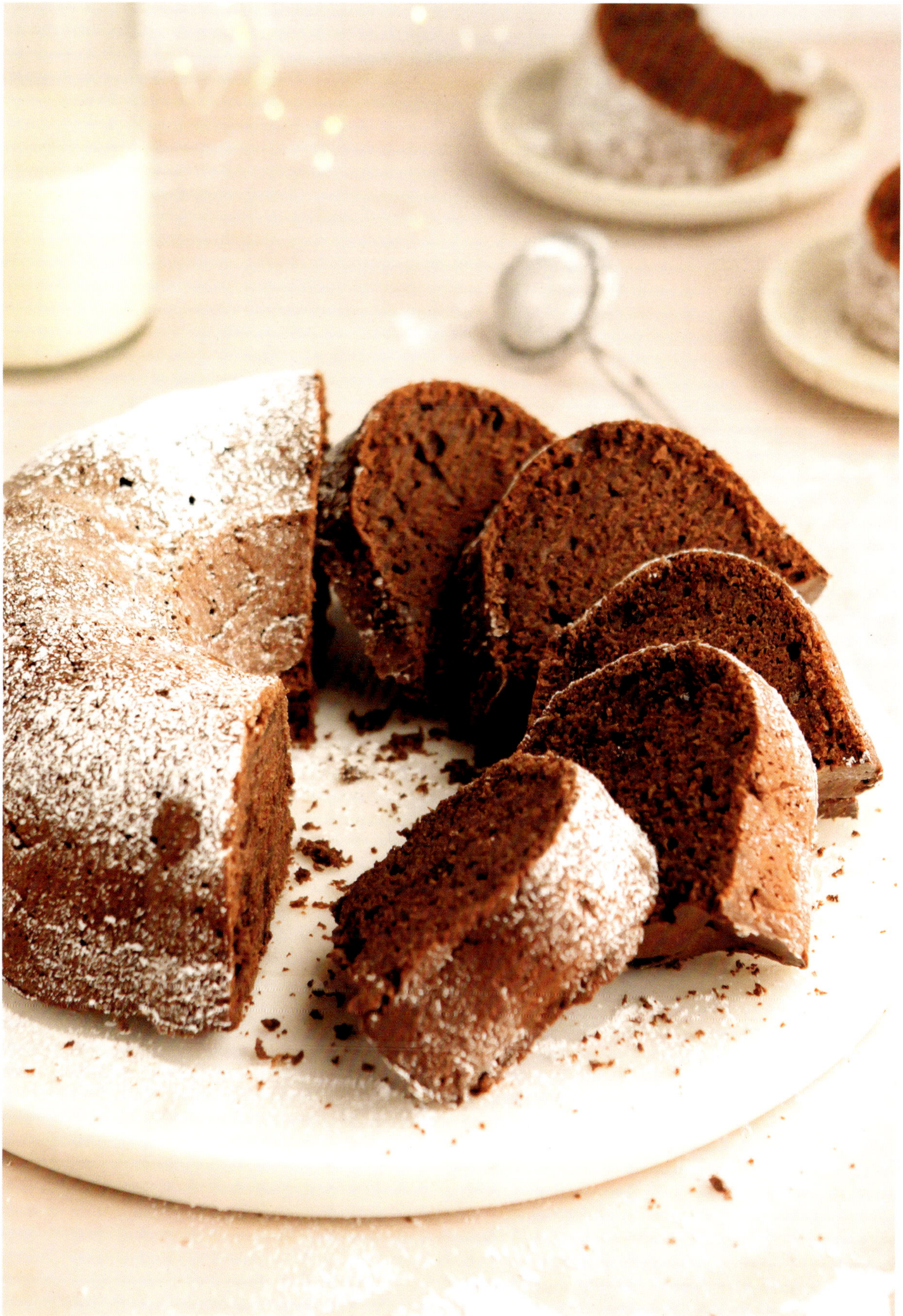

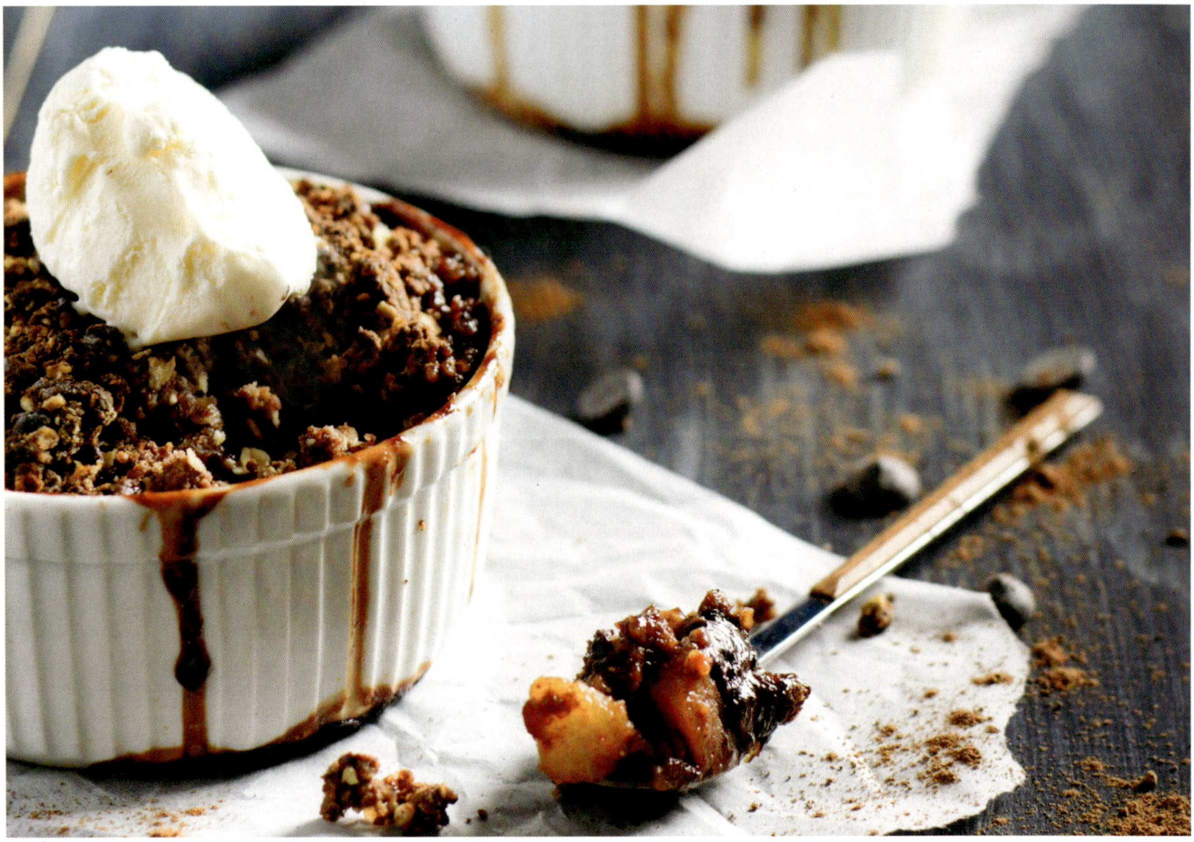

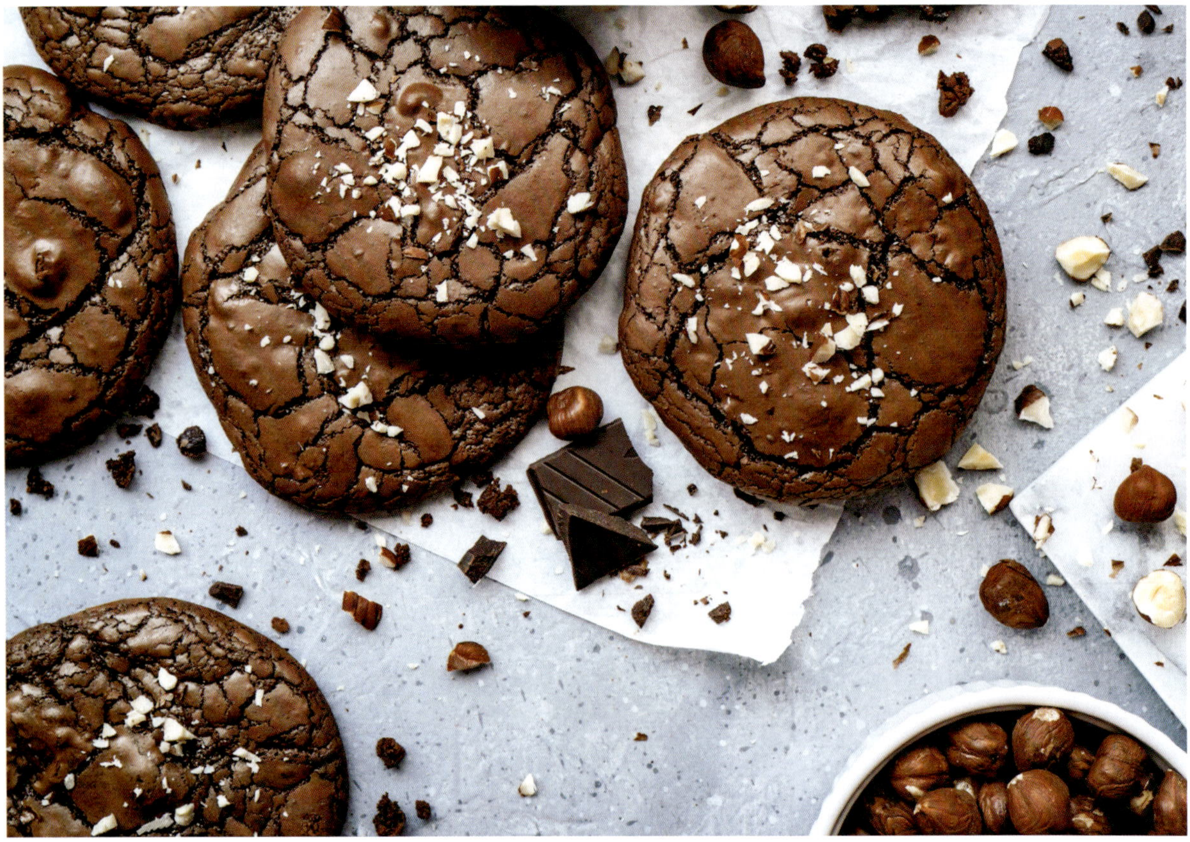

Pear & Banana Chocolate Crumble

SERVES 4
PREP + COOK TIME: 45 MINS

4 small pears, diced
2 bananas, sliced
90g dark chocolate, chopped
¼ cup (60ml) coconut oil, melted
¼ cup (80g) maple syrup
1⅓ cups (120g) rolled oats
¾ cup (80g) almond meal
Pinch of salt
Vanilla ice cream to serve

Preheat the oven to 180°C.

Divide the fruit evenly between four ramekins.

Spread half of the chopped chocolate over the fruit.

In a large bowl, mix together the coconut oil, maple syrup, oats, almond meal and salt. Fold in the remaining chocolate and stir to combine.

Sprinkle the crumble with your hands over the fruit.

Bake for 30 minutes in the middle of the oven until the crumble is golden brown. Serve warm with ice cream.

Chocolate Hazelnut Cookies

MAKES 15
PREP + COOK TIME: 25 MINS

2½ cups (310g) plain flour
1 tsp bicarbonate of soda
½ tsp salt
¾ cup (90g) cocoa powder
225g butter, room temperature
1 cup (220g) white sugar
1 cup (200g) brown sugar
2 eggs
1 tsp vanilla extract
1 cup (170g) chocolate chips
1 cup (140g) hazelnuts, chopped
½ tsp salt
2 tbsps finely chopped hazelnuts to serve (optional)

Preheat oven to 180°C. Line a baking tray with greaseproof paper.

Sift flour into a medium bowl and add bicarb, salt and cocoa. Set aside.

With an electric mixer, cream butter and sugars together on a medium speed until smooth. Add in eggs, one at a time, beating for 30 seconds after each addition. Then add vanilla extract and mix to combine.

Gradually add flour mixture and beat on low speed until just incorporated. Stir in the chocolate chips and hazelnuts.

Scoop the dough into rounded tablespoons and place on the prepared baking tray, about 5cm apart. Sprinkle each cookie with salt.

Bake for 10 minutes, or until cookies are firm, but still soft in the centre.

Remove from oven and cool on baking tray for 3 minutes before moving to a wire rack to cool completely. Decorate with chopped hazelnuts, if desired.

3

Cinnamon & Caramel

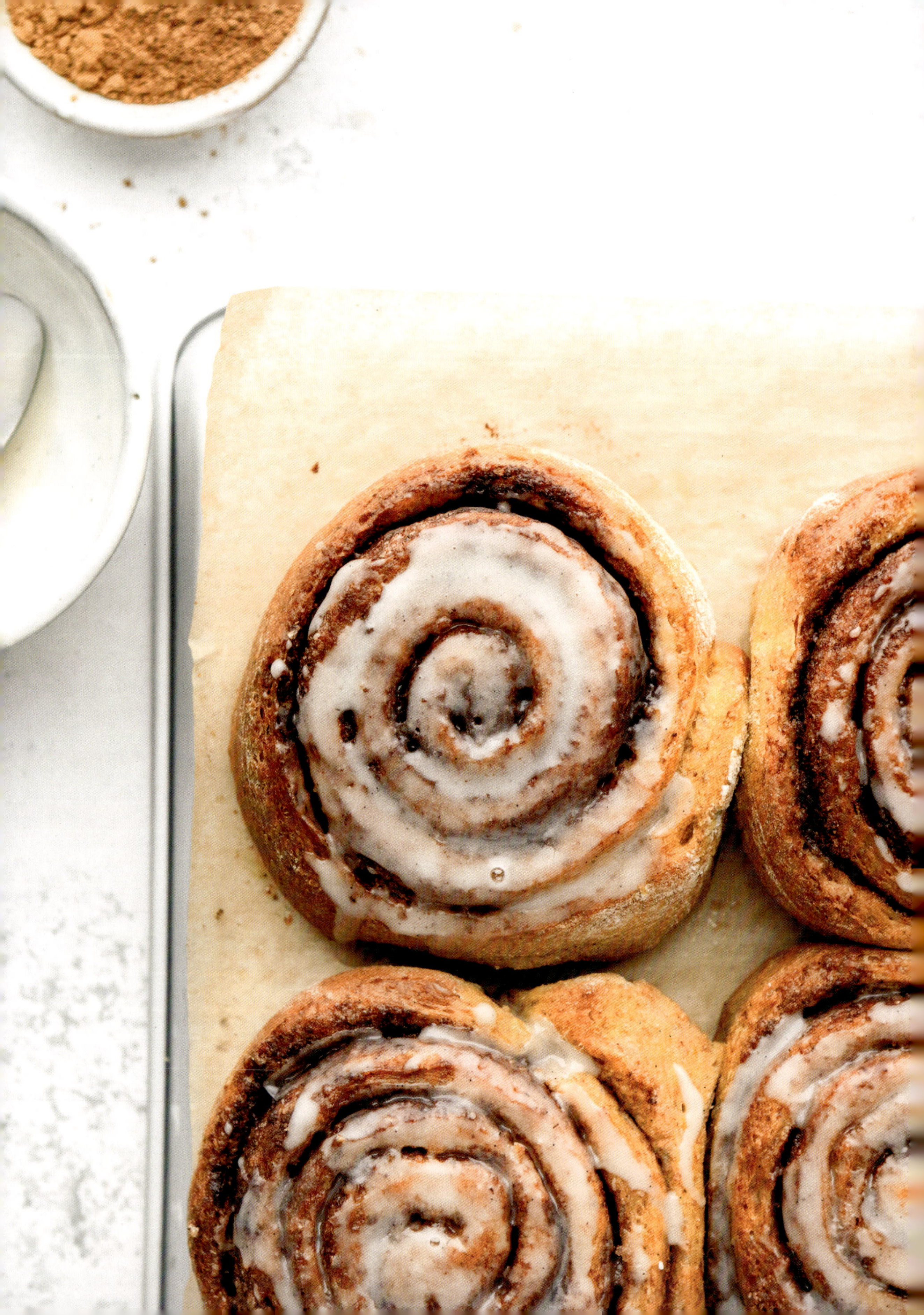

Cinnamon Scrolls

MAKES 9
PREP + COOK TIME: 30 MINS + 1-2 HOURS PROVING

¾ cup (185ml) milk
2¼ tsps active yeast
¼ cup (55g) sugar
1 egg + 1 egg yolk, room temperature
60g butter, melted
3 cups (375g) bread flour
¾ tsp salt
Vanilla glaze (see next recipe)

FILLING
60g butter, softened
⅔ cup (125g) brown sugar
1½ tbsps cinnamon

Heat milk until just lukewarm. Transfer to a mixing bowl and sprinkle yeast on top. Add in sugar, egg, egg yolk and melted butter. Mix well to combine. Stir in flour and salt with a wooden spoon until a dough begins to form.

Mix with a dough hook for about 8 minutes, or turn out onto a lightly floured surface and knead with your hands for about 8 minutes until smooth and elastic. Transfer dough ball to an oiled bowl, cover with a tea towel and leave in a warm place for 1-1½ hours, or until doubled in size.

Transfer risen dough to a well-floured surface and roll out into a 35 x 23cm rectangle. Spread softened butter over dough, leaving a 1cm margin down the edge of one of the long sides, furthest from you.

Mix together brown sugar and cinnamon. Sprinkle over the buttered dough.

Tightly roll dough up, starting from the long side closest to you. Cut into 3cm sections with a serrated knife. Place scrolls in a greased 23cm square cake tin. Cover with a tea towel and set aside in a warm place to rise again for 30-45 minutes.

Preheat oven to 175°C. Remove tea towel and bake cinnamon scrolls for 20-25 minutes or until golden brown on the edges. Allow them to cool for 5-10 minutes before drizzling with the glaze.

Vanilla Glaze

SERVES 9
PREP + COOK TIME: 5 MINS
GLUTEN FREE

2 cups (310g) icing sugar
2 tbsps butter, melted
2 tsps vanilla
4 tbsps cream

Mix together icing sugar, melted butter, vanilla and cream in a large bowl until smooth.

Napoleon Cake

SERVES 16
PREP + COOK TIME: 1 HOUR 15 MINS

7 egg yolks
1½ cups (330g) sugar
⅔ cup (80g) plain flour
6 cups (1.5L) milk
1 tbsp vanilla extract
200g unsalted butter, chopped
1kg puff pastry sheets
1 tsp cinnamon

In a bowl, whisk together egg yolks and sugar using an electric mixer. Add flour, then whisk in ½ cup of milk.

Heat remaining milk over low heat to a gentle simmer, stirring continuously. Slowly pour hot milk into egg mixture while whisking. Cook mixture over low-medium heat, stirring, until custard thickens. Remove custard from heat. Mix in vanilla extract. Add butter and allow to melt, stirring until smooth. Pour custard into a glass baking dish and cover with plastic wrap. Allow custard to cool at room temperature.

Preheat oven to 200°C. Roll out puff pastry sheets into 30 x 40cm rectangles, dusting with flour as needed. Pierce all over with a fork to prevent bubbles from forming as they bake. Bake each puff pastry layer for 7-9 minutes until lightly golden. Remove from the oven, place a 25cm dish on top and cut around it with a sharp knife collecting all scraps to a bowl for use later. Allow to cool.

Spread 4 large tablespoons of custard over the first pastry layer and top with another piece of pastry. Repeat with remaining custard and pastry, finishing with a layer of custard on top.

Top with crumbs made from baked pastry scraps. To make these place any scraps and the cinnamon in a food processor and process until crumbly.

Refrigerate cake for 48 hours and serve chilled.

Peanut Butter Caramel Brownies

MAKES 16
PREP + COOK TIME: 40 MINS

70g butter
190g dark chocolate
⅓ cup (70g) white sugar
⅔ cup (125g) brown sugar
2 eggs
1 tsp vanilla extract
1 cup (125g) plain flour
⅓ cup (35g) cocoa powder
⅓ cup (80g) peanut butter
½ cup (60g) roasted peanuts

BROWNIE CARAMEL TOPPING

⅓ cup (65g) brown sugar
25g butter, melted
2 tbsps milk

Preheat the oven to 160°C and line a 23cm square baking tin with greaseproof paper.

Melt the butter and dark chocolate together in a heatproof bowl over a pan of simmering water.

In another bowl beat together the sugars, eggs and vanilla extract until fluffy. Pour the chocolate mixture into the egg mixture and stir together until smooth. Add the flour and cocoa and stir to combine. Add the peanut butter and fold through with a metal spoon. Pour the mixture into the prepared tin.

Bake for 20-25 minutes until just firm on top. Allow to cool in the tin for 5 minutes, before transferring to a wire rack.

To make the topping, place brown sugar and butter in a saucepan over medium-high heat. When the butter melts add the milk and bring to a boil. Boil for 2 minutes then remove from the heat. Set aside to cool.

Pour the caramel topping over the brownie and sprinkle with roasted peanuts before slicing and serving.

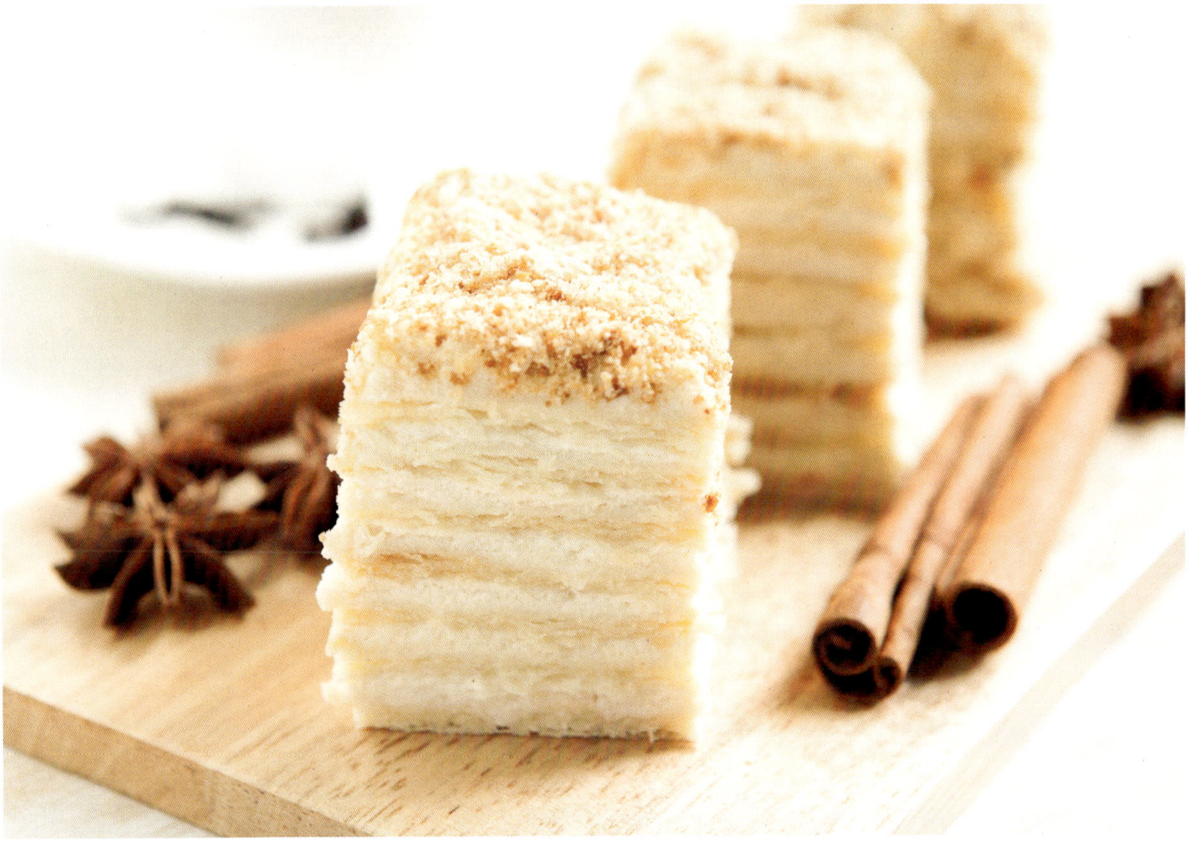

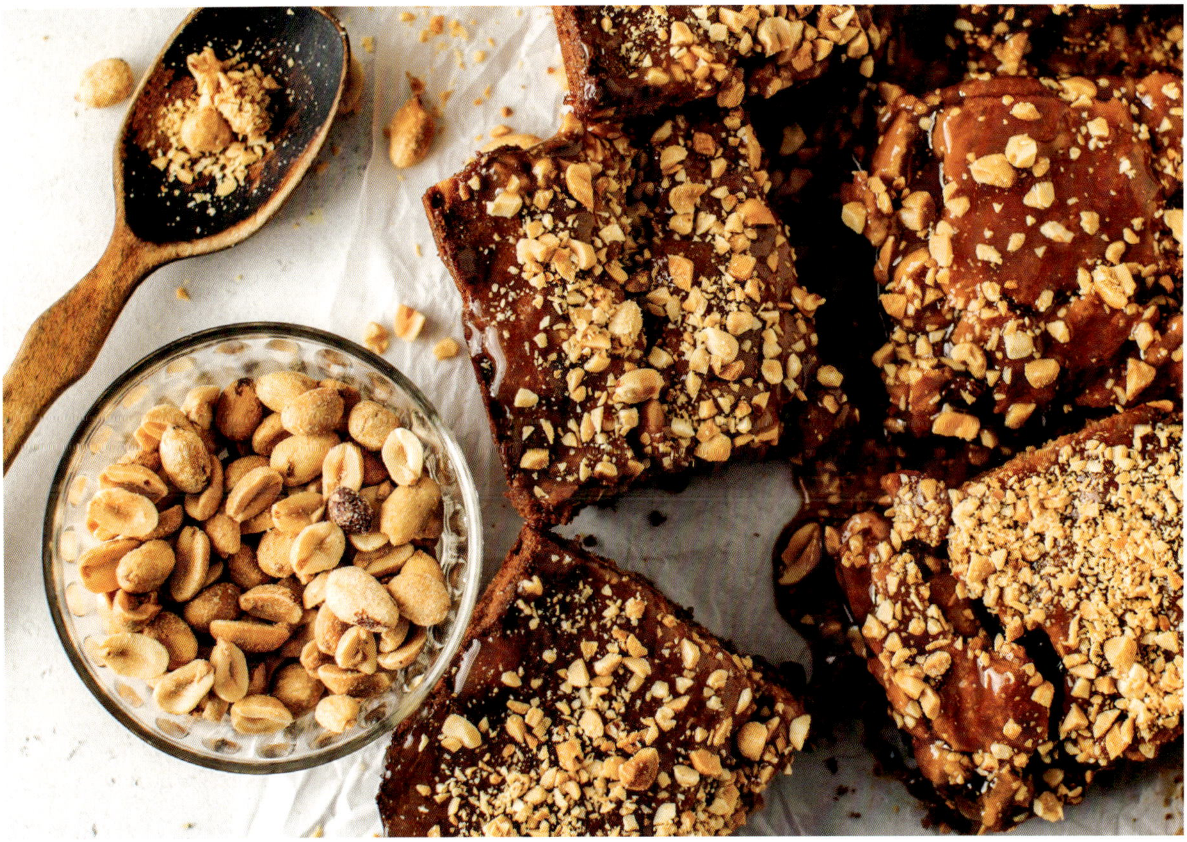

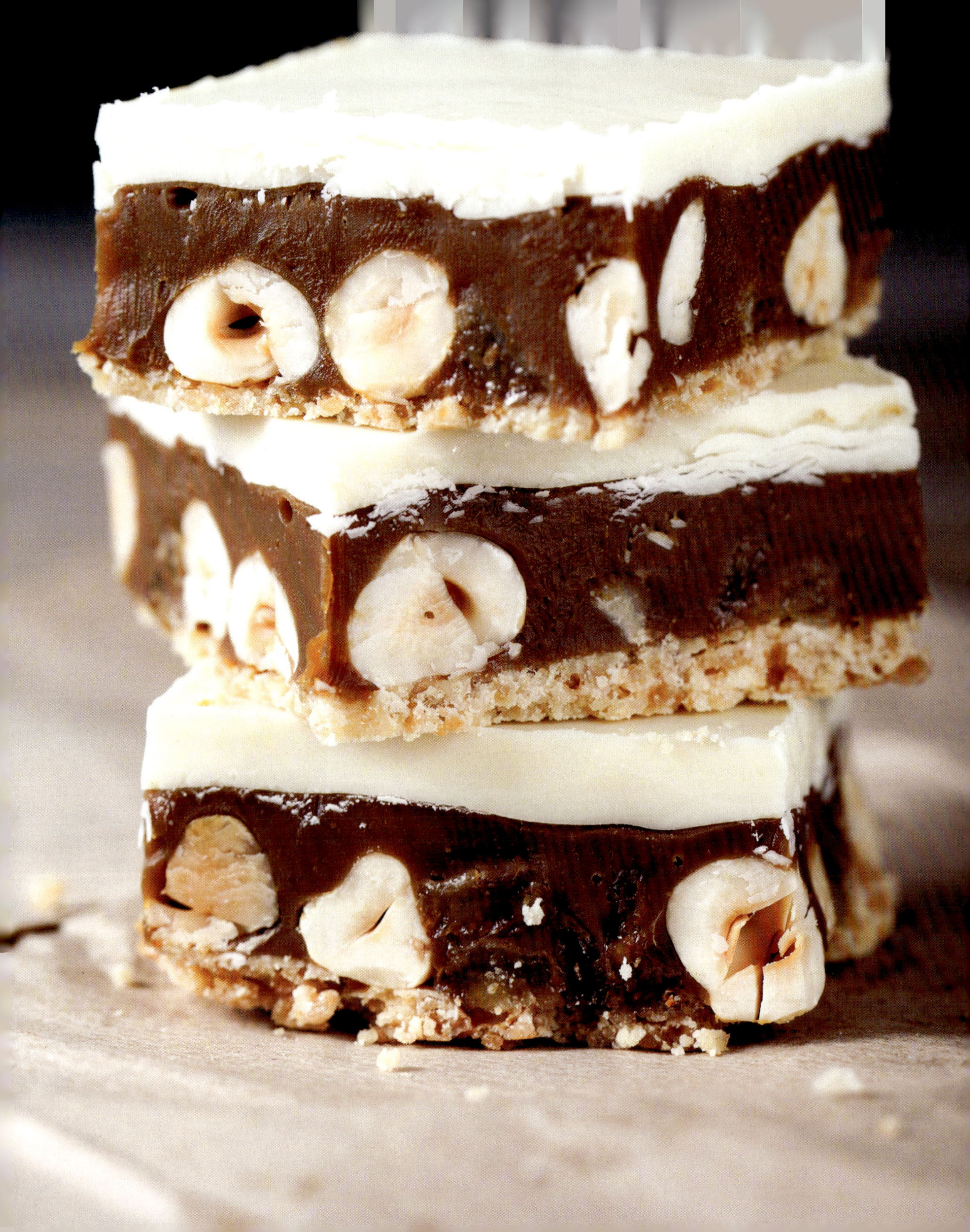

Hazelnut Caramel White Chocolate Slice

MAKES 16

PREP + COOK TIME: 45 MINS + 3 HOURS CHILLING

BASE

250g shortbread biscuits or other sweet biscuits

120g butter, melted

FILLING

1 cup (120g) roasted hazelnuts

1 x 400g can sweetened condensed milk

125g butter

⅓ cup (70g) caster sugar

⅓ cup (115g) golden syrup

TOPPING

250g white chocolate, chopped

1 tbsp melted butter

Preheat oven to 180°C. Line a 20cm square cake tin with greaseproof paper.

Arrange the hazelnuts on a baking tray and roast for 10 minutes. Transfer roasted nuts to a clean tea towel and gently rub off the skins. Set aside.

Crush the biscuits into fine crumbs in a food processor. Add melted butter and pulse to combine.

Press into an even layer in the base of the tin. Chill in the fridge while you make the caramel.

Mix together the condensed milk, butter, sugar and golden syrup in a saucepan over a low heat. Stir continuously for 15 minutes until the mixture is thick and becomes a dark golden colour. Let the caramel cool slightly then pour into the tin over the biscuit base. Press the roasted hazelnuts into the caramel.

Return to the fridge to set.

Melt white chocolate and butter in a microwave in 20-seconds bursts or in a heatproof bowl over a pan of simmering water. Stir until just melted.

Pour chocolate mixture over the hazelnut caramel then transfer to the fridge for 3 hours to set, before cutting into squares.

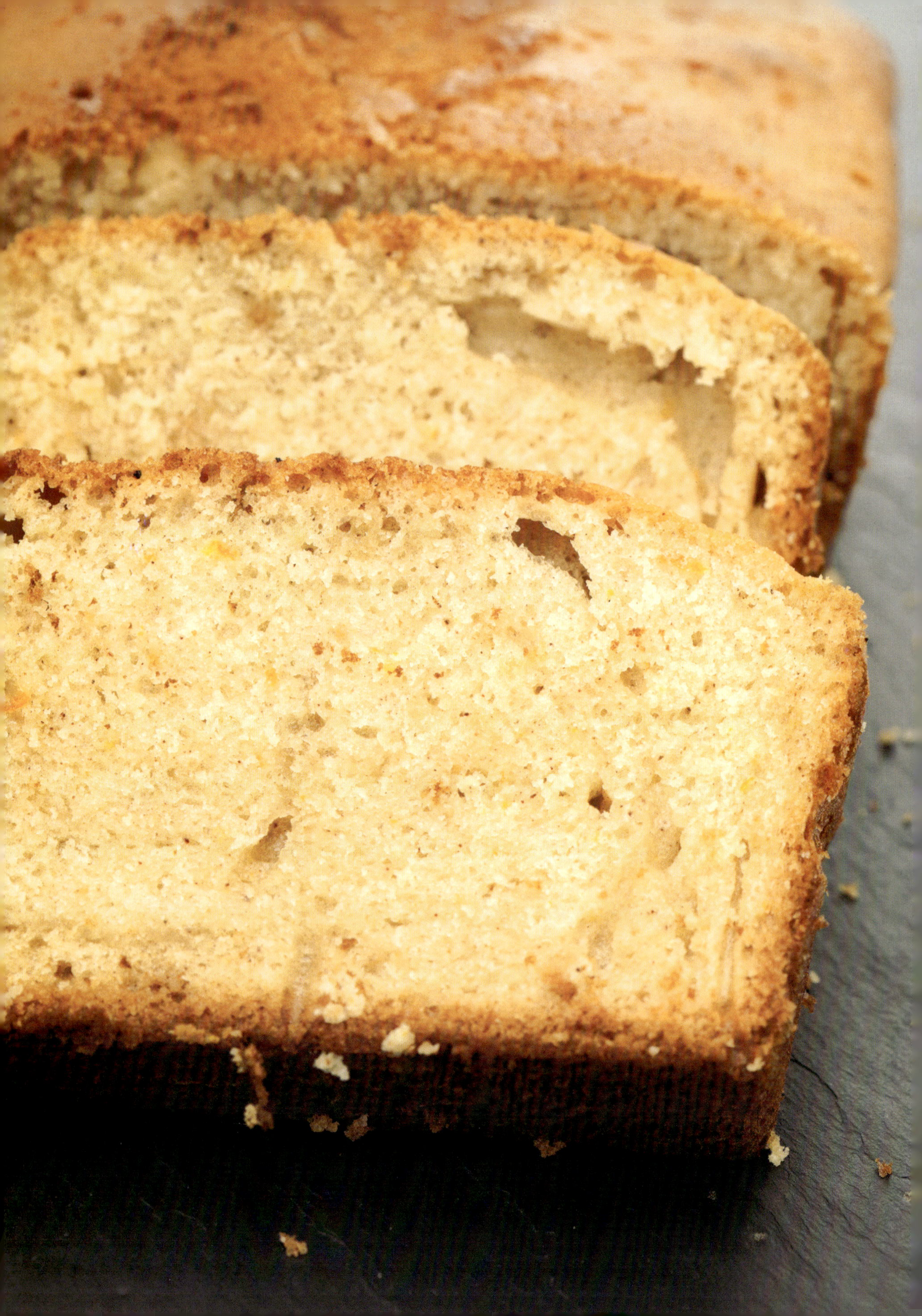

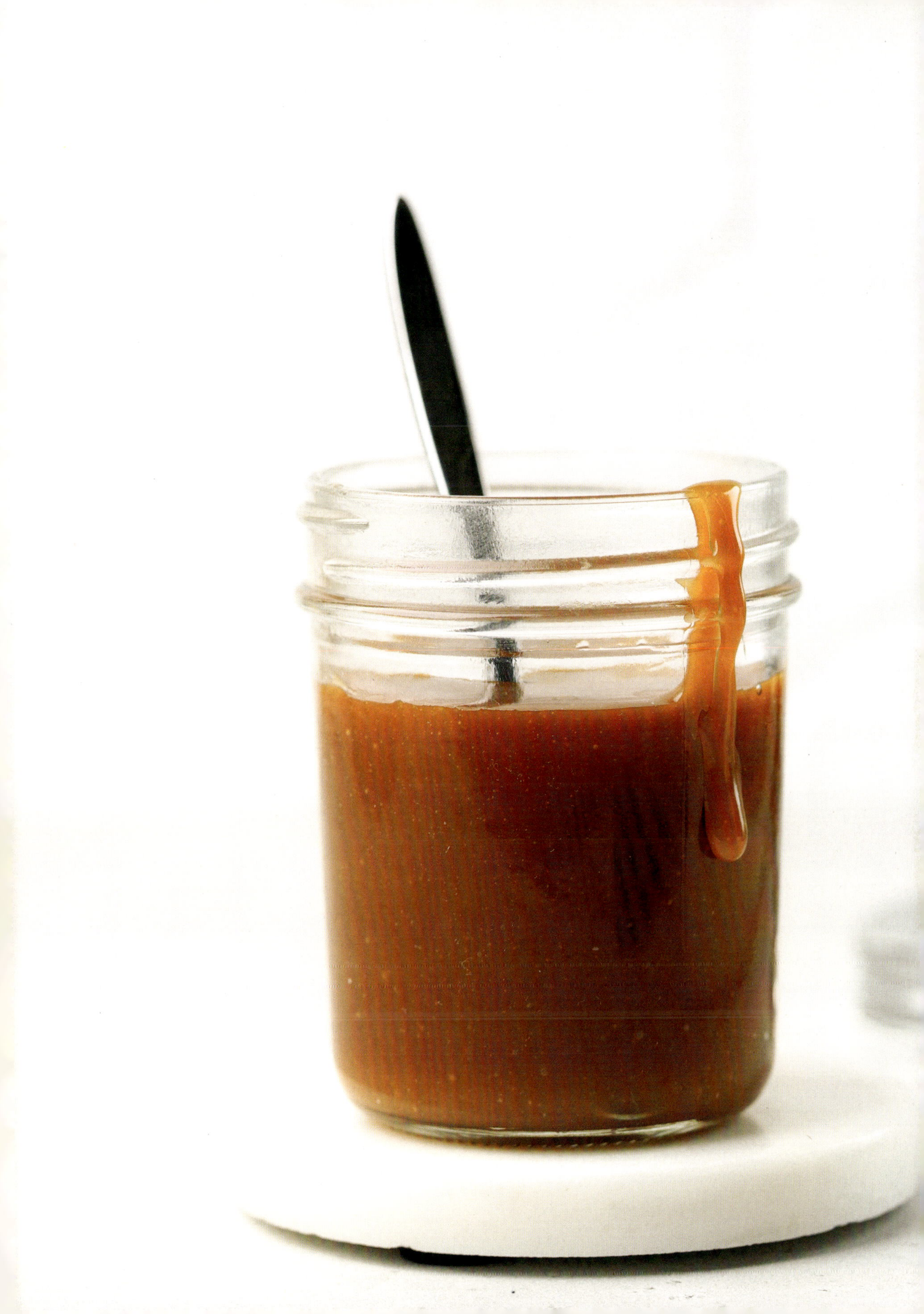

Orange Cinnamon Cake

SERVES 10
PREP + COOK TIME: 2 HOURS 30 MINS
GLUTEN FREE • DAIRY FREE

CAKE

2 oranges (500g), skin on
3 eggs
½ cup (100g) brown sugar
1¼ cups (150g) almond meal
½ cup (60g) buckwheat flour
1 tsp baking powder

SYRUP

2 cups (500ml) orange juice
⅓ cup (65g) brown sugar
2 cinnamon sticks

Place oranges in a small saucepan, cover with water and weigh down to submerge. Bring to a simmer over high heat and cook for 1 hour or until very soft. Drain and cool slightly. Place in a food processor and process until smooth.

Preheat oven to 180°C. Line a 20 x 30cm slice tin with greaseproof paper.

Whisk eggs and sugar in the bowl of an electric mixer on high speed for 6-8 minutes or until thick and tripled in volume. Fold through orange puree, almond meal, flour and baking powder until combined. Pour into the tin and bake for 30 minutes or until a skewer comes out clean when inserted.

While the cake is baking, place orange juice, sugar and cinnamon in a small saucepan over high heat and cook for 12-15 minutes until slightly reduced.

Remove and discard cinnamon sticks and pour half the syrup over the hot cake in the tin. Allow to cool slightly.

Remove the cake from the tin, place on a serving plate and top with the remaining syrup.

Caramel Sauce

MAKES 1 CUP
PREP + COOK TIME: 20 MINS
GLUTEN FREE

1 cup (220g) sugar
6 tbsps salted butter, room temperature, diced
½ cup (120ml) thickened cream, room temperature
1 tsp salt

Heat sugar in a heavy-bottomed pan over medium heat, stirring constantly until the sugar melts into a thick, amber-coloured liquid. Immediately stir in the butter until melted and combined. Take care as the caramel bubbles when the butter is added.

Slowly pour in the cream, stirring constantly as you do so. When all the cream is added stop stirring and allow to boil for 1 minute. Remove from heat and stir in the salt. Allow to cool slightly before using. Caramel thickens as it cools.

Caramel Fudge

SERVES 12
PREP + COOK TIME: 15 MINS + CHILLING
GLUTEN FREE

125g butter
1 x 400g can sweetened condensed milk
2 tbsps golden syrup
1 cup (200g) brown sugar
120g white chocolate, chopped into pieces

Line a 25cm square tin with greaseproof paper. Melt butter in a medium saucepan over low heat. Add condensed milk, golden syrup and brown sugar. Stir over low heat until it comes to the boil, then simmer for 10 minutes, stirring constantly.

Remove from heat, stir in white chocolate and mix until smooth. Pour into prepared tin and allow to cool. Refrigerate for at least 2 hours to firm before cutting into squares.

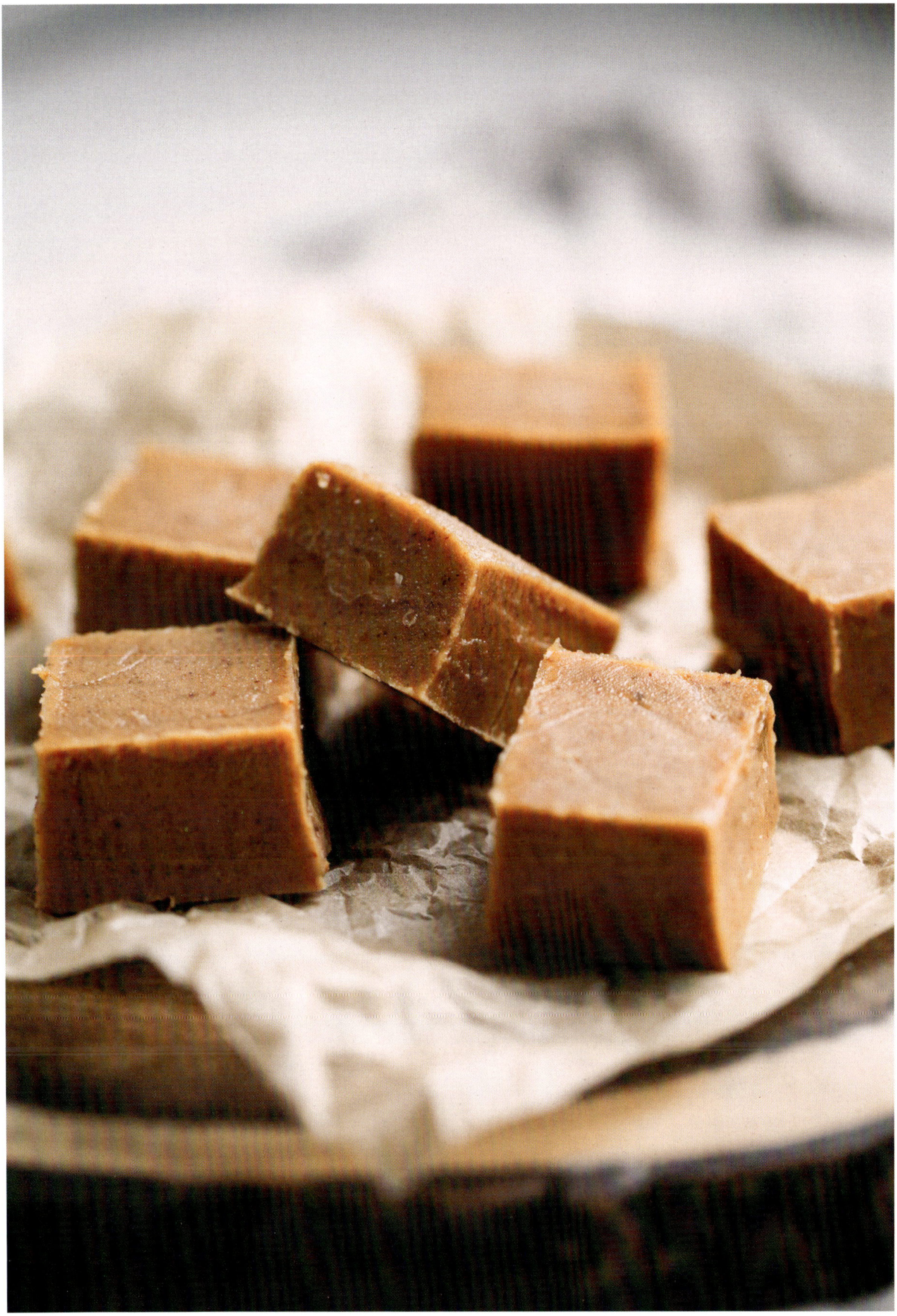

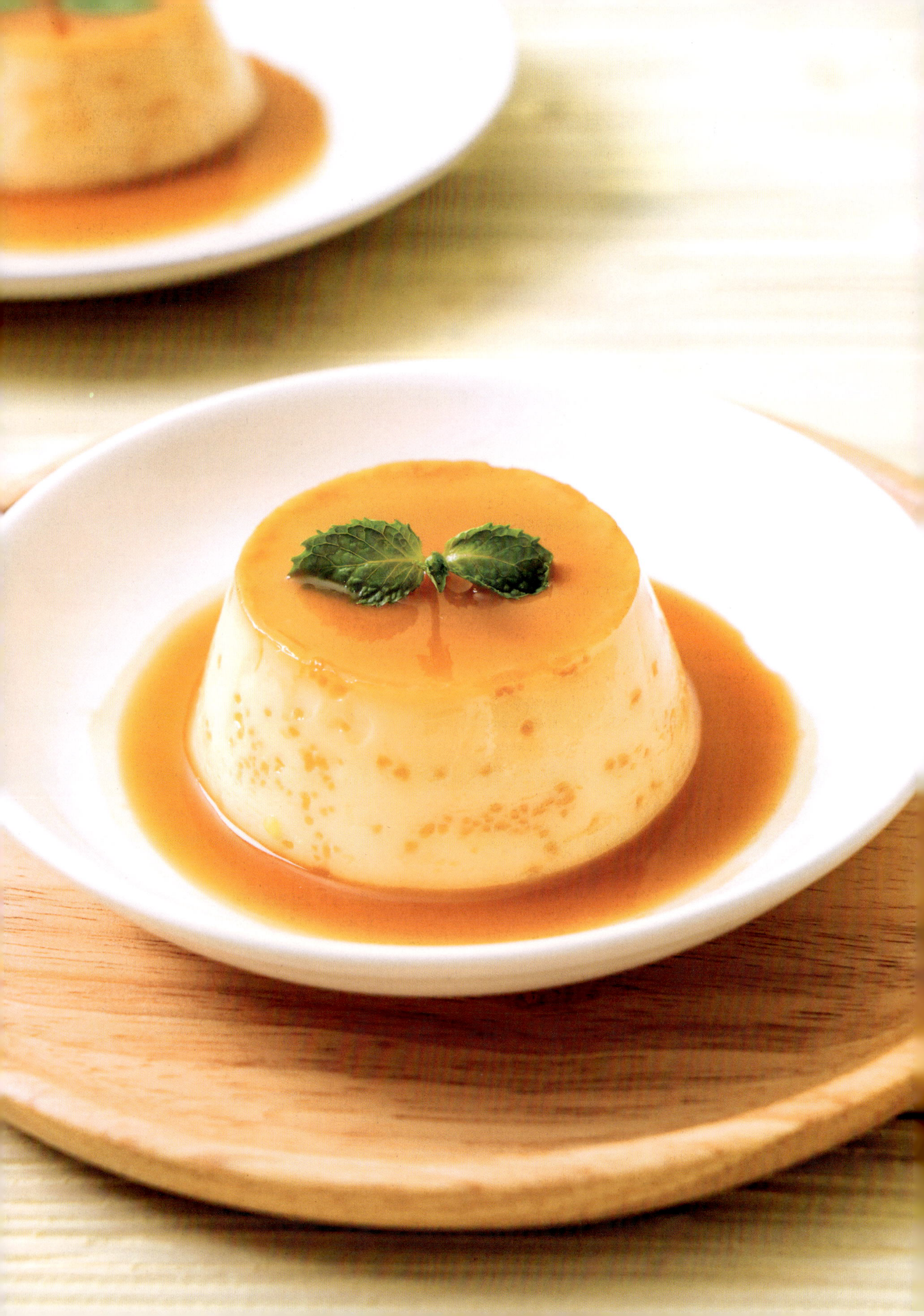

Creme Caramel

SERVES 4
PREP + COOK TIME: 1 HOUR 30 MINS + 4 HOURS CHILLING
GLUTEN FREE

SAUCE

½ cup (100g) sugar
3 tbsps water

CUSTARD CREAM

2 cups (500ml) milk
1 vanilla bean, split
2 large eggs
3 egg yolks
⅓ cup (70g) sugar

Preheat the oven to 170°C. Grease four individual ramekins.

Put the sugar and water in a saucepan on medium heat and cook undisturbed until the sugar begins to melt. Reduce heat to low and stir occasionally until sugar is fully dissolved and syrup is light brown. Immediately pour the caramel into the ramekins.

Pour the milk into a medium saucepan over medium-low heat. Add the vanilla bean and allow the milk to heat to simmering point, where bubbles just begin to appear, but not boiling. Cover and remove from the heat. Set aside for 15 minutes to cool slightly.

Whisk the eggs, yolks and sugar vigorously in a medium bowl until pale and creamy.

Remove the vanilla bean from the milk, scraping out the seeds and adding to the milk. Pour the warm vanilla milk into the egg yolk mixture and whisk gently to combine. Pour custard into the ramekins.

Place ramekins into a deep-sided baking dish, and pour hot water into the dish until it is three-quarters up the sides of the ramekins.

Place in the oven and bake for 40 minutes or until set. Remove from the oven and allow to cool completely in the dish, then refrigerate for 4 hours or overnight.

Run a knife around the edge of the ramekins then turn onto serving plates.

Sharlotka

SERVES 10
PREP + COOK TIME: 1 HOUR 10 MINS

3 apples
Juice of 1 lemon
1 tsp cinnamon
1¼ cups (155g) plain flour
1½ tsps baking powder
4 eggs, room temperature
Pinch of salt
1 cup (220g) sugar
¼ cup (60ml) sour cream
1 tsp vanilla extract

Preheat oven to 175°C. Grease a 23cm springform cake tin.

Cut two apples into small dice. Place them into a bowl and sprinkle with the lemon juice and cinnamon. Stir to coat evenly and set aside.

In a bowl, mix the flour and baking powder. Set aside.

In another large bowl, add the eggs and salt. Beat with an electric hand mixer until well combined. Add sugar about ¼ cup at a time, mixing continuously as you do so. Continue mixing for another 5 minutes until the mixture is pale and thick. Add sour cream and vanilla extract and beat to incorporate. Sift the flour into the egg mixture a little at a time, and gently fold in with a spatula.

Pour a third of the batter into the cake tin and spread with a spatula. Add half of the diced apples and gently press into the batter. Add another third of the batter to cover the apples, then repeat with another layer of apple and another layer of batter. Slice the remaining apple into very thin wedges and arrange on top of the cake.

Place in the oven and bake for 50-60 minutes or until a toothpick inserted in the centre of the cake comes out clean. Allow to cool before removing from the tin.

Banana Tarte Tatin

SERVES 6
PREP + COOK TIME: 40 MINS

50g butter
⅓ cup (75g) firmly packed brown sugar
¼ cup (60ml) thickened cream
¼ tsp cinnamon
4 small bananas, sliced lengthwise
1 sheet frozen puff pastry, thawed
1 egg, beaten lightly

Preheat oven to 220°C.

Place butter, brown sugar, cream and cinnamon in an ovenproof frying pan, over medium-low heat. Stir until sugar dissolves, then bring to a boil. Reduce heat and simmer, uncovered, for 2 minutes. Remove from the heat.

Very carefully arrange the sliced bananas on top of the caramel. DO NOT touch the caramel with your fingers!

Cut a 24cm circle from the pastry sheet. Place pastry over banana, and tuck edges down the insides of the frying pan. Brush pastry with beaten egg.

Transfer the frying pan to the oven and bake for 15-20 minutes or until pastry is browned.

Carefully turn tart onto a serving plate and serve immediately.

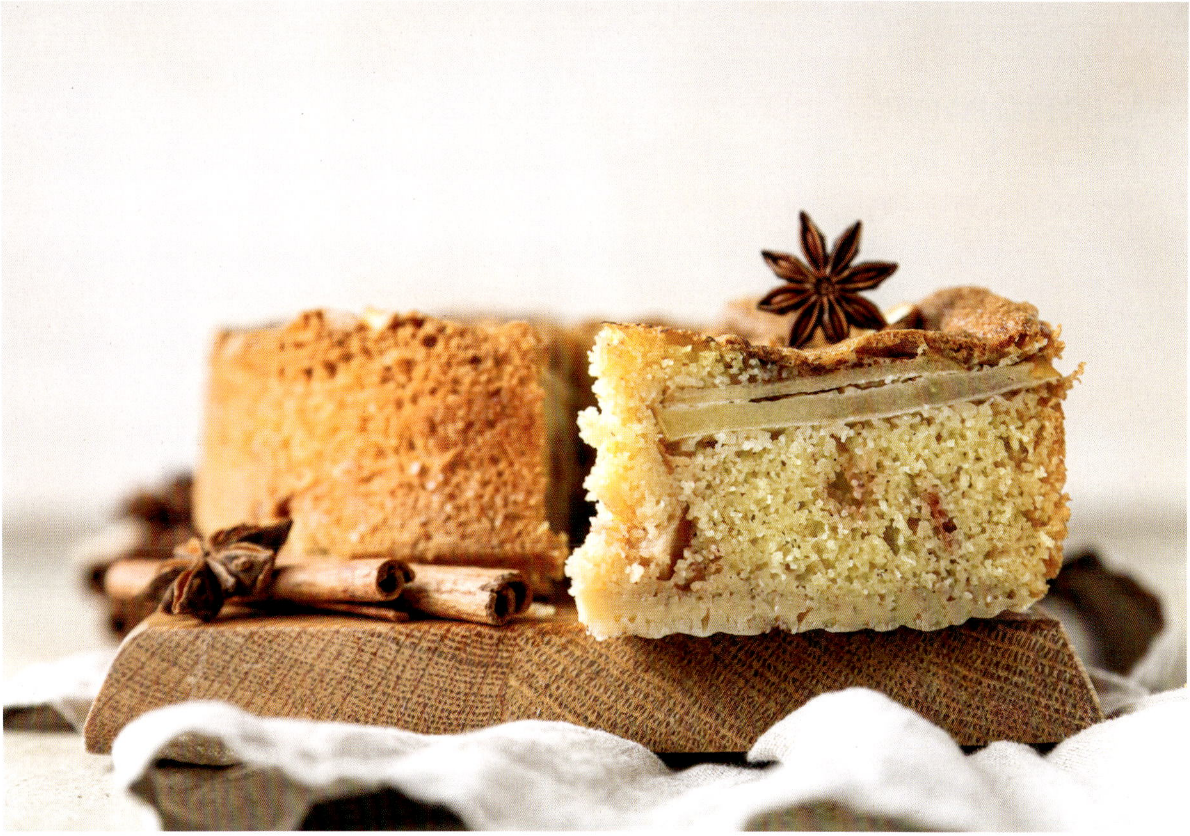

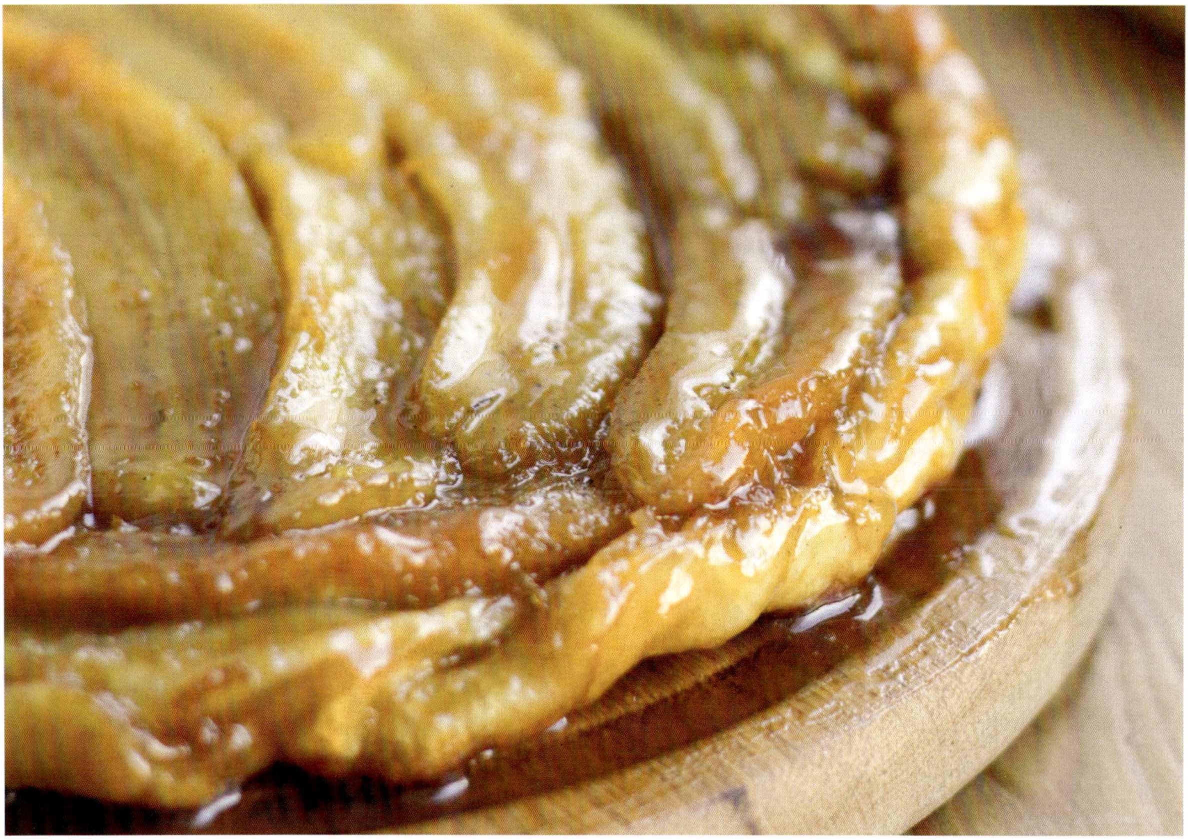

Cinnamon French Toast

SERVES 6-8
PREP + COOK TIME: 15 MINS

4 eggs
½ cup (125ml) milk
¼ tsp salt
2 tsps cinnamon
⅔ cup (140g) sugar
6 tbsps butter
8 thick slices white bread, preferably stale
Maple syrup to serve (optional)

Combine eggs, milk and salt in a large mixing bowl. Combine cinnamon and sugar on a plate. Melt 4 tablespoons butter in a large frying pan over medium-high heat. Quickly dip bread slices into egg mixture, shake off excess and cook in pan. Cook each side until golden. While still hot, transfer slices to the plate with cinnamon sugar and coat each side.

Melt the last 2 tablespoons butter and cook remaining slices before coating in cinnamon sugar.

Serve immediately with maple syrup if desired.

Baklava

SERVES 16
PREP + COOK TIME: 1 HOUR 10 MINS

BAKLAVA
3 cups (375g) walnuts, finely chopped
1 cup (125g) pistachios, finely chopped
½ cup (60g) almonds, finely chopped
½ cup (110g) caster sugar
2 tsps allspice
2 tsps ground cardamon
2 tsps cinnamon
16 sheets filo pastry
125g butter, melted

SYRUP
1 tbsp butter
1 tbsp caster sugar
½ cup (180g) honey
2 tbsps lemon juice

Preheat oven to 180°C and grease an 18 x 28cm slice tin.

In a medium bowl, mix together walnuts, half the pistachios, almonds, sugar and the spices.

Layer four sheets of filo pastry in the tin, brushing each one with melted butter before placing the next one on top. Trim off any overhanging pastry. Spoon out a portion of the nut mixture into the tin and flatten with the back of the spoon before adding another layer of pastry. Repeat, until you have a top layer of pastry and all the nut mixture has been used up. Brush the top with melted butter and cut baklava into 16 small rectangles with a sharp knife. Bake for 25 minutes or until turning golden.

For the syrup, heat butter, sugar, honey and lemon juice in a saucepan over medium-high heat. Stir for 5 minutes until sugar dissolves. Reduce to a simmer and cook for a further 10 minutes until the mixture has thickened.

Pour the syrup over the baklava and let it cool. Sprinkle the remaining pistachios over the top.

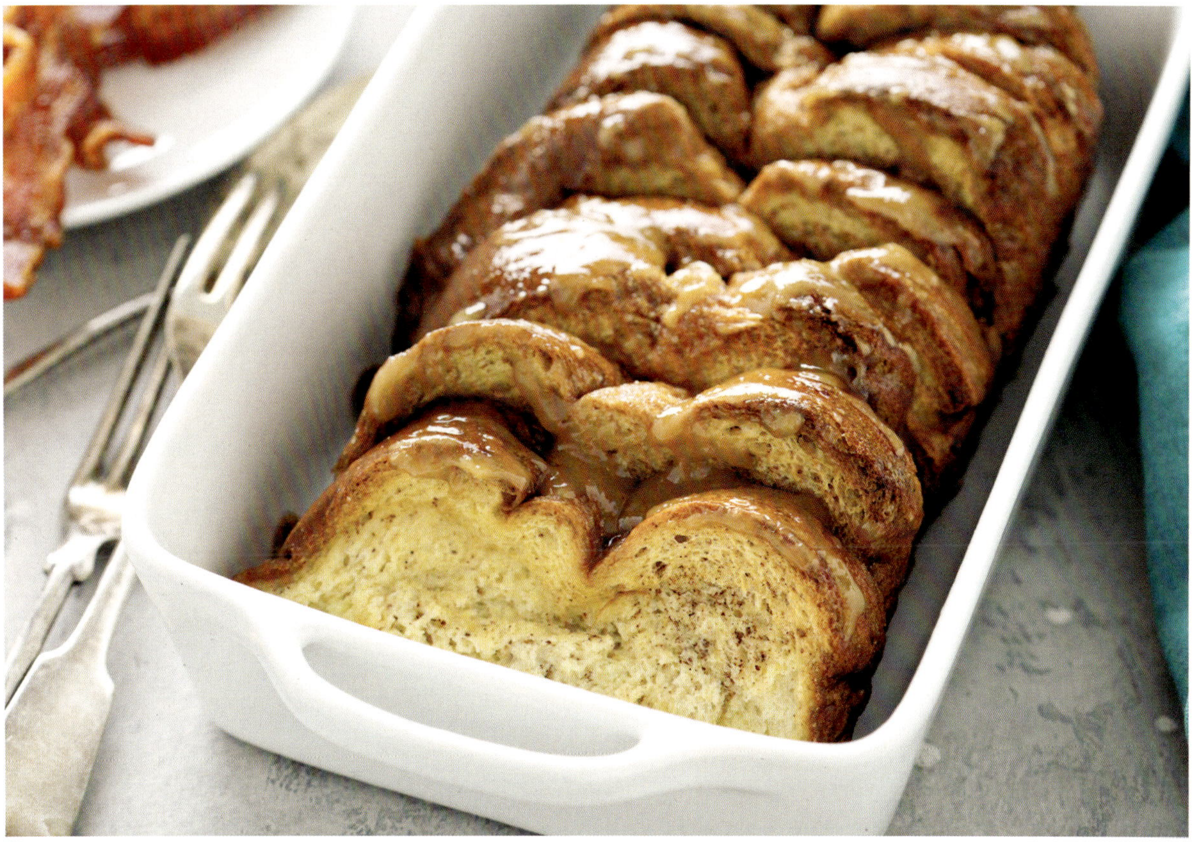

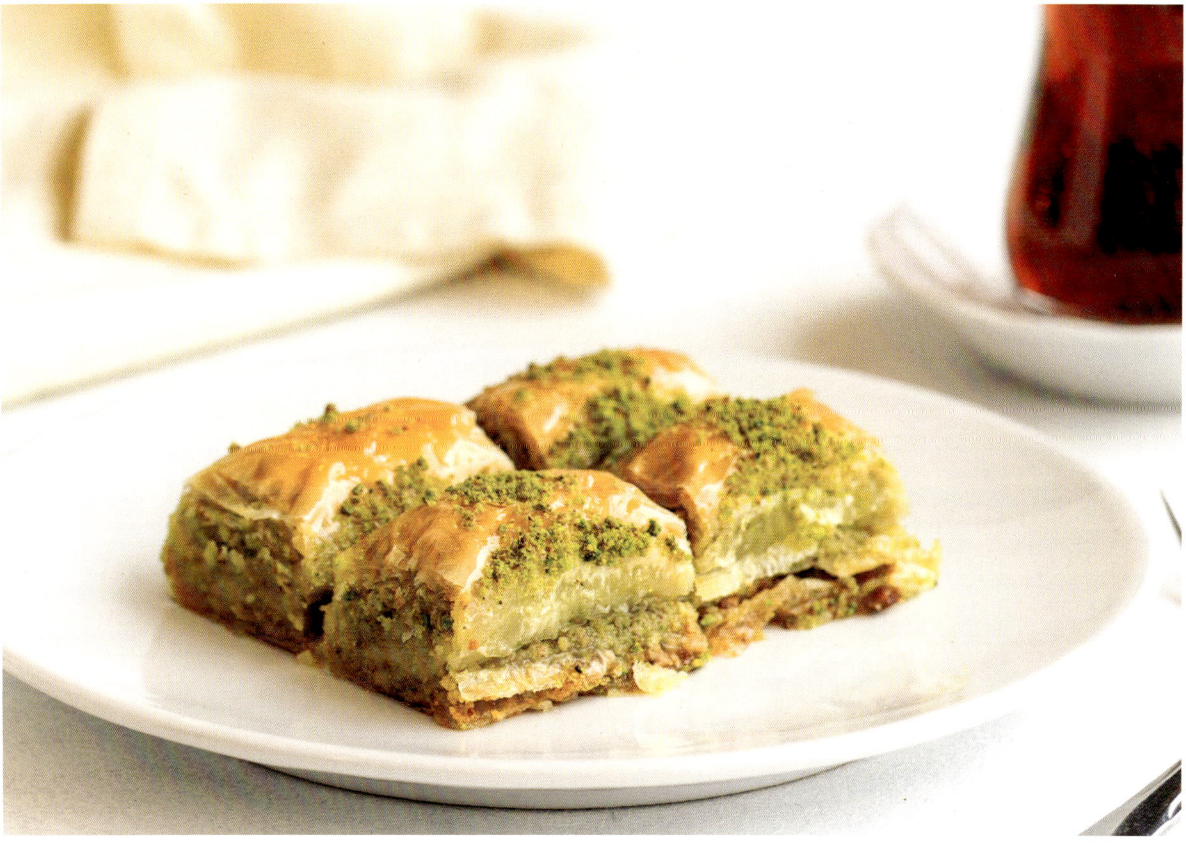

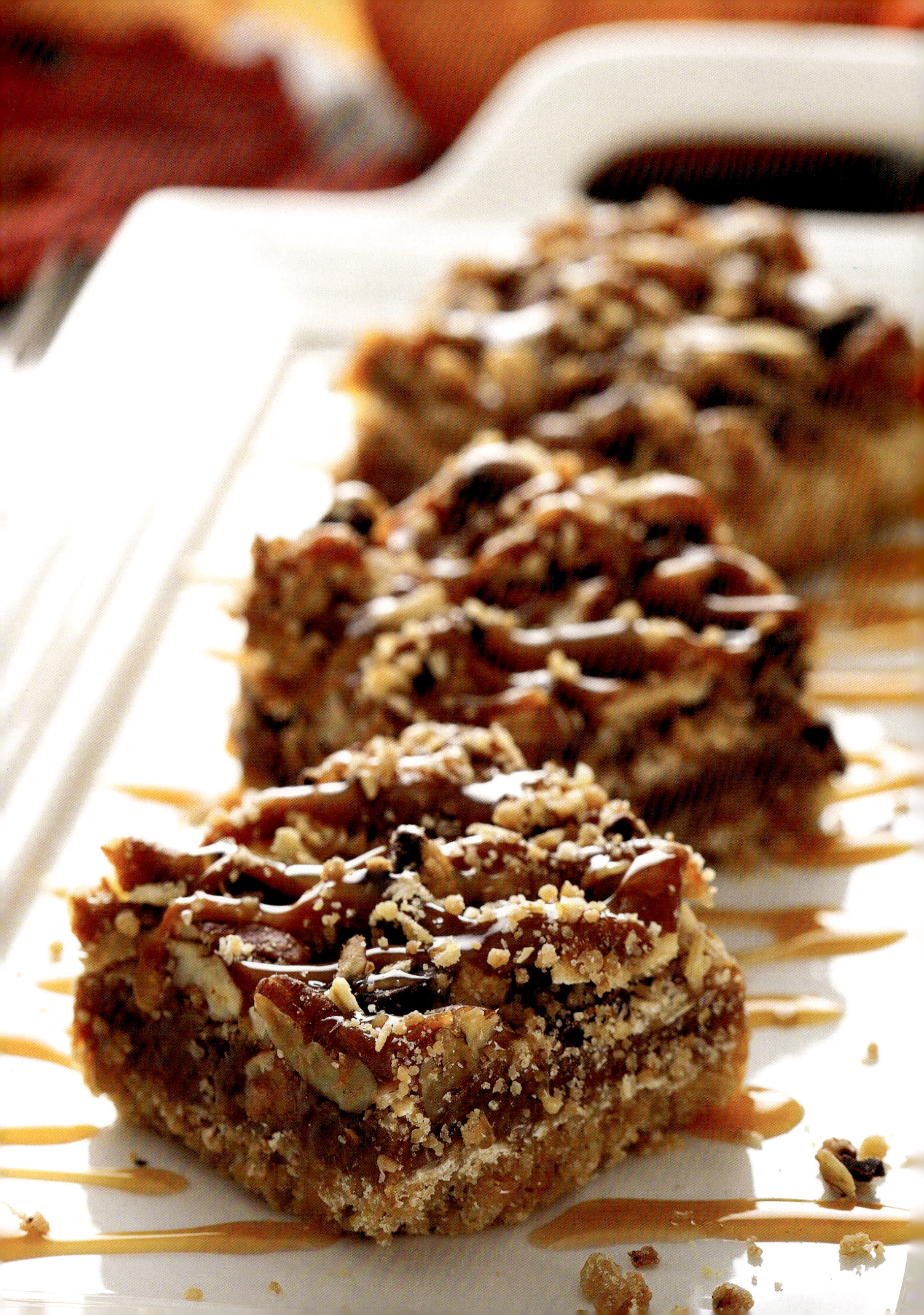

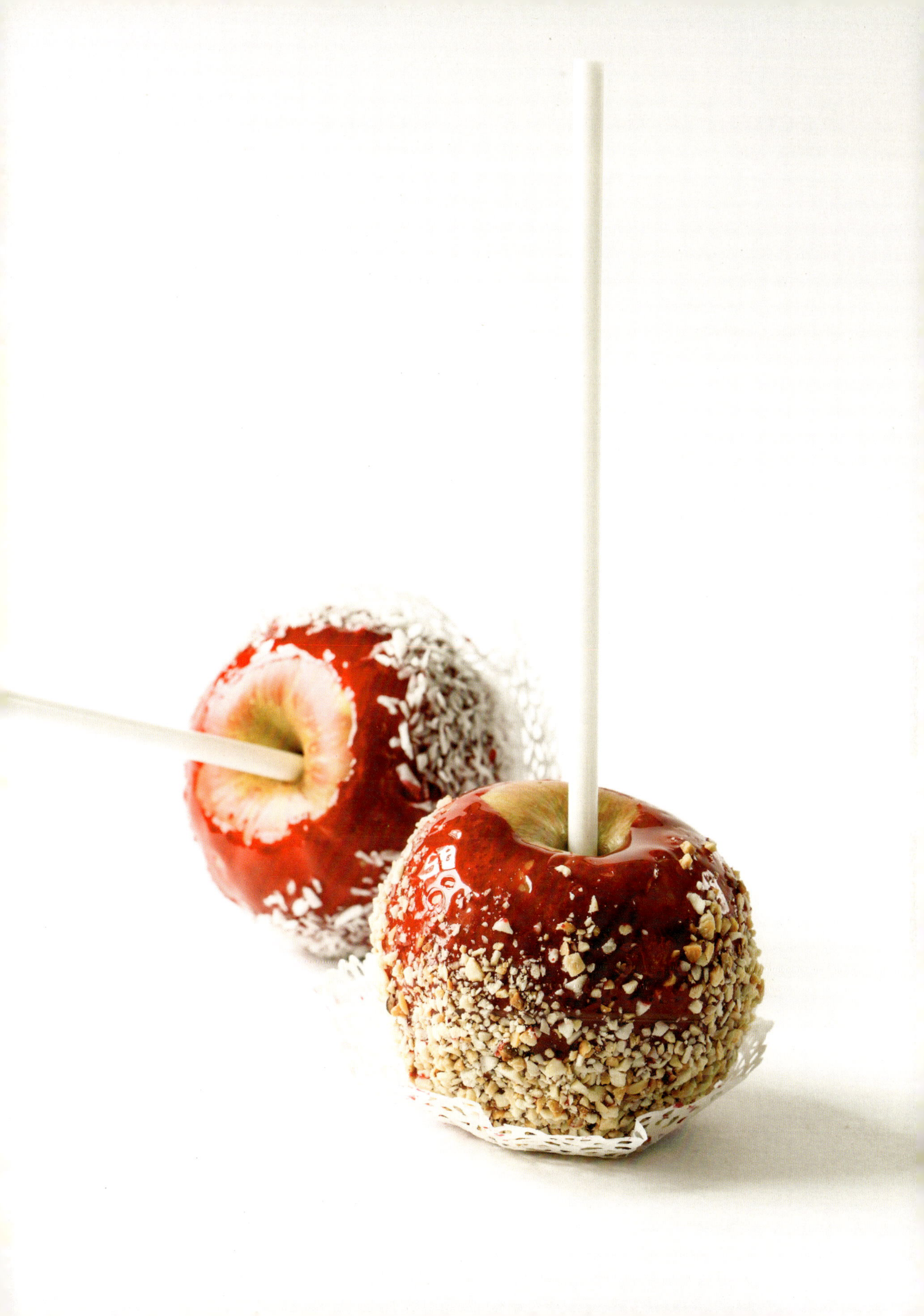

Pecan Pie Bars

MAKES 20
PREP + COOK TIME: 1 HOUR

BASE

2 cups (250g) plain flour

2 tbsps cornflour

1 cup (200g) brown sugar

115g butter, melted

FILLING

170g butter

1 cup (200g) brown sugar

½ cup (180g) honey

1 cup (250ml) thickened cream

1 tsp vanilla extract

2 cups (240g) pecan halves

TOPPING

¼ cup (30g) toasted pecans

1 tsp salt

Caramel sauce for drizzling (optional; see recipe page 80)

Preheat oven to 175°C. Grease and line a 25 x 35cm baking dish with greaseproof paper.

In a large mixing bowl, combine the ingredients for the base. Beat with an electric hand mixer until the mixture resembles fine crumbs. Press into the prepared baking dish. Bake for 8 minutes, then set aside to cool.

In a large saucepan over medium heat, stir together the butter, sugar and honey. Cook, stirring constantly, for 7-8 minutes until thick and bubbly. Pour in the cream and continue to cook, stirring, for 10 minutes. Remove from the heat and stir in the vanilla and pecans. Pour the mixture over the crust. Spread with a spatula.

In a food processor, add the toasted pecans and salt. Process until finely chopped. Sprinkle over the caramel mixture. Bake for 15 minutes until caramel is bubbly.

Allow to cool completely, then slice and drizzle with caramel sauce, if desired.

Toffee Apples

MAKES 12
PREP + COOK TIME: 30 MINS + SETTING
GLUTEN FREE • DAIRY FREE

12 small red apples, washed in boiling water to remove wax coating, stalks removed

3 cups (660g) caster sugar

¾ cup (185ml) warm water

¼ cup (60ml) liquid glucose

1 tsp white vinegar

½ tsp red food colouring

Chopped nuts or desiccated coconut (optional)

Line two large baking trays with greaseproof paper. Push 1 lollypop stick or wooden skewer into the top of each apple. Place sugar, warm water, glucose and vinegar in a heavy-based saucepan over low heat. Cook, stirring, for 5-7 minutes or until sugar dissolves. Increase heat to medium-high and bring to the boil. Cook, without stirring, for 15-20 minutes or until toffee reaches 150°C. Remove from heat. Add red food colouring. Dip an apple into the toffee, tilting pan to coat. Dip in nuts or coconut, if desired. Place on prepared baking tray. Repeat with remaining apples. Stand for 20 minutes to set.

Baked Pears

SERVES 2
PREP + COOK TIME: 30 MINS
GLUTEN FREE

2 pears, halved and cored

2 tsps cinnamon + more to serve

2 tsps maple syrup

1 cup (250ml) yoghurt

3 tbsps roughly chopped walnuts

Preheat oven to 175°C. Place pears cut-side down in a large roasting pan. Sprinkle cinnamon and maple syrup on top. Bake for 25 minutes. Serve pears on top of yoghurt with chopped walnuts and an extra sprinkle of cinnamon.

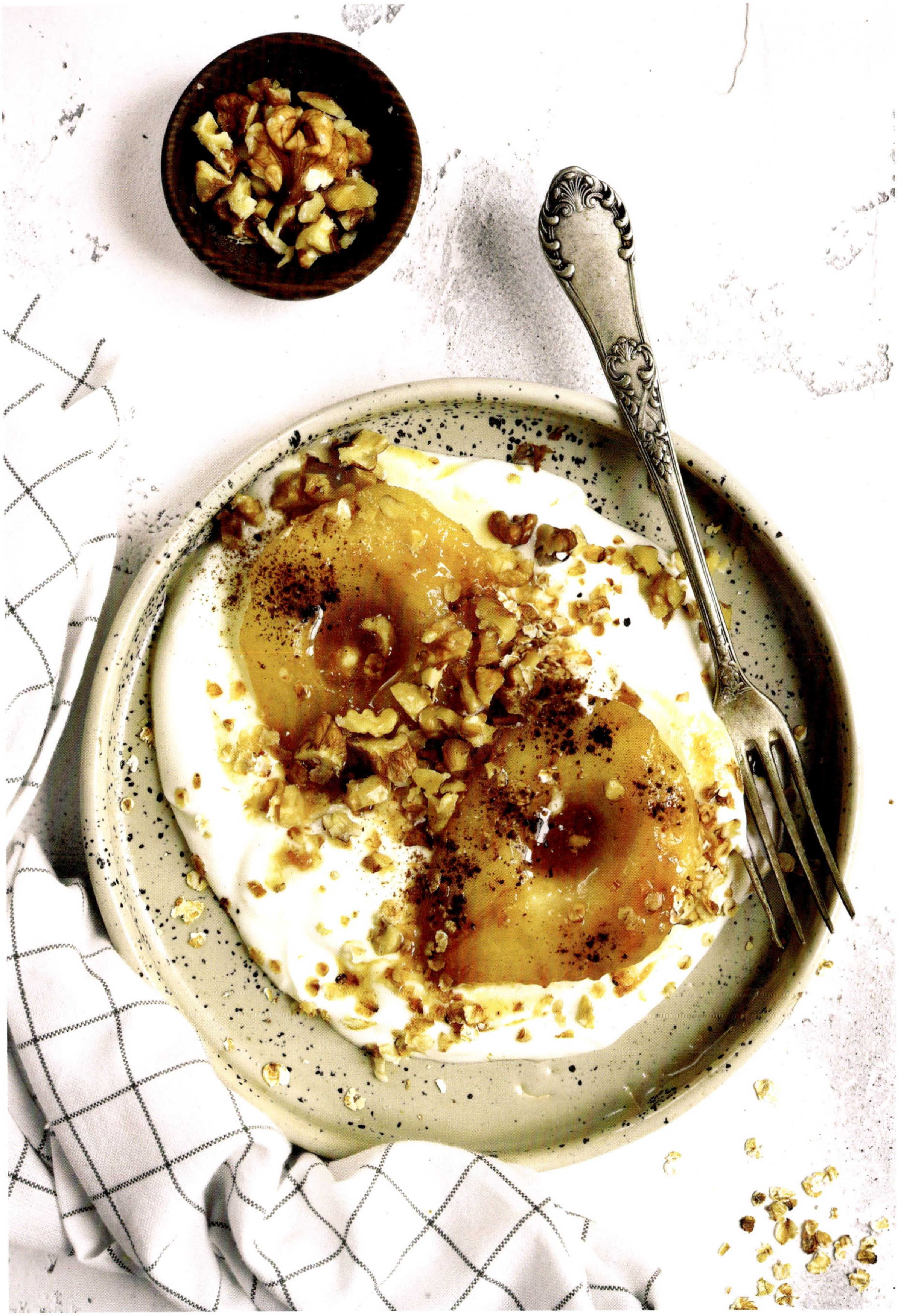

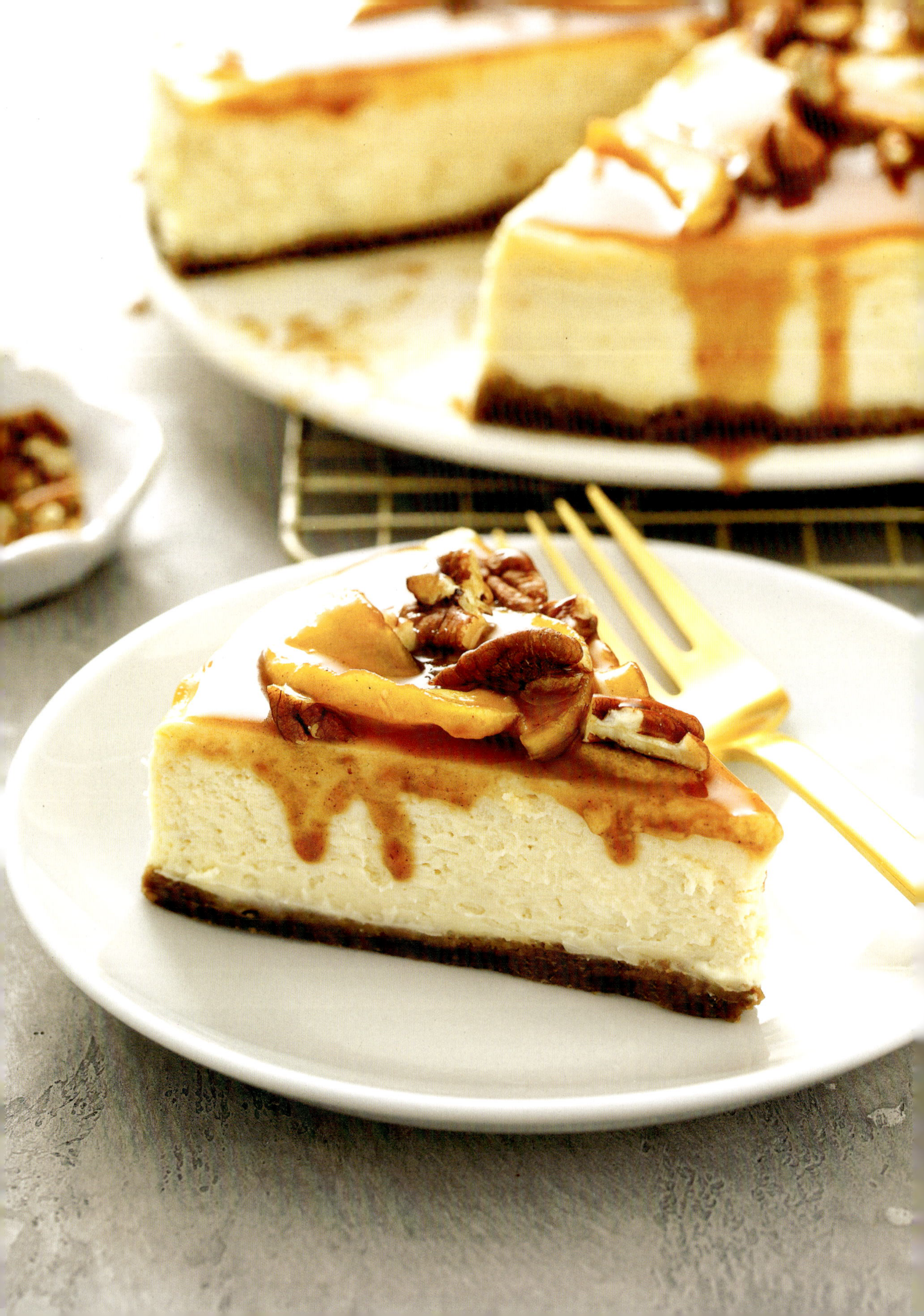

Apple Caramel Cheesecake

SERVES 12
PREP + COOK TIME: 2 HOURS 45 MINS + 1 HOUR COOLING AND 6 HOURS CHILLING

BASE
1½ cups (150g) crushed digestive biscuits
60g butter, melted
2 tbsps packed brown sugar
½ tsp cinnamon

FILLING
4 x 225g packets cream cheese, softened
1¼ cups (275g) packed brown sugar
1 tsp vanilla extract
1 cup (250ml) sour cream, room temperature
4 eggs, room temperature

TOPPING
2 Granny Smith apples, peeled and thinly sliced
¾ cup (90g) coarsely chopped pecans
1 tsp cinnamon
½ cup (110g) packed brown sugar

CARAMEL SAUCE
1 cup (220g) sugar
¼ cup (60ml) + 2 tbsps water
60g butter, diced
½ cup (125ml) thickened cream, warmed
½ tsp fine salt

Preheat oven to 160°C. Grease a 23cm springform cake tin. Wrap with a triple layer of foil around the bottom and up the outside of the pan to prevent water leaking in from a water bath.

In a medium bowl, mix together the biscuit crumbs, melted butter, brown sugar and cinnamon. Pour into the prepared tin and firmly press with the back of a spoon. Bake for 10-12 minutes until dark golden brown and fragrant. Set aside to cool while preparing the filling.

Beat the cream cheese with an electric mixer until smooth. Add the brown sugar and vanilla and beat well to combine. Add the sour cream and mix well. Add the eggs, one at a time, mixing well after each addition until the batter is smooth. Pour the batter over the cooled crust. Set aside.

In a large bowl, combine the apples, pecans, cinnamon and brown sugar. Gently spoon over the cheesecake batter in an even layer.

Transfer the filled springform pan into a roasting pan. Pour enough boiling water into the roasting pan to reach halfway up the sides of the cheesecake tin.

Transfer to the oven, and bake for 1¾-2 hours until set. Turn off the oven. Leave the cheesecake inside to cool for 1 hour. Transfer to a wire rack to cool for completely, then cover and refrigerate for at least 6 hours.

In a heavy-bottomed saucepan, bring the sugar and water for the sauce to a simmer over medium-high heat without stirring. Allow the mixture to boil without whisking, just swirling the saucepan occasionally, until it reaches an amber colour. Remove from the heat and immediately whisk in the butter, followed by the cream. Return to the heat and continue to whisk until smooth. Stir in the salt.

Pour caramel sauce over the cheesecake to serve.

Pumpkin & White Chocolate Cookies

MAKES 40
PREP + COOK TIME: 40 MINS

2 cups (250g) plain flour
1 tsp bicarbonate of soda
1 tsp cinnamon
⅛ tsp nutmeg
⅛ tsp ground ginger
170g unsalted butter, room temperature
⅔ cup (140g) white sugar
⅔ cup (140g) packed light brown sugar
1 large egg
⅔ cup (150g) mashed cooked pumpkin
1¼ cups (110g) rolled oats
1 cup (155g) white chocolate chips
1 cup (155g) caramel choc chips

Preheat oven to 175°C. Line two baking trays with greaseproof paper.

Whisk together the flour, bicarb and spices in a large bowl.

In a separate large bowl, use an electric mixer to cream together the butter and sugars until light and fluffy. Add the egg and mashed pumpkin and stir to combine.

Pour the wet mixture into the flour mixture and stir to incorporate. Add the oats, white chocolate chips and caramel choc chips. Stir to combine. Cover and refrigerate for at least 10 minutes or overnight.

Scoop heaped tablespoons of the mixture onto the baking trays, leaving 5cm between each one.

Bake for 13-15 minutes until light golden brown. Cool on trays for 10-15 minutes before transferring to a wire rack to cool completely.

Millionaire's Shortbread

MAKES 16
PREP + COOK TIME: 1 HOUR + 1 HOUR CHILLING

SHORTBREAD
2 cups (250g) plain flour
⅓ cup (75g) caster sugar
175g butter, softened

CARAMEL
100g butter
½ cup (100g) muscovado sugar
1 x 400g can condensed milk
2 tbsps golden syrup
1 tsp vanilla

TOPPING
200g dark chocolate, roughly chopped
3 tbsps cream

Heat the oven to 180°C. Grease and line a 22cm square cake tin with greaseproof paper.

To make the shortbread, mix flour and caster sugar in a bowl. Rub in butter with your fingertips until the mixture resembles fine breadcrumbs. Knead the mixture until it forms a dough, then press into the base of the prepared tin. Prick lightly with a fork and bake for 20 minutes or until firm to the touch and very lightly browned. Leave to cool in the tin.

To make the caramel, place butter, sugar, condensed milk, golden syrup and vanilla in a pan over medium-low heat. Cook, stirring continuously until the sugar dissolves. Bring to a gentle boil, whisking constantly, for about 6 minutes until the caramel is thick. Pour over the shortbread and leave to cool.

For the topping, melt chocolate and cream slowly in a bowl over a pan of simmering water. Pour over the cold caramel and refrigerate for about 1 hour to set.

Cut into squares with a hot knife.

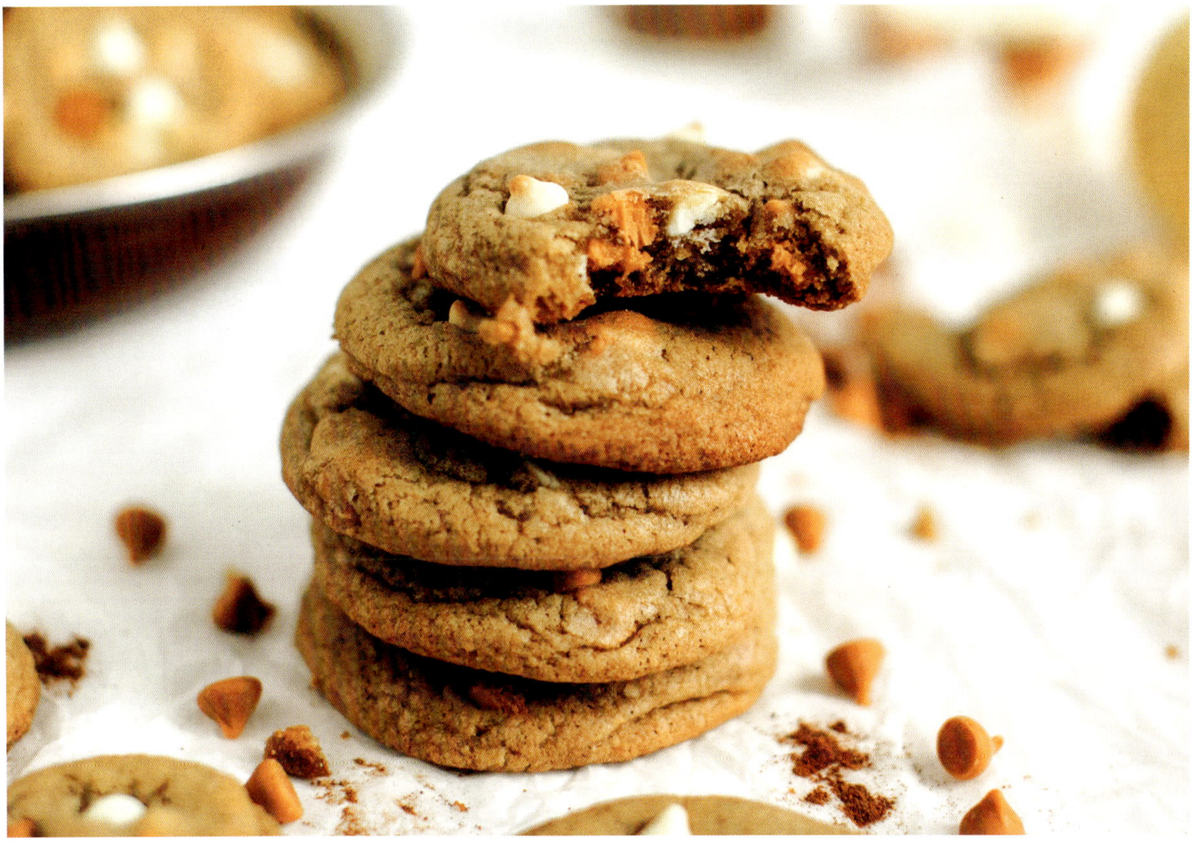

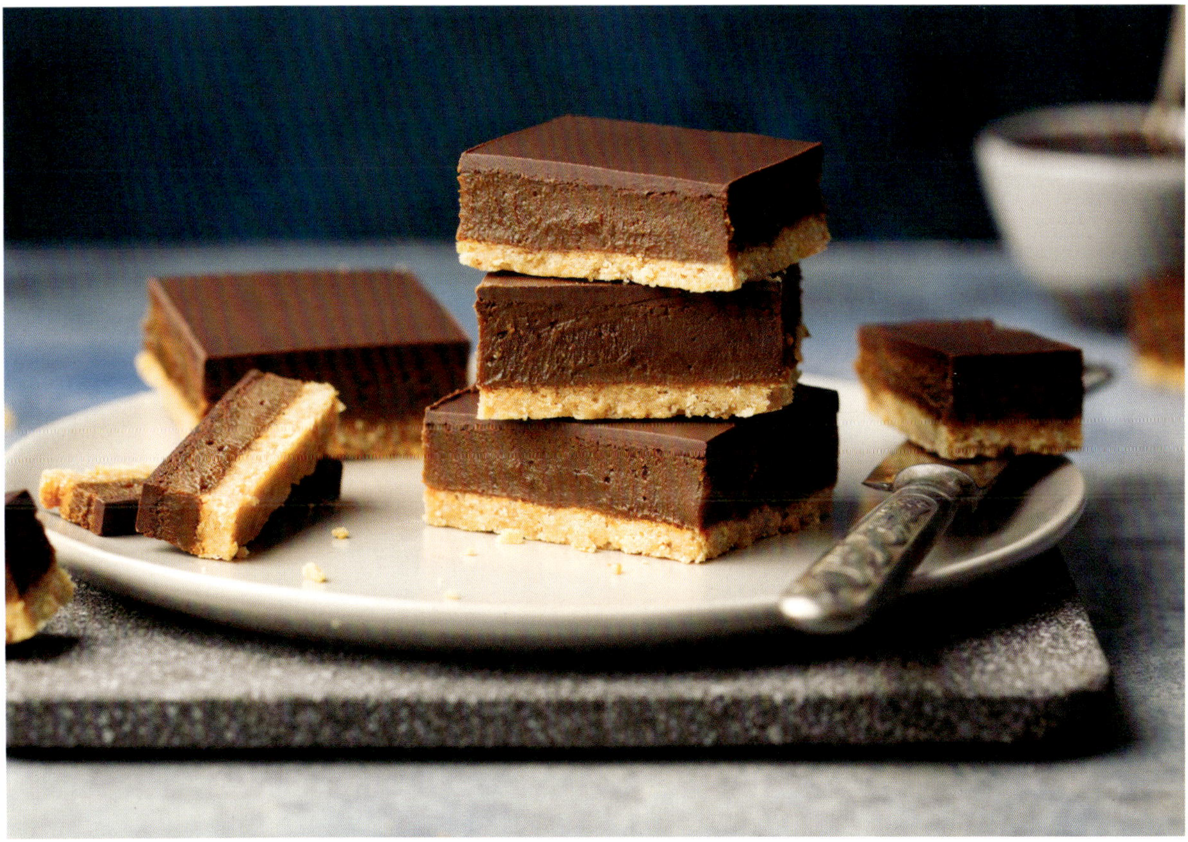

4

Custard & Cream

Tiramisu

SERVES 6
PREP + COOK TIME: 30 MINS + 4 HOURS CHILLING

3 eggs, separated
½ cup (110g) caster sugar
½ tsp vanilla extract
1 cup (250g) mascarpone
1¼ cups (310ml) strong brewed black coffee
2 tbsps Marsala or coffee liqueur
200g savoiardi or sponge finger biscuits
Cocoa powder for dusting

Beat egg yolks and sugar with an electric mixer until pale and thick. Add vanilla and mascarpone, and beat until smooth. Set aside.

In a clean bowl with clean beaters, whisk the egg whites until stiff peaks form.

Add half the mascarpone mixture into the egg whites and gently fold through. Add the remaining mascarpone mixture and fold through until just combined.

Mix coffee and Marsala or liqueur together in a medium bowl. Quickly dip half the biscuits, one at a time, in the coffee mixture, then place in a 20cm square dish, covering the base.

Spread over half the cream mixture, then top with another layer of coffee-dipped biscuits. Spread with remaining cream.

Cover and refrigerate for at least 4-5 hours, preferably overnight.

Dust with cocoa powder just before serving.

Portuguese Custard Tarts

MAKES 12
PREP + COOK TIME: 1 HOUR + 1 HOUR CHILLING

2 egg yolks + 1 whole egg
½ cup (110g) caster sugar
1½ tbsps cornflour
1¼ cups (310ml) milk
1 cup (250ml) thickened cream
2 tsps vanilla extract
2 sheets frozen puff pastry, thawed
2 tsps cinnamon
1 tbsp caster sugar

Whisk egg yolks, egg, sugar and cornflour in a medium saucepan until well combined. Slowly add milk, cream and vanilla, stirring all the time.

Cook custard over low heat, stirring constantly with a whisk until it begins to thicken. Remove from heat. Transfer to a bowl and refrigerate for 1 hour.

Preheat oven to 210°C. Grease a 12-hole muffin tin.

Place one pastry sheet on a floured bench top. Sprinkle with cinnamon and sugar then top with the other pastry sheet. Fold into quarters then roll out to approximately 3mm thick. Cut out 10cm circles.
Press the pastry rounds into muffin tin holes.

Spoon the cooled custard into the pastry. Bake for 30 minutes or until the pastry is crisp and the custard golden on top.

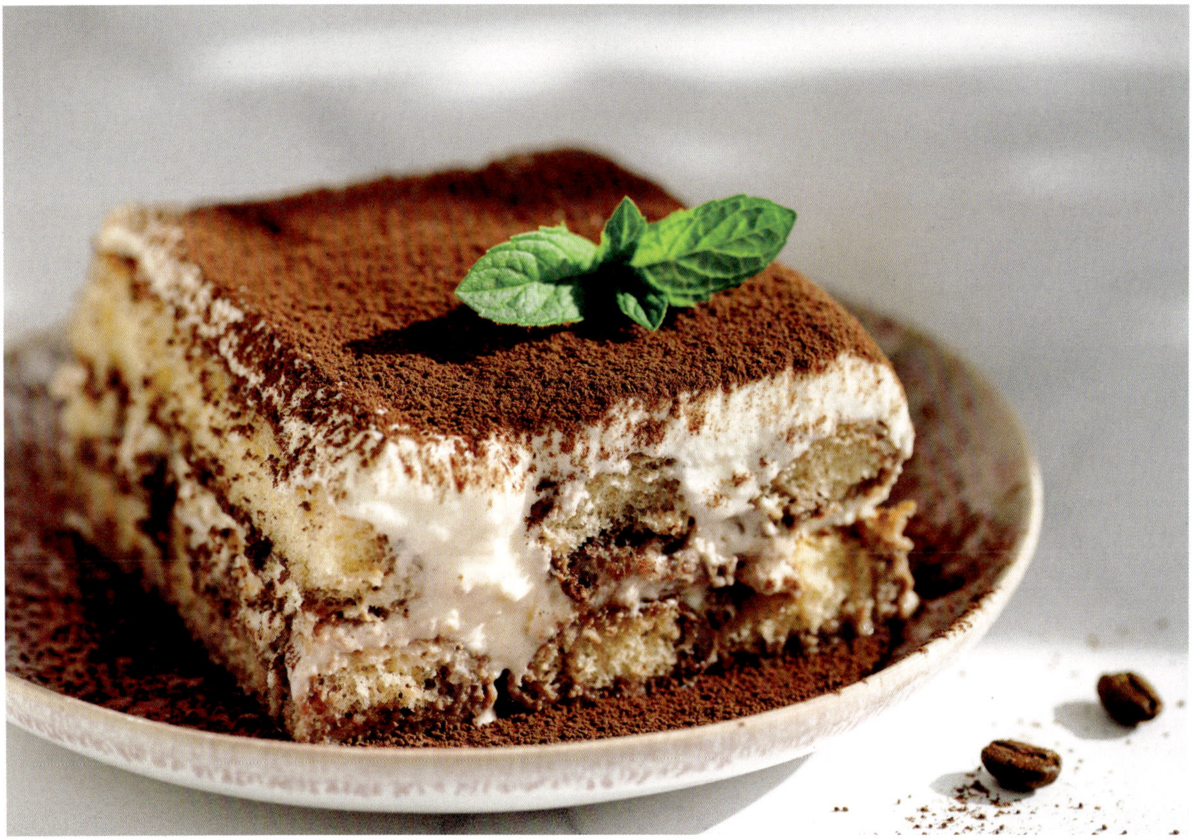

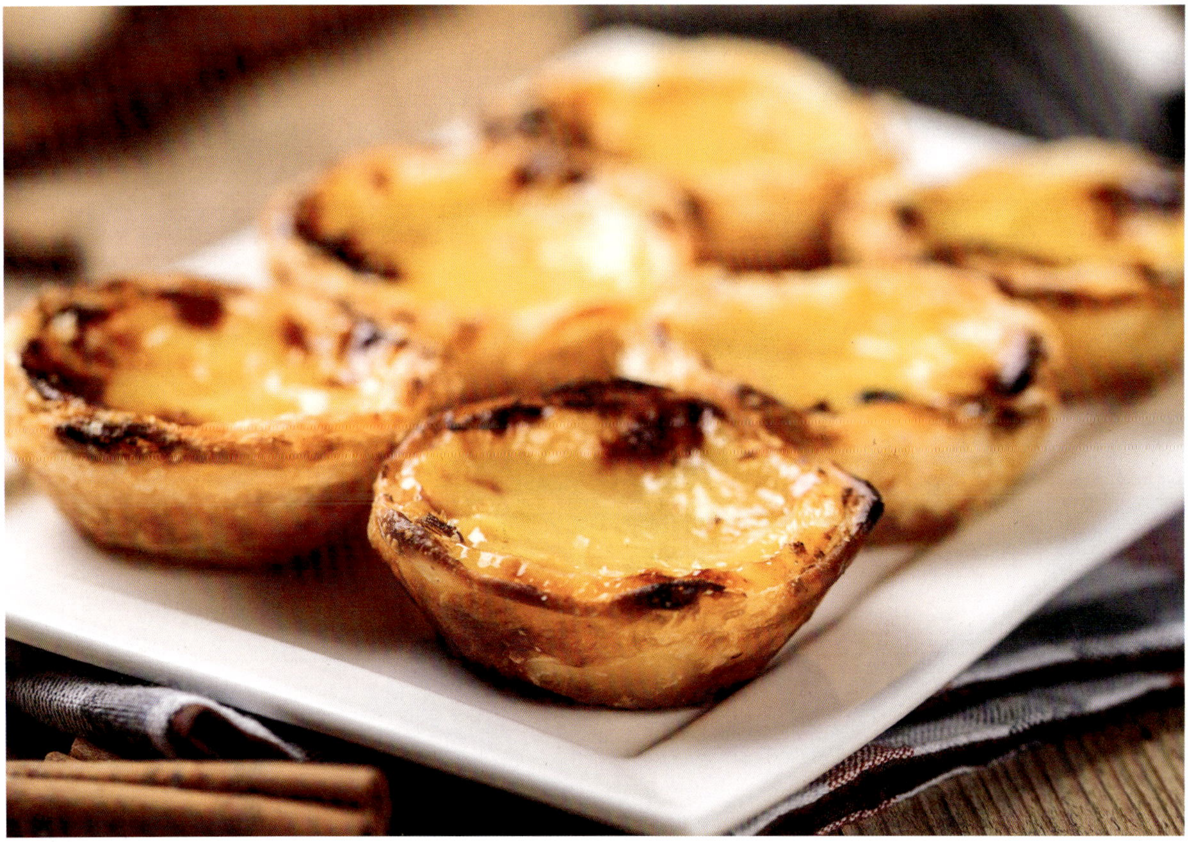

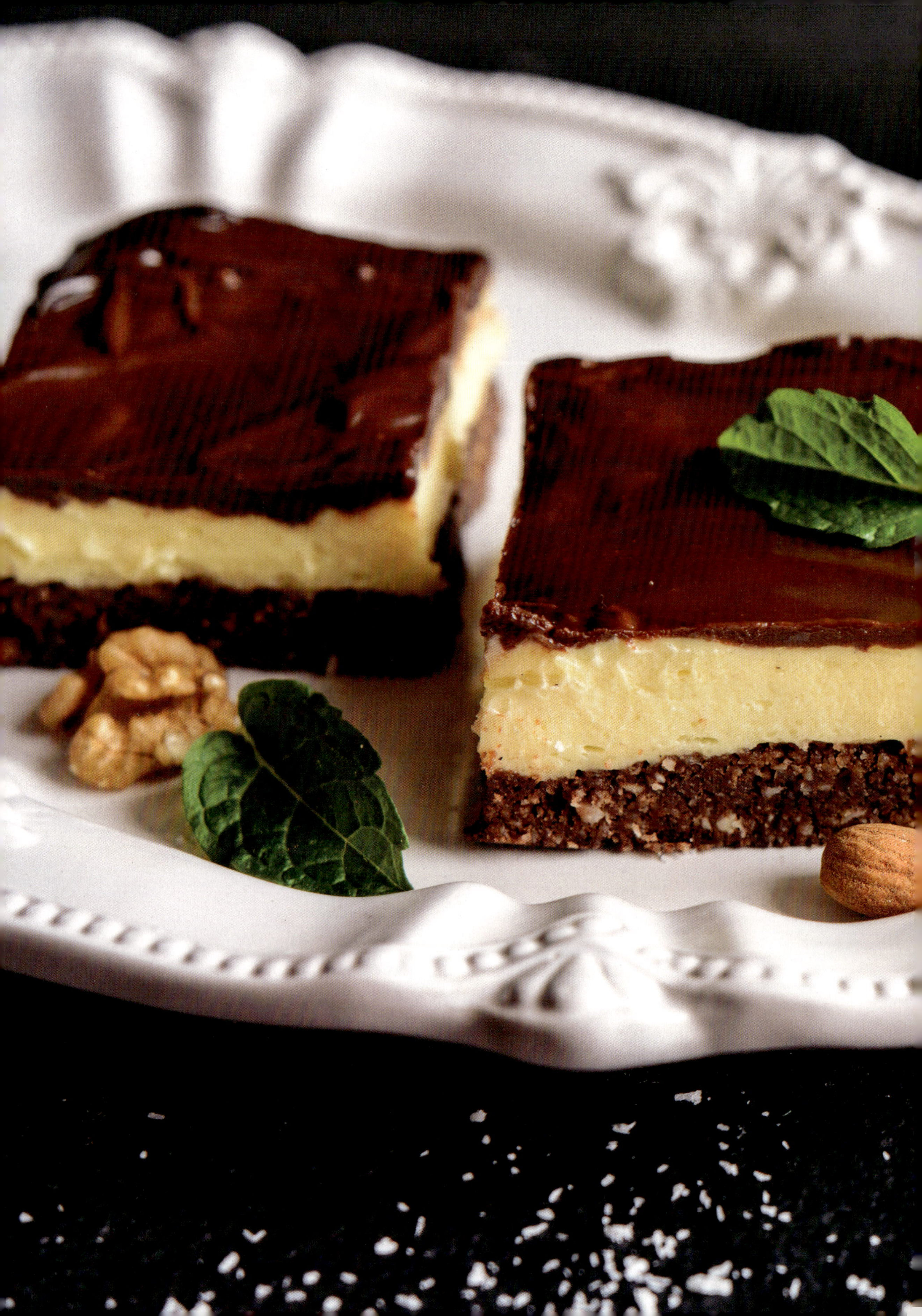

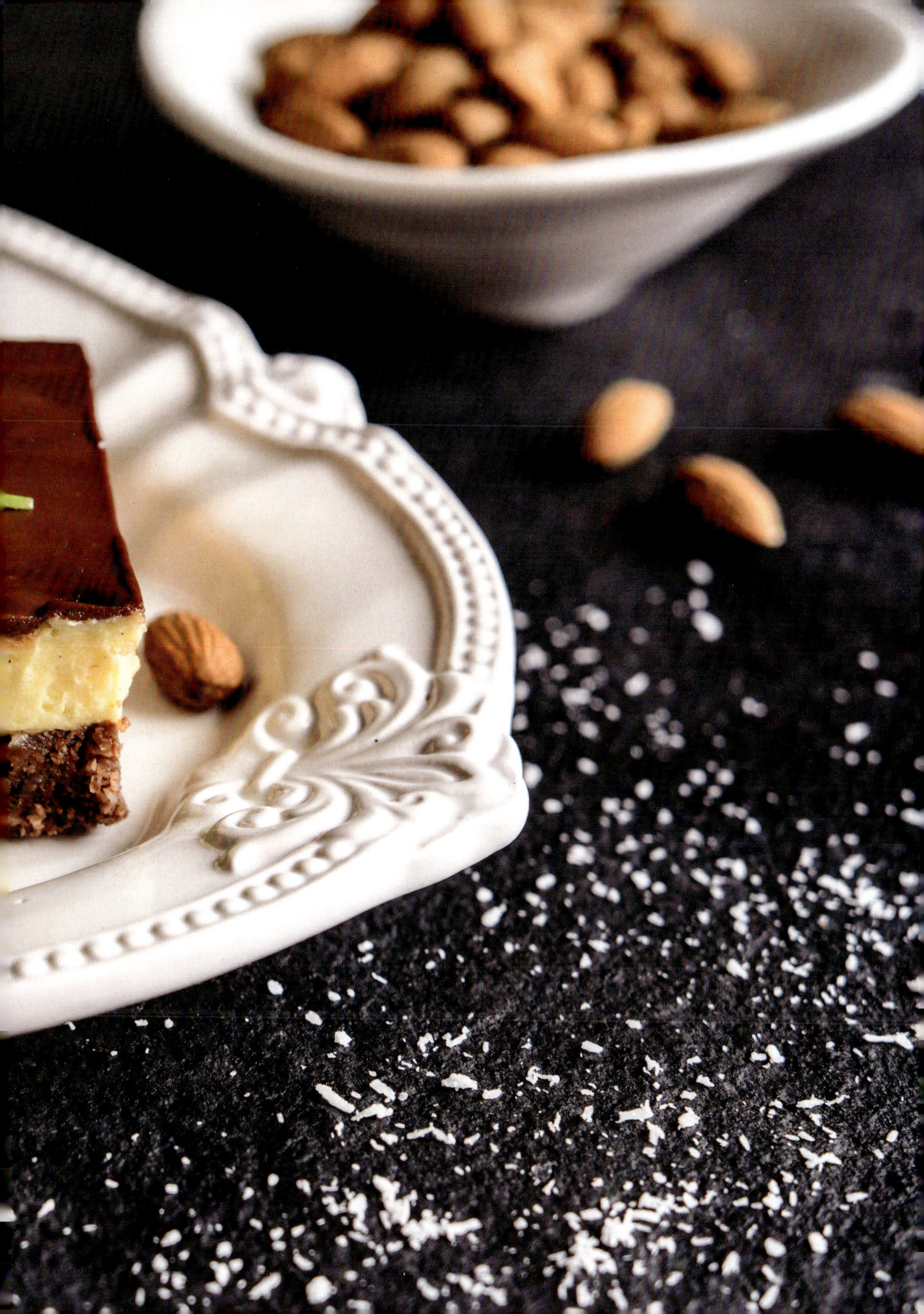

Nanaimo Bars

MAKES 16
PREP + COOK TIME: 45 MINS

BASE

½ cup (113g) unsalted butter, diced
¼ cup (50g) sugar
5 tbsps cocoa powder
⅛ tsp salt
1 large egg, lightly beaten
1¾ cups (180g) crushed digestive biscuits
¼ cup (30g) almonds, finely chopped
¼ cup (30g) walnuts, finely chopped
1 cup (90g) desiccated coconut

FILLING

Easy custard cream (see next recipe)

TOP LAYER

125g dark chocolate, chopped
2 tbsps unsalted butter

Grease and line a 22cm square cake tin with greaseproof paper.

Melt butter in large heatproof bowl over a pan of simmering water. Remove from heat, add in sugar, cocoa powder and salt and whisk well to combine. Slowly pour in the egg, whisking vigorously while you do so. Return bowl to the pan over simmering water and cook until the mixture thickens. Remove from heat and add in biscuit crumbs, nuts and coconut. Mix well. Press mixture into prepared baking dish. Place in the freezer for 10 minutes.

Spread custard cream evenly over the chilled base. Transfer to the freezer.

Melt chocolate and butter in a heatproof bowl set over a pan of simmering water. Stir until smooth. Spread over filling layer then chill to set. Cut into squares to serve.

Easy Custard Cream

SERVES 16
PREP + COOK TIME: 10 MINS
GLUTEN FREE

1¾ cups (210g) icing sugar
½ cup (113g) unsalted butter, softened
2 tbsps custard powder (gluten-free if required)
2½ tbsps thickened cream

Mix all the ingredients with an electric mixer until very pale and fluffy. Use immediately when preparing Nanaimo bars or chill for at least 2 hours to thicken for other uses.

Creme Anglaise

MAKES 2½ CUPS
PREP + COOK TIME: 45 MINS
GLUTEN FREE

1 cup (250ml) full-cream milk
1 cup (250ml) double cream
2 vanilla beans, split lengthwise, seeds scraped
6 large egg yolks
½ cup (110g) sugar

Heat milk, cream, vanilla bean and seeds in a saucepan until just bubbling. Cover pan, turn off heat and set aside for 20 minutes.

Whisk yolks and sugar together in a bowl or jug. Whisking constantly, drizzle in one-quarter of the warm milk. Pour the egg and milk mixture into the pan with the remaining milk. Remove vanilla bean and return pan to medium-low heat. Cook, stirring continuously, for 10-15 minutes until the mixture thickens enough to coat the back of a spoon. Immediately pour into a cold bowl to halt the cooking process.

Serve warm or chilled.

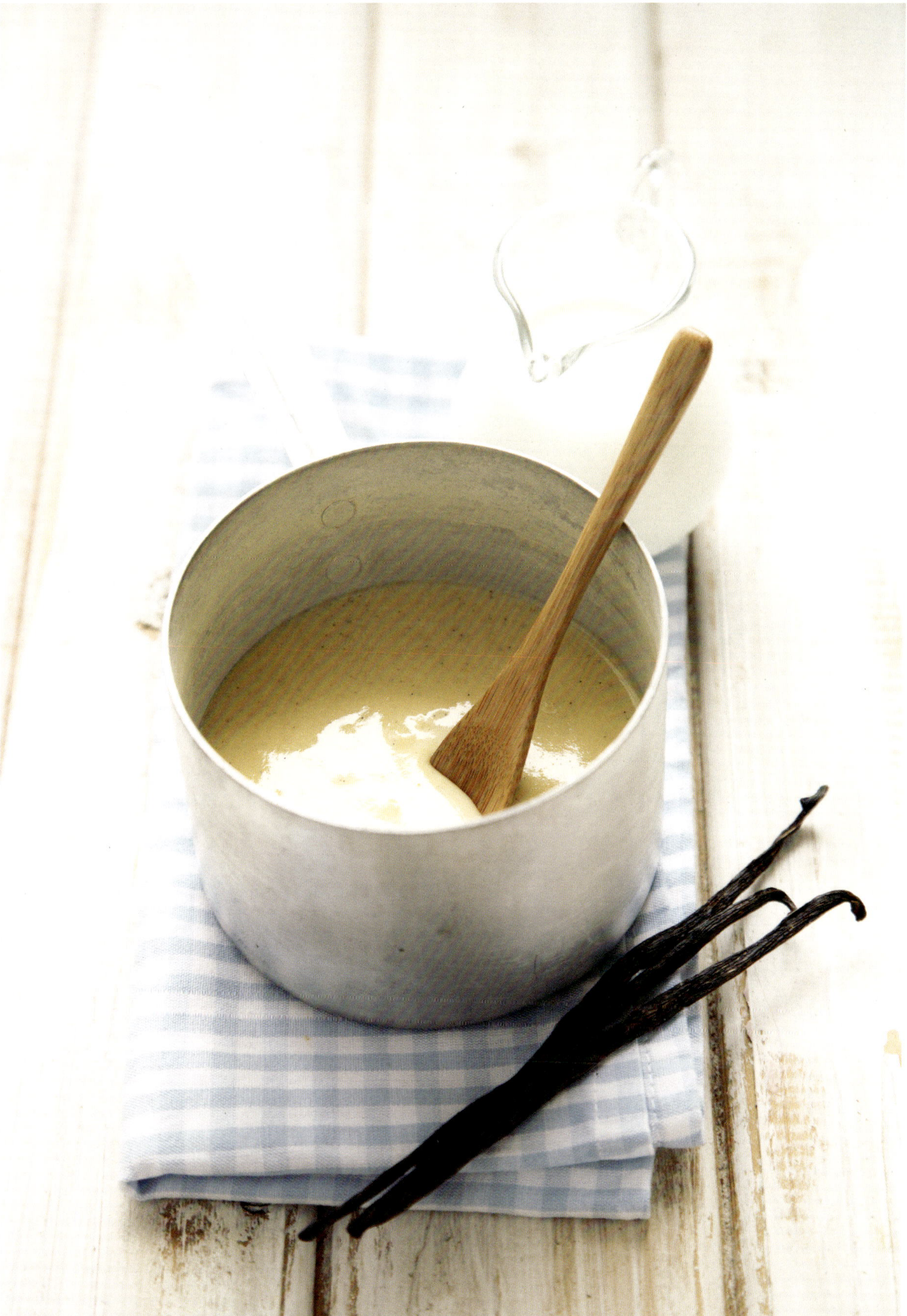

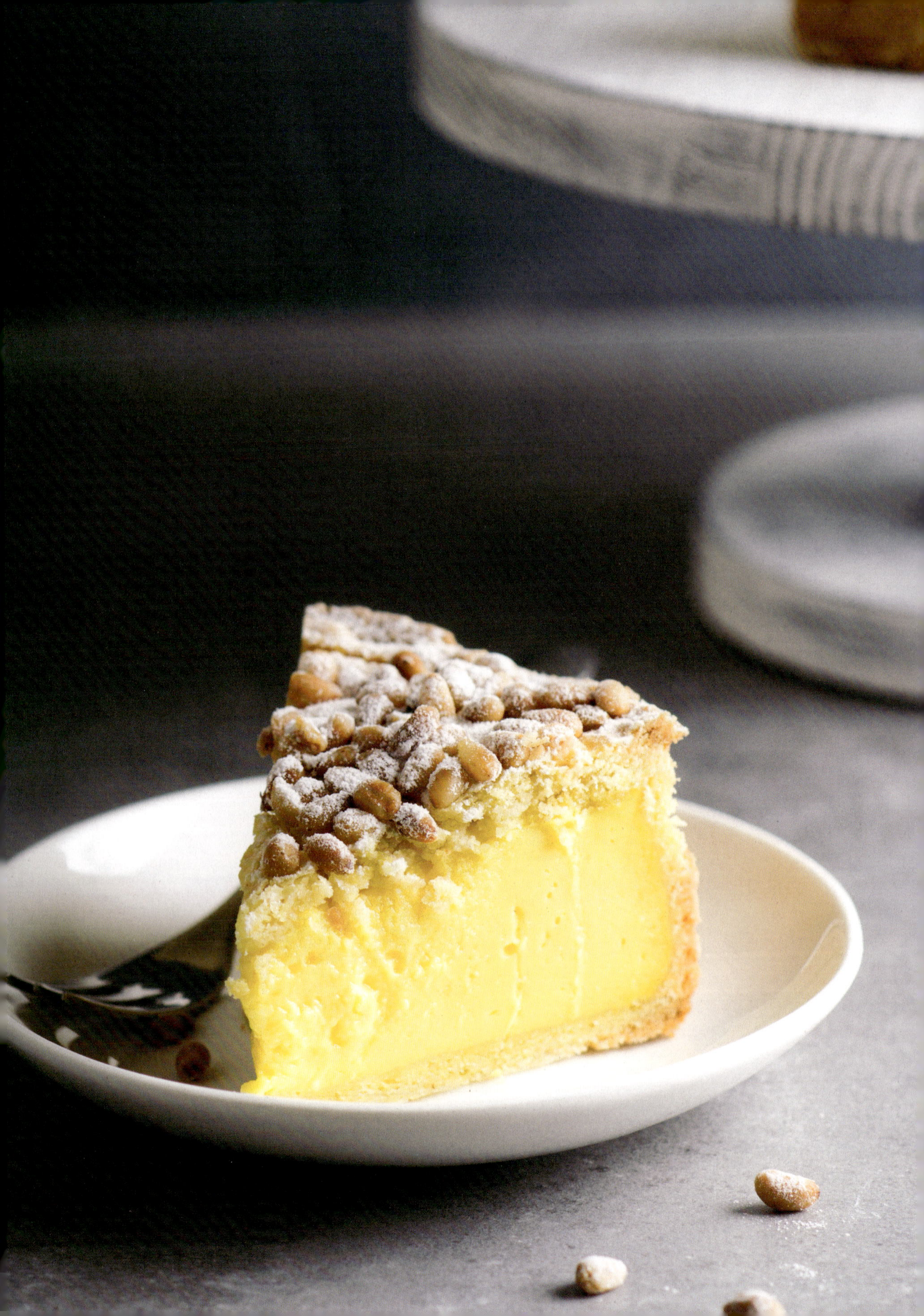

Sweet Shortcrust Pastry

MAKES 1 QUANTITY
PREP + COOK TIME: 15 MINS + CHILLING

2 cups (250g) plain flour
½ cup (80g) caster sugar
¼ tsp baking powder
Pinch of salt
Zest of 1 lemon
120g butter, chilled and cubed
1 large egg

Sift the flour into a large bowl then add the sugar, baking powder, salt and lemon zest; stir to combine.

Add the butter and rub into the flour with the tips of your fingers. Add the egg and cut it into the flour mixture with a spatula or knife to form rough crumbs.

Bring the mixture together with your hands to form a smooth dough. Transfer to a lightly floured surface and gently knead the pastry until it becomes smooth. Wrap in greaseproof paper or plastic wrap and place in the fridge for 30-60 minutes before use.

Torta Della Nonna

SERVES 12
PREP + COOK TIME: 1 HOUR 20 MINS + 2½ HOURS CHILLING

2⅓ cups (590ml) milk
1 tsp vanilla bean paste
5 egg yolks
⅓ cup (70g) sugar
¼ cup (40g) cornflour
1 quantity sweet shortcrust pastry (see previous recipe)
⅓ cup (45g) pine nuts
Icing sugar for dusting

Heat the milk and vanilla in a saucepan until just warm. Remove from the heat and set aside.

In a bowl whisk together egg yolks and sugar until just combined, then whisk in the cornflour. Slowly pour the warm milk into the bowl with the eggs, whisking constantly as you do so. Pour the mixture back into the saucepan and heat over low heat for 10 minutes, stirring constantly with a wooden spoon until very thick. Pour into a bowl and cover with plastic wrap. Allow to cool then transfer to the fridge for 1 hour to chill.

Grease a 23cm pie dish.

Roll out the pastry on a floured surface to ½cm thickness. Line the base and sides of the pie dish with pastry. Trim the edges with a sharp knife and prick the base with a fork. Chill in the fridge for at least 30 minutes.

Preheat the oven to 180°C.

Soak the pine nuts in water for 5 minutes.

Fill the chilled pastry case with the cooled pastry cream, spreading it out evenly. Scatter over the pine nuts then bake for 50 minutes or until slightly golden on top.

Allow to cool completely, then chill in the fridge for at least 1 hour before serving.

Dust with icing sugar to serve.

Rhubarb Frangipane Tart

SERVES 12
PREP + COOK TIME: 2 HOURS

1 quantity sweet shortcrust pastry (see recipe page 105)

150g butter

¾ cup (165g) caster sugar

1½ cups (180g) almond meal

1 egg

2 tsps grated orange zest

1 tsp almond extract

½ tsp salt

300g rhubarb, cut on the diagonal into 5cm pieces

Icing sugar for dusting

Roll out the shortcrust pastry to ½cm thickness and use to line the base and sides of a 23cm pie dish. Trim the edges with a sharp knife. Transfer to the fridge for 30 minutes.

Preheat oven to 200°C.

Remove the crust from the fridge. Cover with a sheet of greaseproof paper and fill with baking beans or rice. Transfer to the oven and bake for 15 minutes. Remove the paper and baking beans and continue to bake for another 5 minutes. Set aside to cool for 10 minutes.

Reduce oven temperature to 190°C.

Cream together the butter and sugar with an electric hand mixer until light and fluffy. Add the almond meal, egg, orange zest, almond extract and salt, and mix to incorporate. Spoon the filling into the slightly cooled crust and smooth with a spatula. Arrange the rhubarb over the tart and press gently into the frangipane.

Bake tart for 45-55 minutes, until the top is slightly puffy and golden. Allow to cool completely, then dust with icing sugar before serving.

Profiteroles

MAKES 48
PREP + COOK TIME: 1 HOUR 10 MINS

100g unsalted butter

1 cup (250ml) water

1 cup (125g) plain flour

Pinch of salt

4 large eggs, room temperature

TO SERVE (OPTIONAL)

Whipped cream or creme patissiere (see recipe page 120)

Ganache topping (see recipe on p66)

Place butter and water in a saucepan over medium heat. Bring to a rapid simmer. Add flour and salt and stir vigorously with a wooden spoon until the dough comes together and pulls away from the sides of the pan. Remove from heat and let mixture cool for 10 minutes.

Preheat oven to 220°C. Grease and line three baking trays with greaseproof paper.

Add eggs to the batter, one at a time, beating well with a wooden spoon between each addition, until the eggs are absorbed.

Transfer dough into a piping bag fitted with a 1½cm round tip. Pipe 2-teaspoon-sized blobs 5cm apart on the prepared baking trays.

Bake for 15 minutes. Then remove from the oven and pierce with a small sharp knife.

Reduce oven temperature to 180°C.

Return profiteroles to the oven for 5-7 minutes until golden and crisp.

Transfer to a wire rack to cool.

Fill with whipped cream or creme patissiere and top with chocolate ganache.

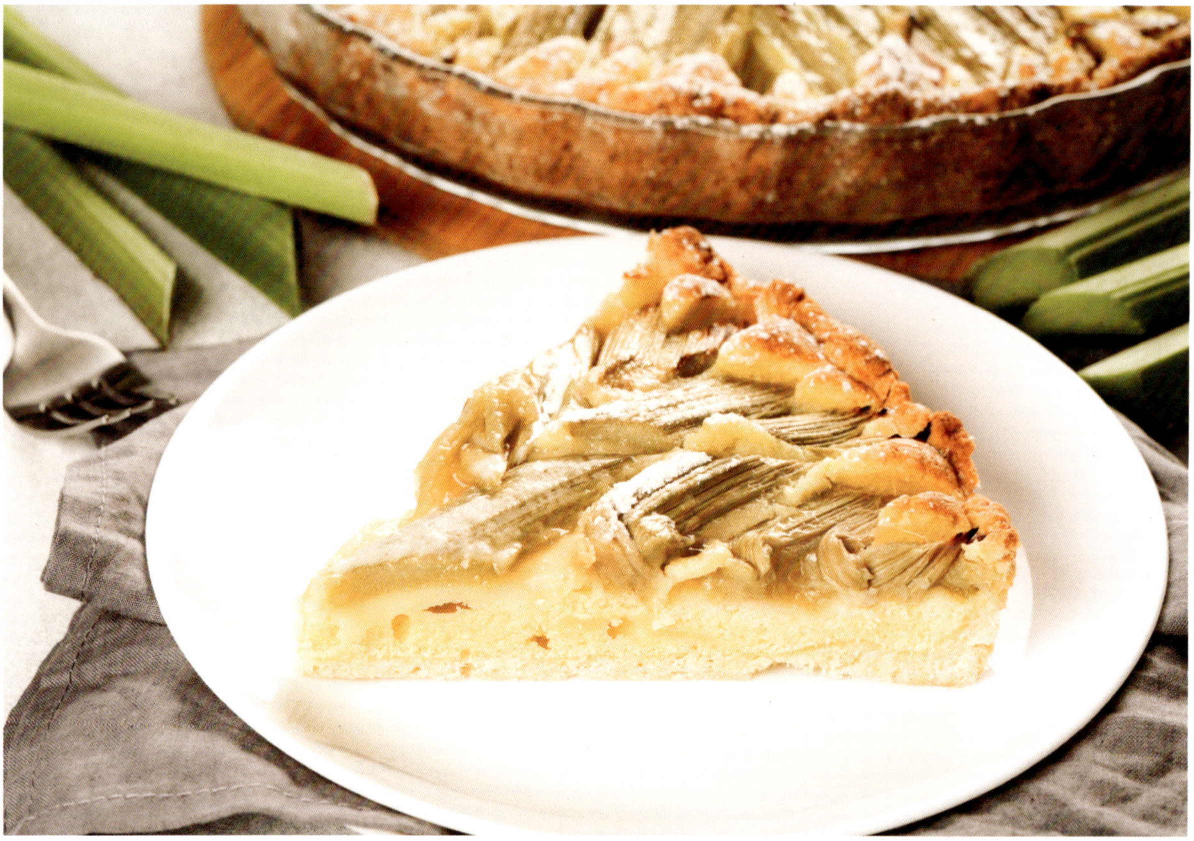

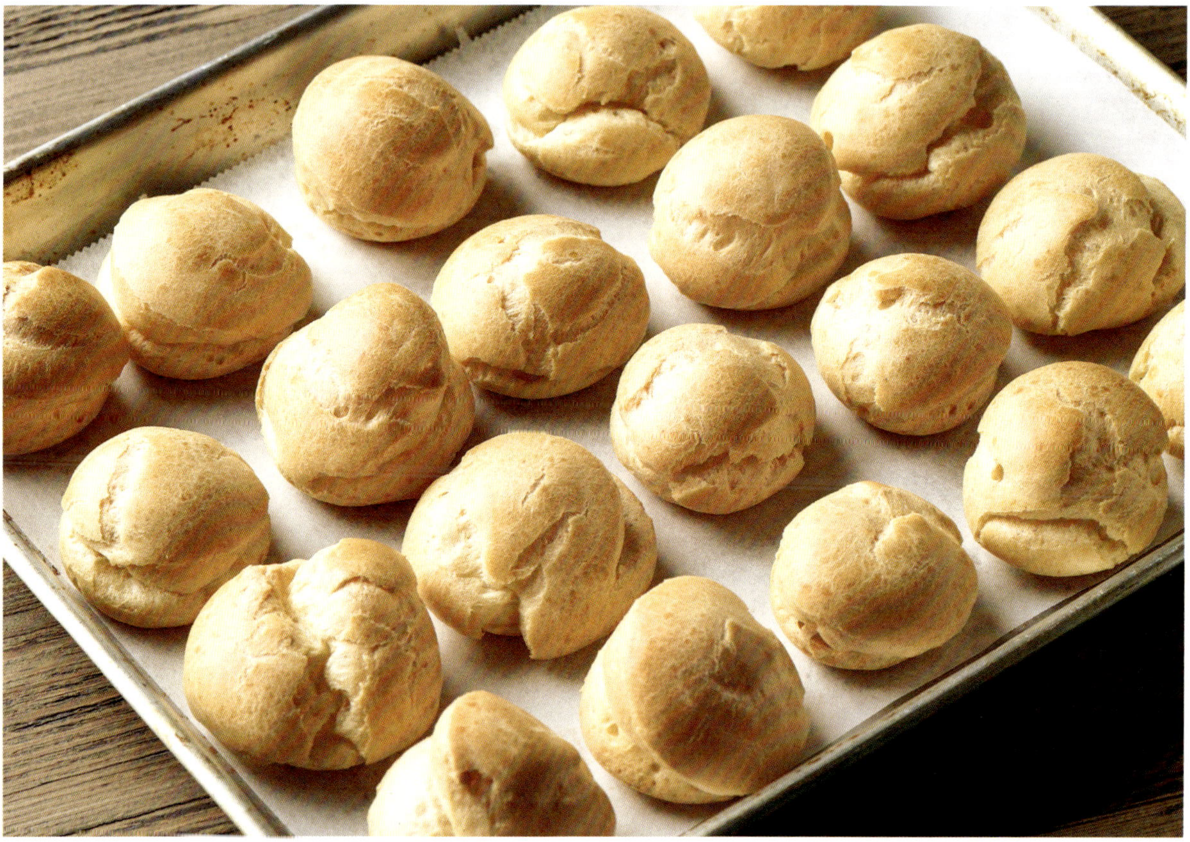

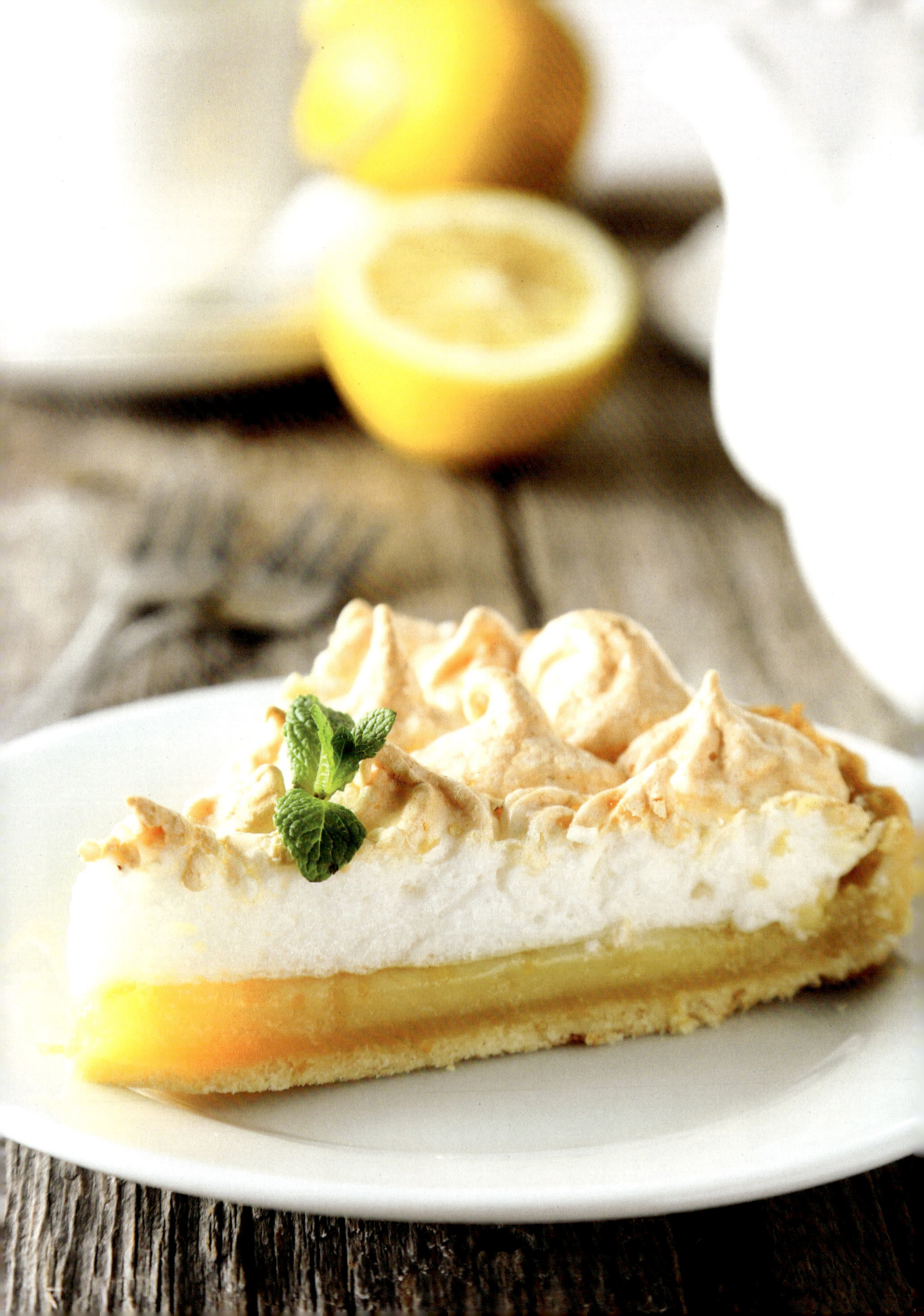

Lemon Meringue Pie

SERVES 10

PREP + COOK TIME: 1 HOUR 15 MINS + 2 HOURS CHILLING

PASTRY

1¾ cups (215g) plain flour

1 tbsp icing sugar

140g butter, chilled and coarsely chopped

1 egg yolk

2 tbsps iced water

FILLING

½ cup (75g) cornflour

1½ cups (330g) caster sugar

½ cup (125ml) lemon juice

1¼ cups (310ml) water

2 tsps finely grated lemon zest

80g butter, coarsely chopped

3 eggs, separated

Rub flour, icing sugar and butter together with fingertips until crumbly. Add egg yolk and iced water. Mix until ingredients come together. Knead dough on a floured surface until smooth. Form into a ball and wrap in plastic wrap. Refrigerate for 30 minutes.

Grease a 23cm fluted flan tin. Roll pastry large enough to line tin. Using a rolling pin, fold pastry into tin. Press pastry gently into the base and sides and trim edge with a sharp knife. Cover with plastic wrap and refrigerate for 30 minutes.

Preheat oven to 200°C. Cover the pastry case with greaseproof paper and cover with baking beans. Blind bake for 15 minutes. Remove paper and beans. Bake for a further 10 minutes until golden. Remove and set aside to cool.

Combine cornflour and 1 cup caster sugar in a medium saucepan. Gradually stir in lemon juice and water and stir until smooth. Cook over a high heat until mixture boils and then thickens. Reduce heat and simmer, stirring, for 1 minute. Remove from heat. Stir in zest and butter and, quickly, stir in egg yolks. Set aside to cool for 10 minutes.

Spoon filling into the pastry case and spread evenly across base. Cover and refrigerate for 2 hours.

Preheat oven to 220°C.

Beat egg whites with an electric mixer until soft peaks form. Slowly add remaining sugar, beating until sugar dissolves and glossy, firm peaks form.

Spread meringue mixture onto lemon filling. Bake for 25 minutes or until meringue is golden brown and filling is set.

Custard Tart

SERVES 6
PREP + COOK TIME: 1 HOUR 30 MINS + CHILLING

- 1 quantity sweet shortcrust pastry (see recipe page 105)
- 1 cup (250ml) thickened cream
- 1 cup (250ml) milk
- 1 vanilla bean, split
- 1 strip lemon zest
- 1 whole nutmeg
- 8 egg yolks
- ½ cup (100g) golden caster sugar
- ¼ cup (30g) toasted flaked almonds

Roll out pastry on a lightly floured surface to ½cm thickness and use to line the base and sides of a 22cm springform tin. Chill for 30 minutes.

Preheat oven to 180°C.

Cover the pastry case with greaseproof paper and cover with baking beans. Blind bake for 20 minutes, then remove the paper and beans and continue to bake for a further 20 minutes until the base is golden brown. Remove from oven and set aside.

Reduce the oven temperature to 140°C.

Bring the cream, milk, vanilla bean, lemon zest and a small grating of nutmeg to the boil. Remove from the heat.

Beat the egg yolks together with the sugar until light and fluffy. Slowly pour the hot milk into the egg mixture, whisking continuously as you do so. Strain custard into a jug, allow to settle for a few minutes, then skim off any froth.

Carefully pour the custard into the tart case, and top with a grating of nutmeg. Bake for 40 minutes or until just set. Remove from the oven, then leave to cool completely. Scatter with flaked almonds to serve.

Three Milk Cake

SERVES 16
PREP + COOK TIME: 1 HOUR 15 MINS + COOLING

- 4 eggs, separated
- Pinch of salt
- 1 cup (200g) caster sugar
- 1 tsp vanilla extract
- 1⅔ cups (200g) plain flour
- 1 tsp baking powder
- ⅓ cup (100ml) milk
- 1 x 410ml can evaporated milk
- ¾ cup (200ml) sweetened condensed milk
- 1¼ cups (300ml) double cream
- 2 tbsps icing sugar
- ¼ cup (20g) toasted coconut flakes

Preheat oven to 180°C. Grease and line a 22cm round cake tin with greaseproof paper.

Whisk egg whites and salt with an electric hand mixer until soft peaks form. Continue mixing as you add ¾ cup caster sugar, a spoonful at a time, until thick and glossy.

In another bowl, mix egg yolks, remaining sugar and vanilla until pale and foamy. Add flour, baking powder and milk. Fold to combine.

Add a third of the egg white to the cake mix, beat to loosen the mixture, then gently fold through the remaining egg whites with a metal spoon.

Pour into prepared tin, smooth the top and bake for 40-45 minutes until a skewer inserted into the centre comes out clean. Leave the cake to cool for 10 minutes in the tin before transferring to a plate. Poke holes over the surface with a skewer.

Mix together evaporated milk, condensed milk and 3 tablespoons of the cream. Pour half the milk mixture over the cake. Leave for 10 minutes, then pour over the remaining milk until it starts to leak a little. Leave to cool.

Whip the remaining cream and icing sugar together until soft peaks form. Spread cream over the cake and sprinkle with coconut flakes.

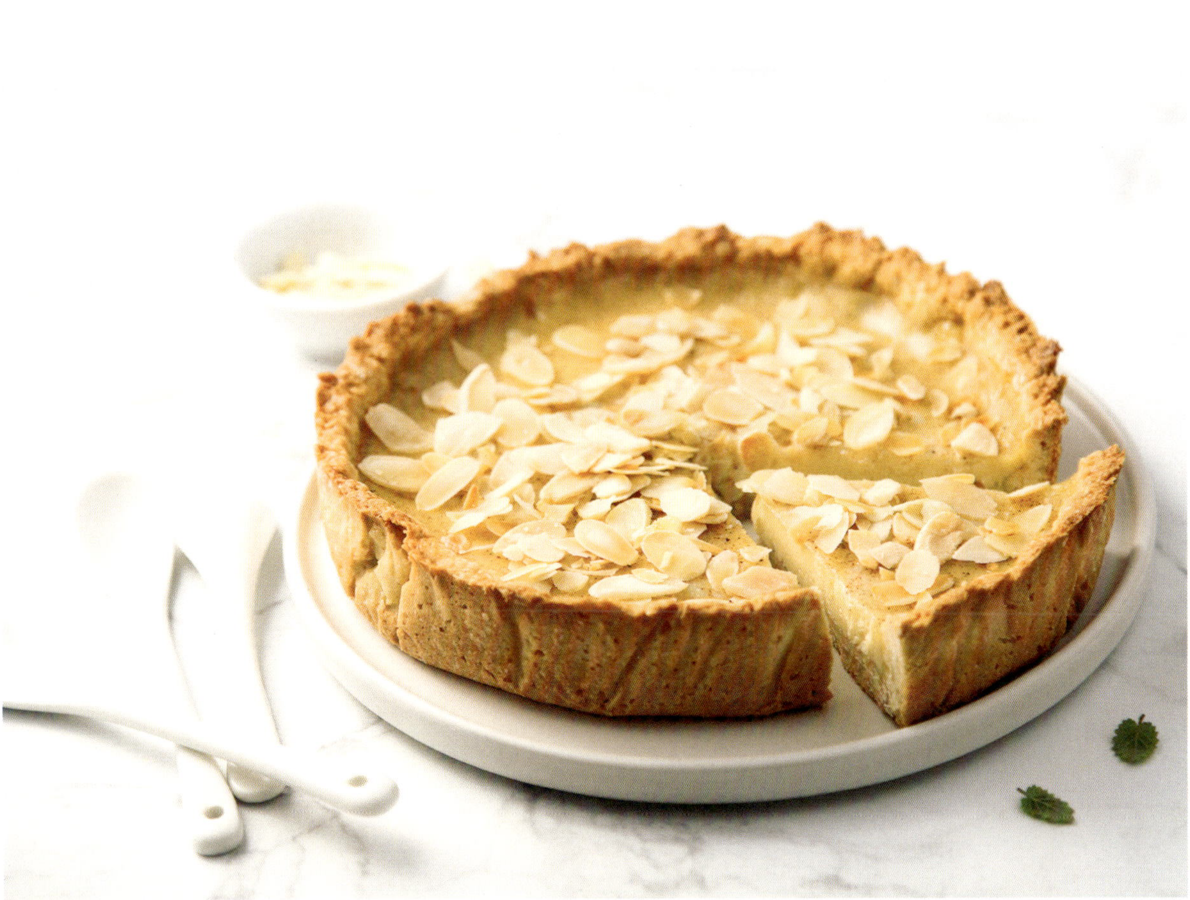

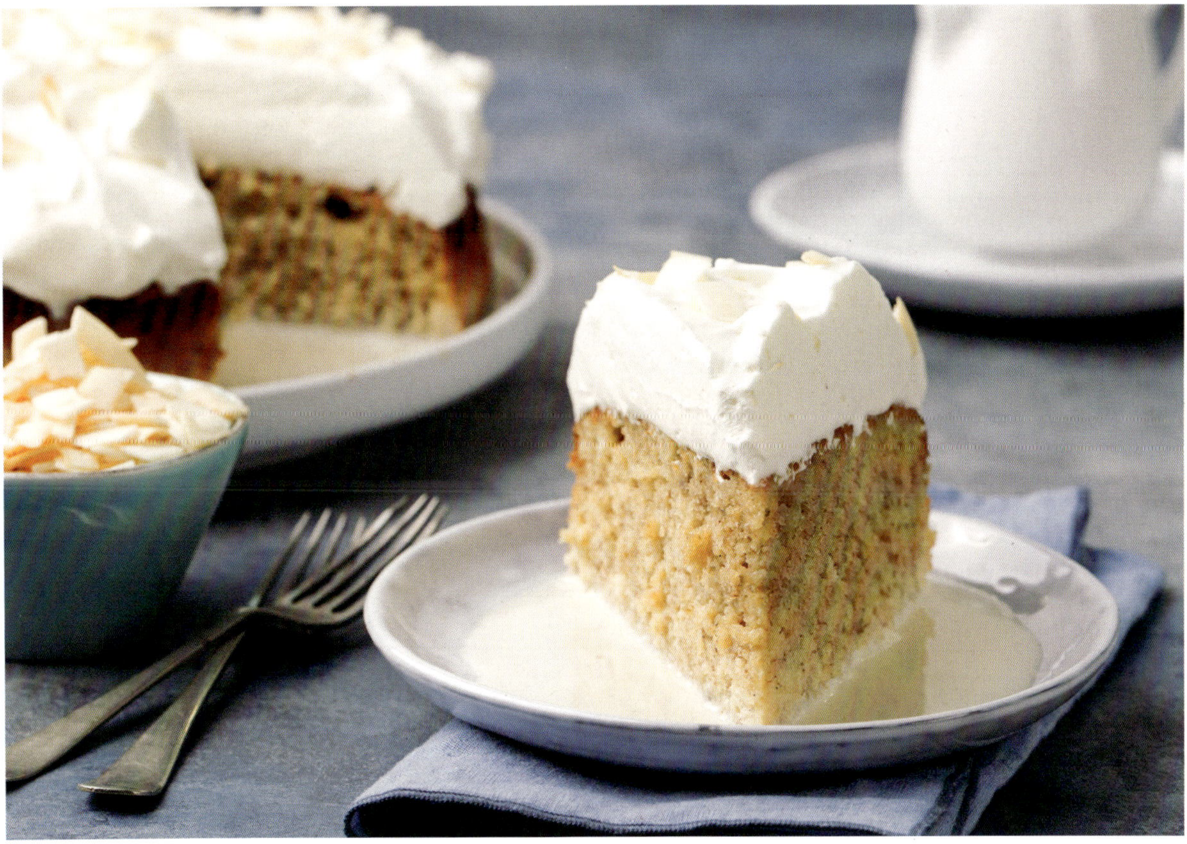

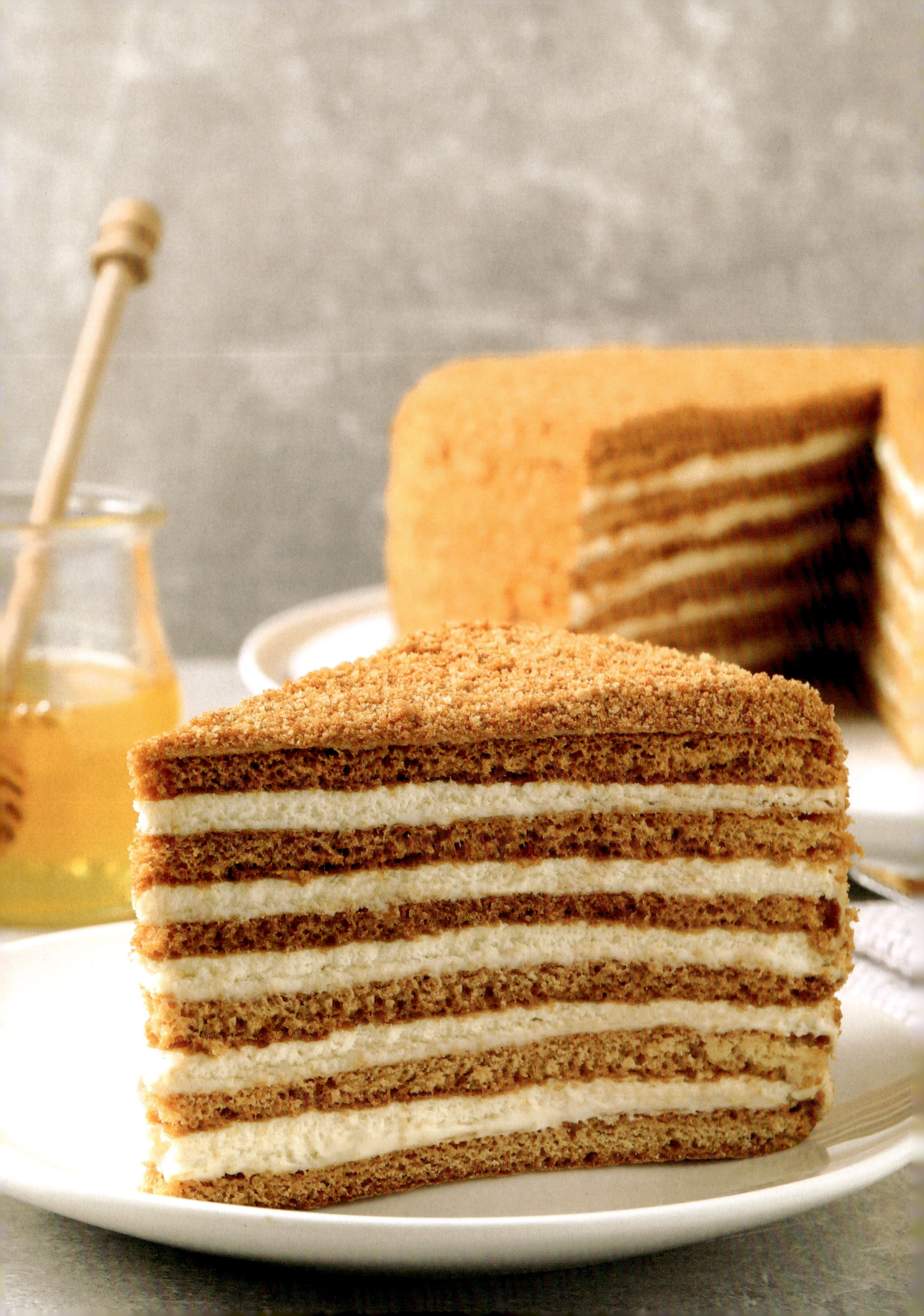

Russian Honey Cake

SERVES 12
PREP + COOK TIME: 1 HOUR 40 MINS + OVERNIGHT CHILLING

BURNT HONEY

¾ cup (260g) honey

3 tbsps cold water

CAKE LAYERS

2½ tsps bicarbonate of soda

1 tsp cinnamon

¾ tsp fine salt

1 cup (220g) sugar

200g unsalted butter, cut into slices

¾ cup (260g) honey

6 large eggs, cold

3¾ cups (465g) plain flour

HONEY CREAM

4 cups (1L) thickened cream, chilled

¾ cup (185ml) sour cream

Pour ¾ cup honey into a deep saucepan over medium heat. Bring to a boil, then boil for 5-10 minutes until dark caramel in colour. Remove from the heat and carefully whisk in the cold water.

Preheat the oven to 190°C. Line a baking tray with greaseproof paper. Draw a circle on the paper by drawing around a 23cm cake tin. Place a mixing bowl and whisk in the fridge.

Combine bicarb, cinnamon and salt in a small bowl. Set aside.

Place sugar, butter, ¾ cup honey and ¼ cup burnt honey in a large metal bowl over a pan of barely simmering water. Heat very gently until butter melts. Whisk in eggs, then whisk in bicarb mixture. Remove from heat. Sift in flour a third at a time, stirring well after each addition, until batter is easily spreadable.

Transfer about ½ cup batter onto the prepared baking tray. Spread to fill the drawn circle using a palette knife or offset spatula. Tap the pan to knock out any air bubbles.

Bake for 6-7 minutes until lightly browned. Remove the cake and greaseproof paper from the pan and let cake layer continue cooling until firm enough to remove paper. Invert cake onto another circle of greaseproof paper.

Continue making and baking circles of cake batter until you have six cake layers, letting each cool on an individual circle of greaseproof paper. Trim edges using a pizza wheel to ensure the circles are the same size. Save scraps in a large bowl for crumb mixture.

Spread any remaining batter onto a lined baking tray. Bake for 10 minutes until edges are dry, Remove from the oven and cut into small pieces Add to the bowl of cake scraps.

Place the cake scraps on a baking tray and return to the oven. Bake for 7-10 minutes until browned. Let cool completely, then transfer to a resealable bag and beat with a rolling pin into fairly fine crumbs. Set aside.

Remove the bowl and whisk from the fridge. Pour in thickened cream and whisk until soft peaks form. Add sour cream and remaining burnt honey; continue whisking until stiff peaks form.

Place a cake layer on a serving plate. Spread a cup of honey cream evenly on top, almost to the edge. Repeat with cake layers and cream, placing the cake layers smooth-side down. Place last cake layer smooth-side up. Spread the top and sides of the cake with honey cream. Cover with crumbs.

Cover with plastic wrap and refrigerate for at least 8 hours before serving.

Matcha Curd Tarts

SERVES 4
PREP + COOK TIME: 25 MINS + COOLING AND CHILLING
GLUTEN FREE

CRUST

1 cup (170g) roasted buckwheat
¼ tsp salt
1½ cups (195g) cashews
8 Medjool dates, pitted
1 tbsp coconut oil
¼ cup (64 g) cashew butter

FILLING

2 eggs
2 egg yolks
⅓ cup (75g) caster sugar
2 tsps finely grated lemon zest
⅓ cup (80ml) lemon juice
75g unsalted butter, chilled and diced
½ cup (125ml) thickened cream
2½ tsps matcha powder + 1 tsp for dusting

For the crust, add the buckwheat and salt to a food processor and blend to a crumb consistency. Add the cashews and blend until a crumb consistency. Add the dates, coconut oil and cashew butter and blend until they form a dough. Press the dough into the base and sides of four individual tart tins. Place in the freezer for 1 hour.

Whisk whole eggs, yolks and sugar in a small heavy-based saucepan until smooth. Add zest, juice and butter, whisking continuously over low heat for 5 minutes or until curd thickens.

Remove from the heat and place in a bowl. Add the matcha and whisk to combine. Set aside to cool to room temperature, then place in the fridge to chill for at least 1 hour.

Spoon curd into the tart shells and dust with more matcha to serve.

Lemon Pudding

SERVES 8
PREP + COOK TIME: 40 MINS

1 cup (220g) caster sugar
125g butter, room temperature
Zest of 1 lemon
4 eggs, separated, room temperature
⅓ cup (80ml) lemon juice
⅔ cup (75g) plain flour
1¼ cups (310ml) milk
Icing sugar for dusting

Preheat oven to 170°C. Grease a 2L ovenproof baking dish.

Cream together caster sugar, butter and lemon zest with an electric mixer until light and fluffy. Add the egg yolks one at a time, beating between each addition. Add lemon juice, flour and milk. Beat to combine.

In another bowl beat the egg whites with clean beaters until stiff peaks form. Add a third of the egg whites to the lemon mixture and fold through with a large metal spoon. Add the remaining egg white and fold through until incorporated.

Pour into the prepared baking dish. Place the dish into a roasting tin and pour in enough boiling water to come halfway up the sides of the baking dish.

Bake for 30 minutes or until lightly golden and firm on the top and soft underneath.

Dust with icing sugar and serve warm.

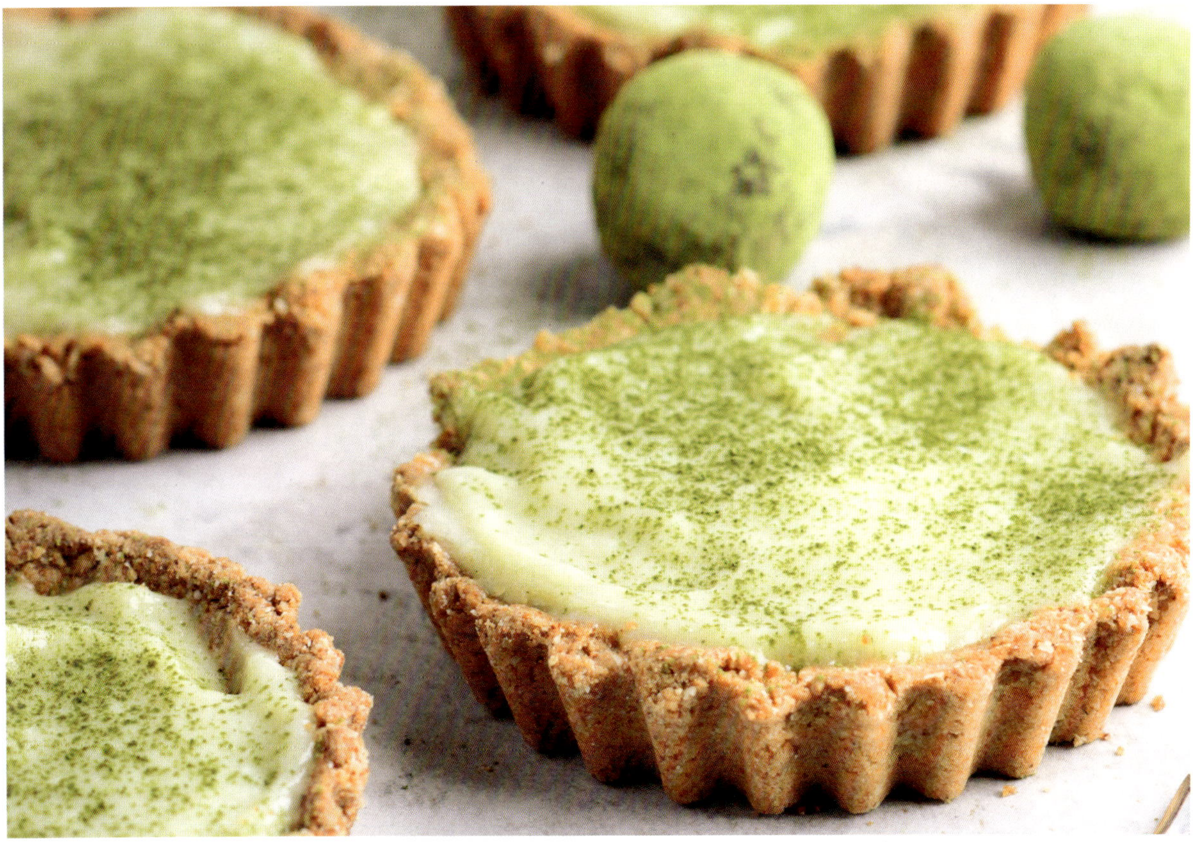

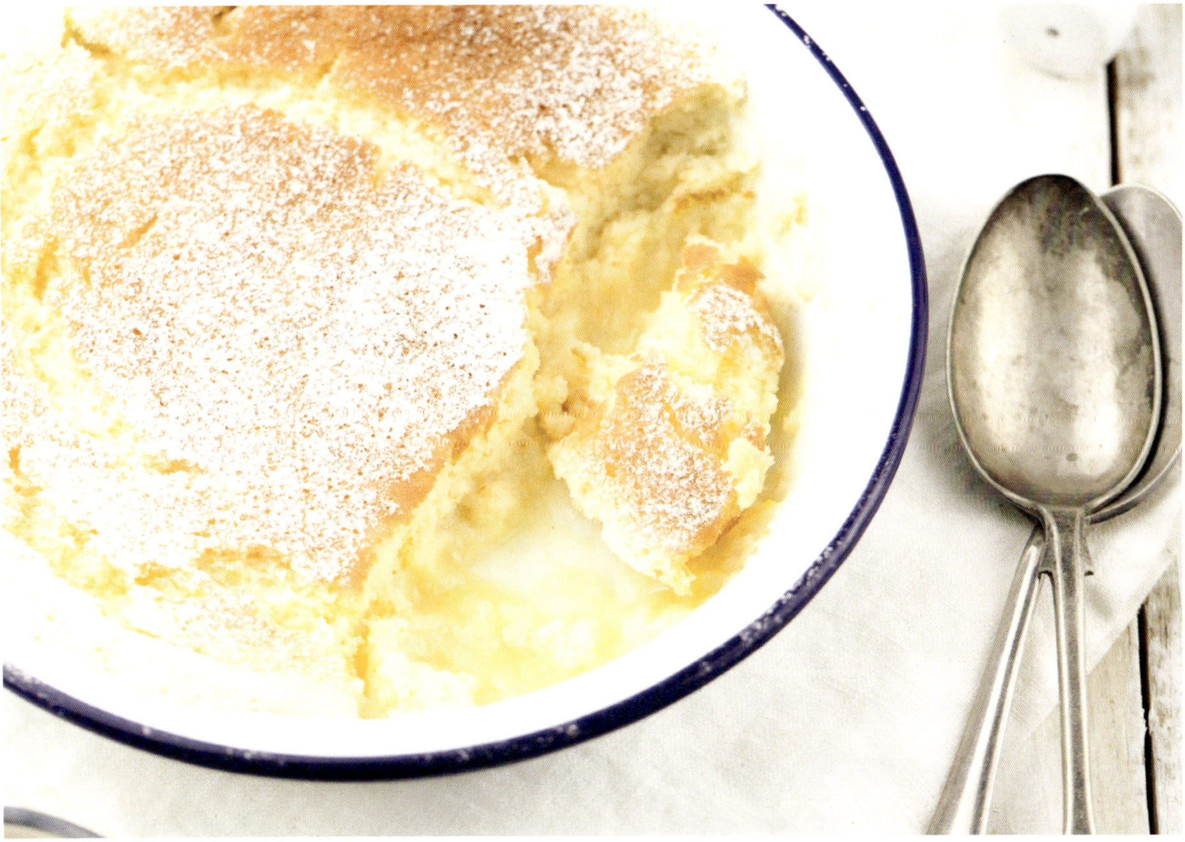

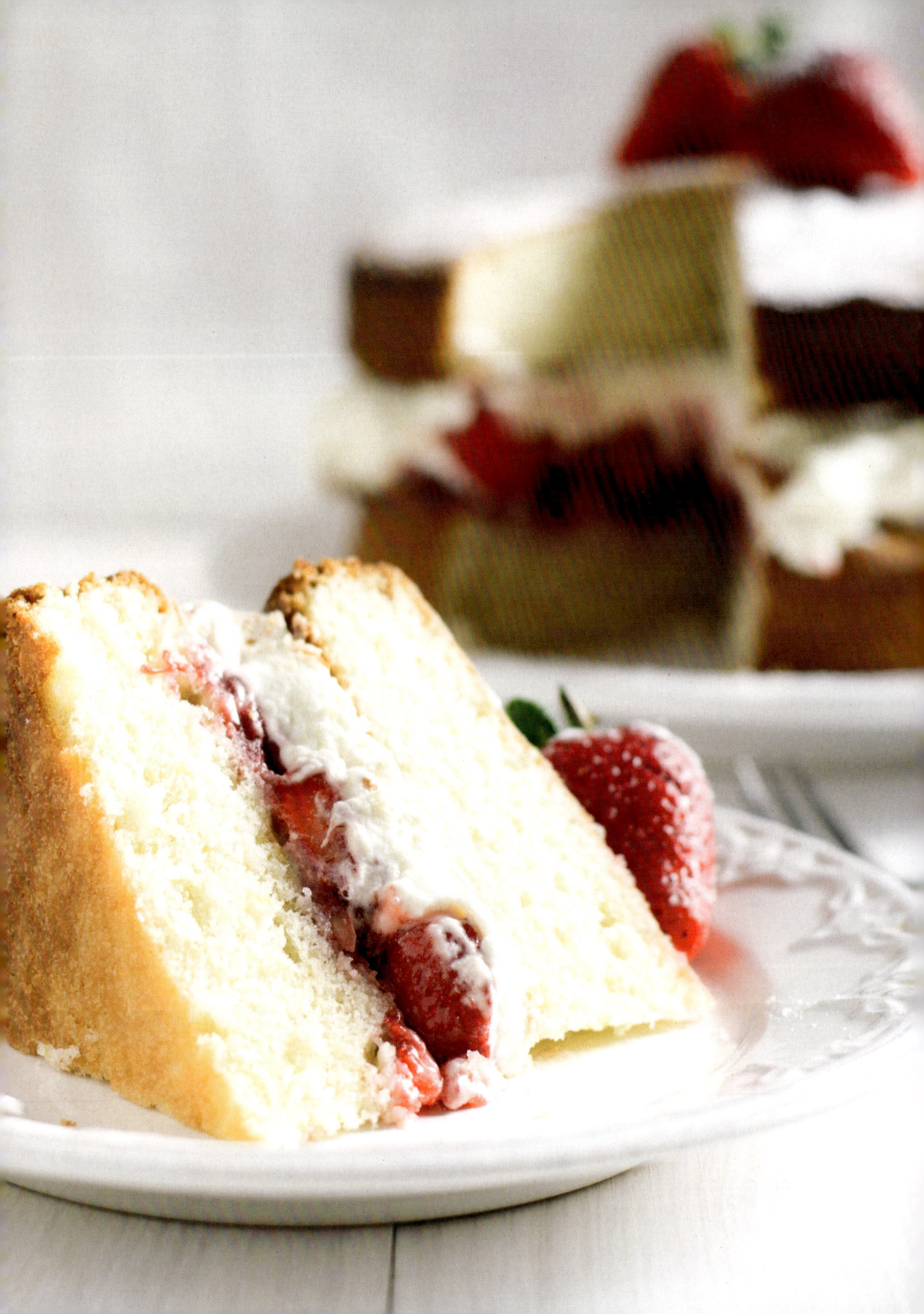

Victoria Sponge Cake

SERVES 10
PREP + COOK TIME: 55 MINS + COOLING

SPONGE
225g unsalted butter, room temperature
1 cup (225g) caster sugar
1¾ cups (225g) plain flour
4 tsps baking powder
1 tsp salt
½ tsp vanilla extract
4 large eggs, room temperature

FILLING
½ cup (170g) strawberry jam
1 cup (200g) fresh strawberries, halved
Chantilly cream (see next recipe)

TO DECORATE
Fresh strawberries, halved
Icing sugar for dusting

To make the sponge, preheat the oven to 180°C and grease and flour two 23cm cake tins.

Cream together the butter and sugar with an electric mixer until light and fluffy.

Sift the flour twice with the baking powder and salt. Add to the butter mixture in thirds, mixing until just incorporated. Add in the vanilla and then add the eggs one at a time, completely mixing each one in before adding the next. Beat for a further 2 minutes until the mixture is smooth and light. Divide the mixture equally between the two cake tins.

Bake for 25 minutes until golden brown and a skewer inserted into the middle comes out clean. Let the cakes cool in the tins for at least 2 minutes before turning out onto a wire rack. Let cool for at least 1 hour before assembling cake.

Spread one cake with jam, then top with sliced strawberries and Chantilly cream. Place the second sponge on top. Decorate with strawberries and dust with icing sugar.

Chantilly Cream

MAKES 3½ CUPS
PREP + COOK TIME: 10 MINS
GLUTEN FREE

3 cups (750ml) thickened cream
½ cup (115g) caster sugar
2 tsps vanilla extract

Whisk the cream together with the sugar until soft peaks form. Mix through the vanilla. Refrigerate until ready to use.

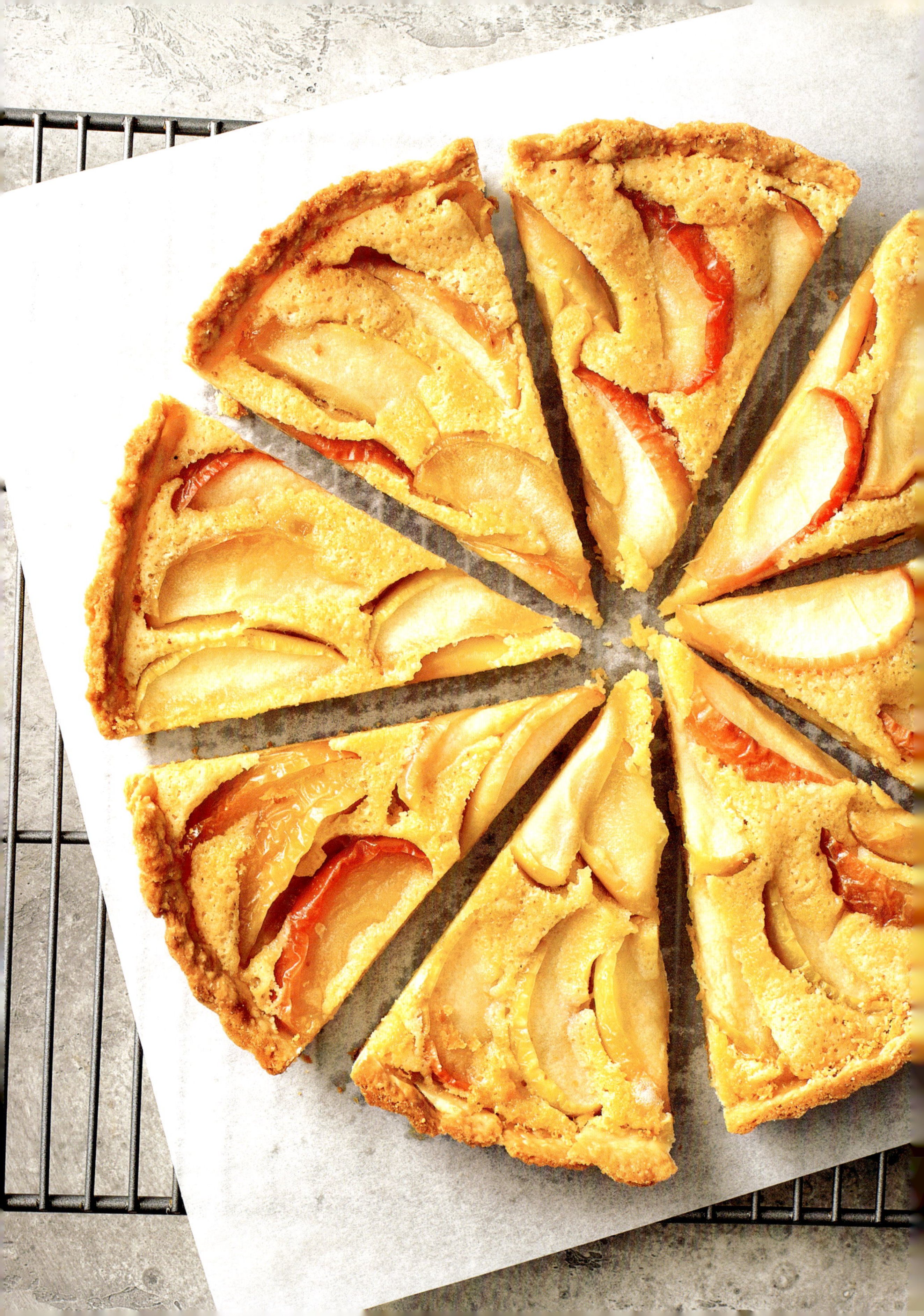

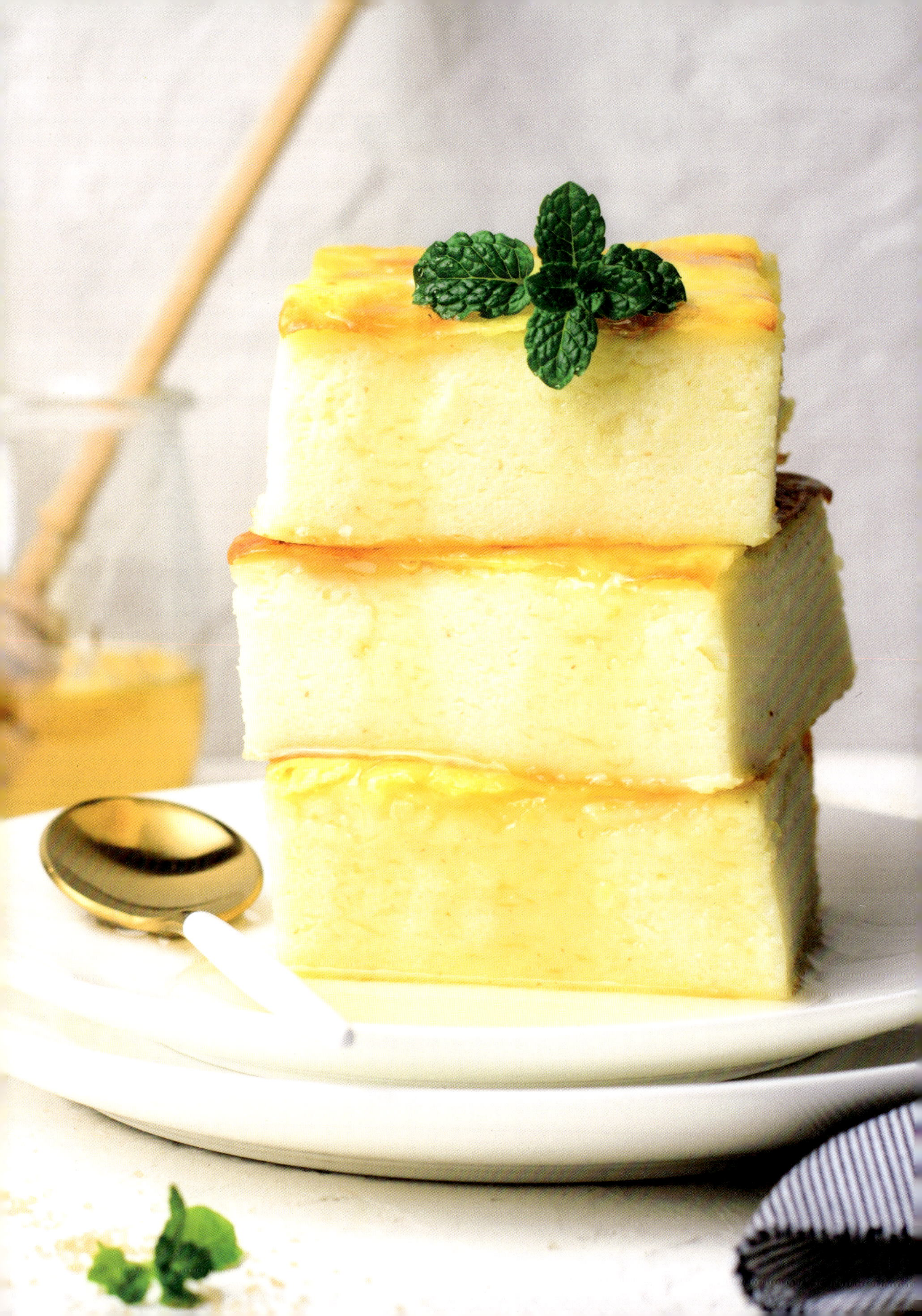

Apple Custard Tart

SERVES 12
PREP + COOK TIME: 1 HOUR 40 MINS

1 quantity sweet shortcrust pastry (see recipe page 105)
2 tbsps cornflour
⅛ tsp salt
⅓ cup (70g) sugar
2 large eggs, room temperature
¾ cup (185ml) cream
½ tsp vanilla bean paste
450g firm apples

Roll the pastry out to ½cm thickness and line the base and sides of a 23cm fluted pie tin. Trim the edges with a sharp knife and pick the base with a fork. Transfer to the fridge for 20 minutes to chill.

Preheat oven to 180°C.

Line the pastry case with greaseproof paper and fill with baking beans or rice. Bake for 20 minutes then remove the paper and baking beans and bake for a further 5 minutes. Remove from oven and set aside to cool.

In a large bowl, whisk the cornflour with the salt and sugar. Whisk in the eggs to make a smooth paste.

In a small saucepan over medium heat, heat the cream until it just starts to boil. Remove from heat and gradually pour into the egg mixture, whisking constantly. Whisk in the vanilla.

Arrange the apple slices in the tart shell. Carefully pour the custard over the apples to just below the top of the tart tin. Bake for 30-40 minutes or until is custard is set and the apples are tender.

Allow to cool for a few minutes before serving. Can be served hot or cold.

Custard Slice

MAKES 12
PREP + COOK TIME: 20 MINS + 5 HOURS CHILLING
GLUTEN FREE

1½ cups (330g) caster sugar
1¼ cups (250g) custard powder
4 cups (1L) thickened cream
1 cup (250ml) milk
2 tsps vanilla bean paste
¼ cup (90g) honey

Line an 18 x 25cm slice tin with greaseproof paper, using enough paper to overhang the sides. Place the sugar and custard powder into a large saucepan and whisk together. Add cream, milk and vanilla and whisk until smooth. Place over low heat and continue to whisk for another 10 minutes until thick. Pour into the prepared tin. Cover with plastic wrap and refrigerate for at least 5 hours until set. Lift out of the tin and drizzle with honey. Slice to serve.

Creme Patissiere

MAKES 2 CUPS
PREP + COOK TIME: 40 MINS + COOLING AND CHILLING
GLUTEN FREE

6 tbsps sugar
3 tbsps cornflour
6 large egg yolks
2 cups (500ml) milk
1 vanilla bean, seeds scraped
3 tbsps unsalted butter, softened

Whisk together sugar, cornflour and egg yolks until smooth and thick. Set aside. Place milk, vanilla bean and seeds in a saucepan. Heat until bubbles appear. Remove from heat and slowly pour into egg yolk mixture, whisking constantly. Return mixture to pan over medium heat and bring to a boil, whisking constantly. Cook for 30 seconds more, remove from heat and whisk in butter. Cool and chill before using.

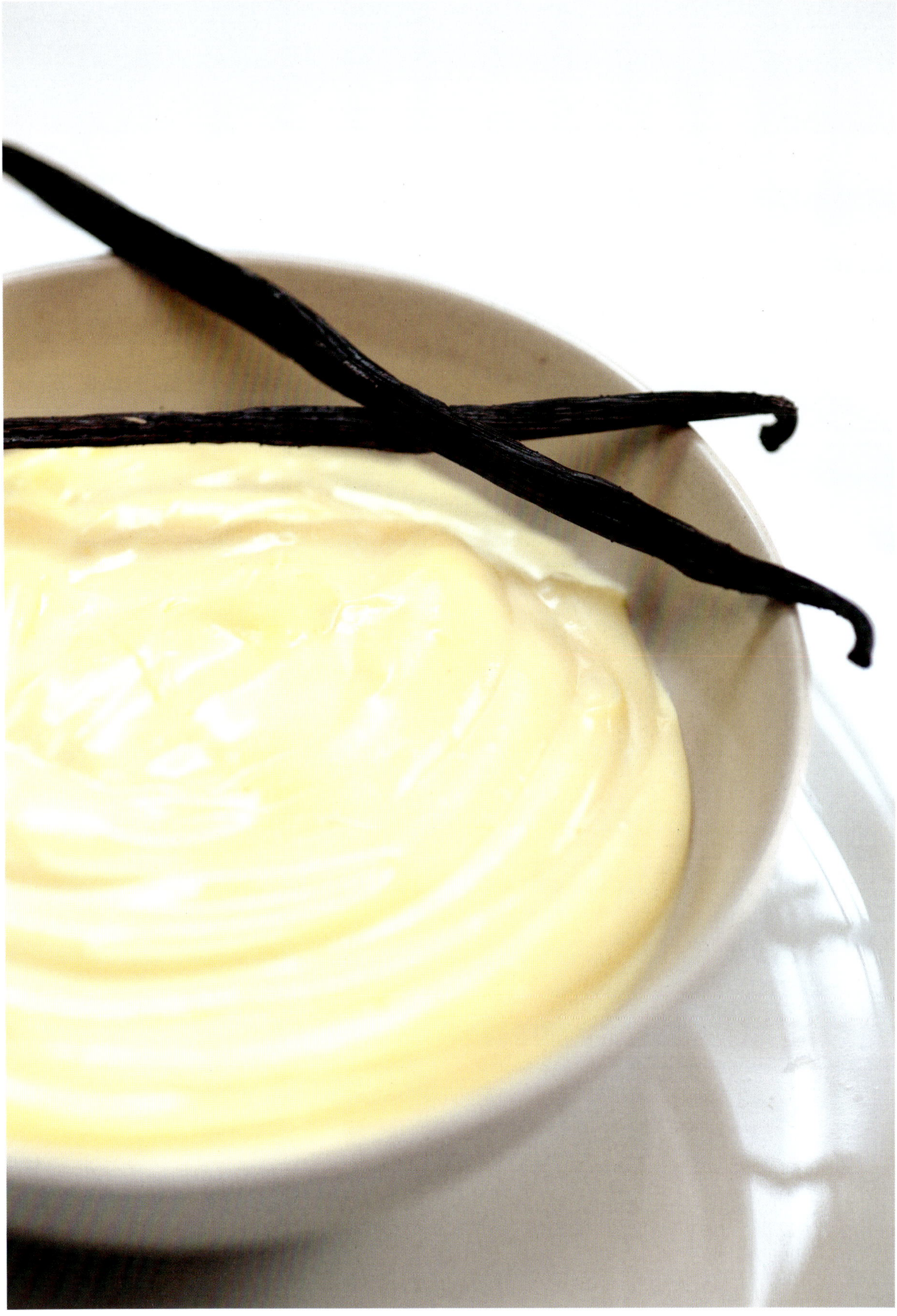

5

Nutty

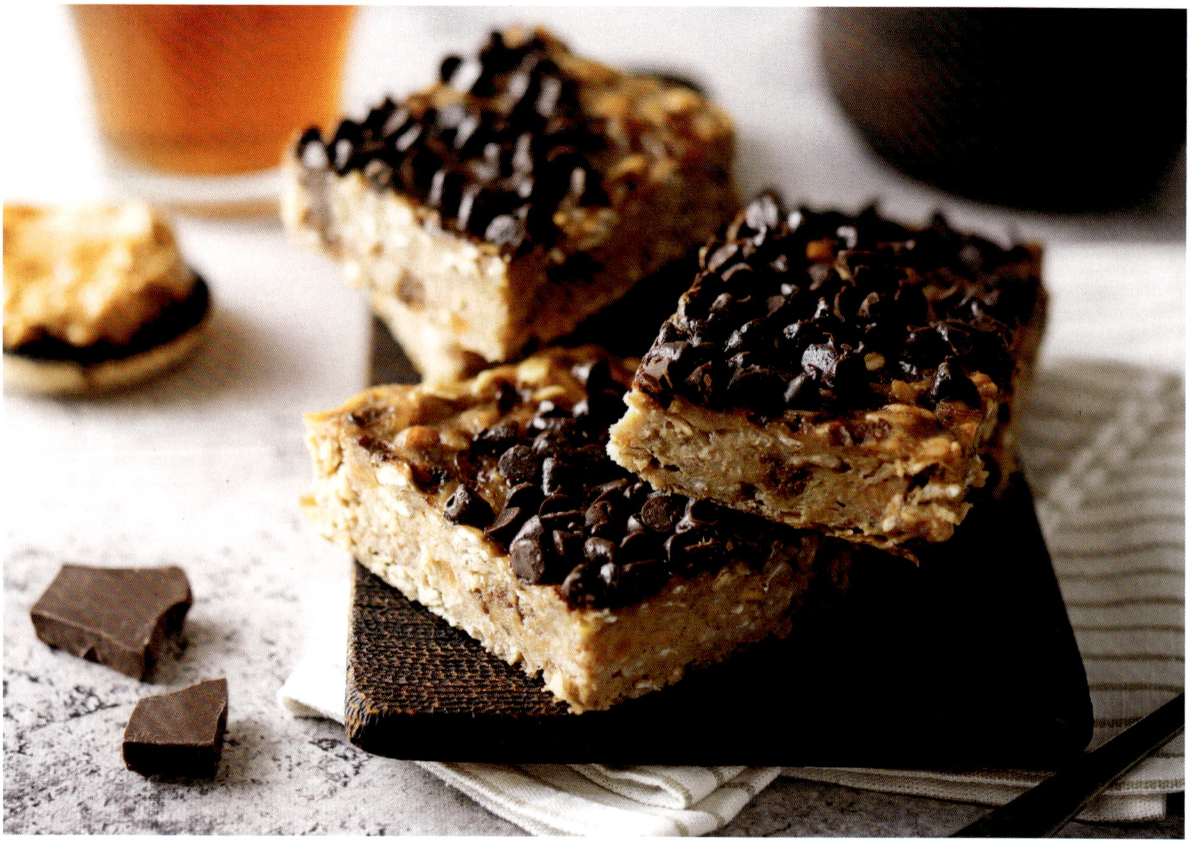

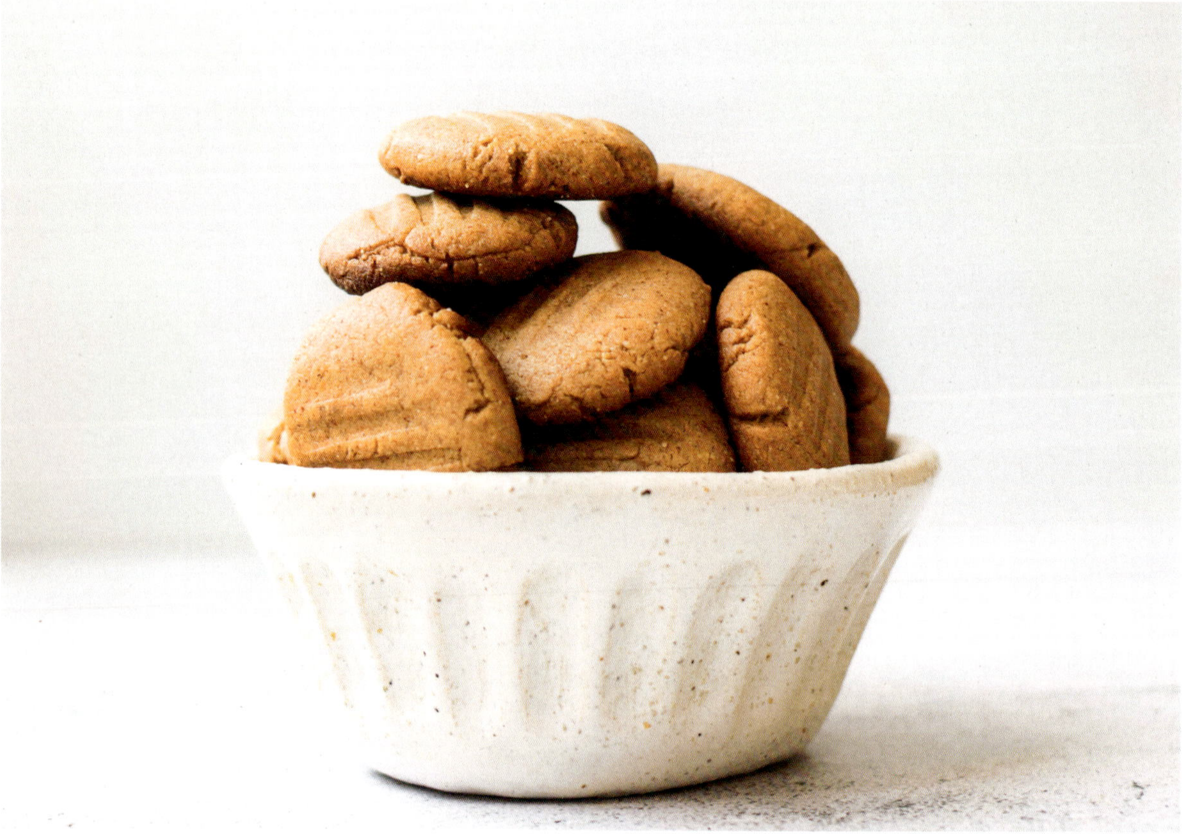

Peanut Butter, Oat & Banana Bars

MAKES 16
PREP + COOK TIME: 40 MINS + COOLING
DAIRY FREE

2 large, ripe bananas (about 1 cup mashed)
1 tsp baking powder
½ tsp salt
1 tsp cinnamon
½ cup (125g) peanut butter
¼ cup (50g) brown sugar
1 egg
½ cup (120ml) almond milk
2½ cups (220g) rolled oats
1 tsp vanilla extract
1 cup (155g) dark chocolate chips

Preheat oven to 175°C. Line a 23cm square cake tin with greaseproof paper, using enough paper to overhang the sides.

In a large bowl mash the bananas. Add the baking powder, salt and cinnamon and mix to combine with an electric hand mixer. Whisk in the peanut butter, followed by the sugar, egg, almond milk, oats and vanilla.

Pour the mixture evenly into the prepared pan and bake for 25-30 minutes or until the centre is set.

Scatter with chocolate chips and cool in the pan at room temperature for 30-60 minutes. Transfer to the fridge for 1 hour until chilled.

Remove from the pan using the paper overhanging the sides then cut into bars.

Peanut Butter Cookies

MAKES 18
PREP + COOK TIME: 25 MINS

1½ cups (185g) plain flour
¾ tsp baking powder
115g unsalted butter, room temperature
½ cup (100g) brown sugar
½ cup (100g) white sugar
1 cup (250g) peanut butter
1 large egg, room temperature
1 tsp vanilla extract

Preheat oven to 175°C. Line a baking tray with greaseproof paper.

Sift flour and baking powder together in a large bowl.

In another bowl cream butter and sugars together with an electric mixer. Add peanut butter and mix to combine. Mix in egg and vanilla extract then add flour mixture and beat to incorporate.

Roll dough into 3cm balls and place on baking tray. Flatten cookies slightly with a fork.

Bake for 10 minutes until golden brown and firm around the edges.

Allow to cool completely on the baking tray.

Pistachio Biscotti

MAKES 15
PREP + COOK TIME: 55 MINS

1½ cups (185g) + 3 tbsps flour
Pinch of salt
½ tsp baking powder
¼ cup (55g) + 2 tbsps sugar
3 tbsps butter, softened
1 large egg
Zest of 1 orange
½ tsp vanilla
½ cup (60g) pistachios, chopped

Preheat oven to 180°C. Line a baking tray with greaseproof paper.

In a mixing bowl whisk together all the flour, the salt and baking powder. Make a well in the middle and add ¼ cup and 1 tablespoon sugar, butter, egg, zest and vanilla. Mix with an electric mixer until combined. Add the pistachios and mix with a wooden spoon to combine.

Move the dough to a flat surface and form into a log about 6cm wide. Scatter with the remaining 1 tablespoon sugar. Place on the prepared baking tray and bake for 20 minutes.

Remove from the oven and allow to cool for 5-10 minutes then slice into 2cm-thick slices. Place the slices cut-side up back on the baking tray and bake again for 15 minutes.

Let cool for 10 minutes on the baking tray before transferring to a wire rack to cool completely.

Pistachio Mousse Cake

SERVES 12
PREP + COOK TIME: 1 HOUR 45 MINS + 4 HOURS FREEZING
GLUTEN FREE

¾ cup (90g) pistachios
½ cup (125ml) water
3 cups (800ml) thickened cream
1¼ cups (300ml) milk
7 egg yolks
¼ cup (55g) caster sugar
300g white chocolate, finely chopped
15g gelatine powder
1 cup (125g) fresh raspberries

Grease a 23cm springform cake tin.

Add pistachios to a pan of boiling water and set aside for 1-2 minutes. Drain then transfer to a clean tea towel and rub off the brown skins. Place the pistachios into a food processor and process for 5-10 minutes until they form a paste. Add ¼ cup water and process until smooth and creamy.

Combine 300ml cream, milk and pistachio puree in a large saucepan over medium heat and bring to a boil, stirring constantly. Remove from heat.

Place egg yolks and sugar in a large bowl and beat until pale and creamy. Pour the pistachio mixture slowly over the egg yolk mixture and stir to combine. Pour the pistachio and egg yolk mixture back into the saucepan and place over very low heat. Cook, stirring continuously, for 5-6 minutes until the mixture coats the spoon.

Place white chocolate in a large bowl and pour over the hot pistachio and egg yolk mixture. Mix the gelatine with ¼ cup water into a smooth paste and pour over the mixture. Stir for 2 minutes. Cool the mixture, stirring every 10 minutes, for 1 hour. Whisk the remaining cream to soft peaks and fold into the cooled mixture.

Pour into the prepared tin and scatter with raspberries. Cover and freeze for at least 4 hours. Remove from freezer 40 minutes before serving.

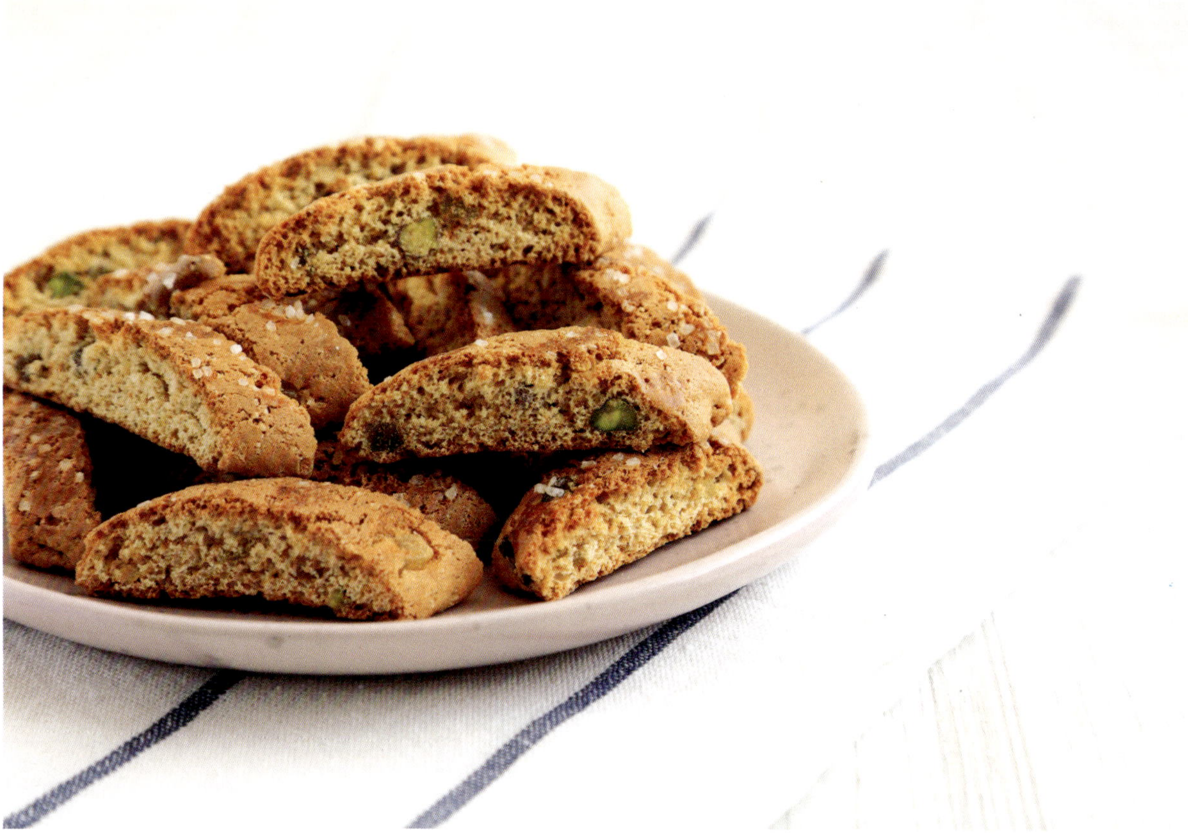

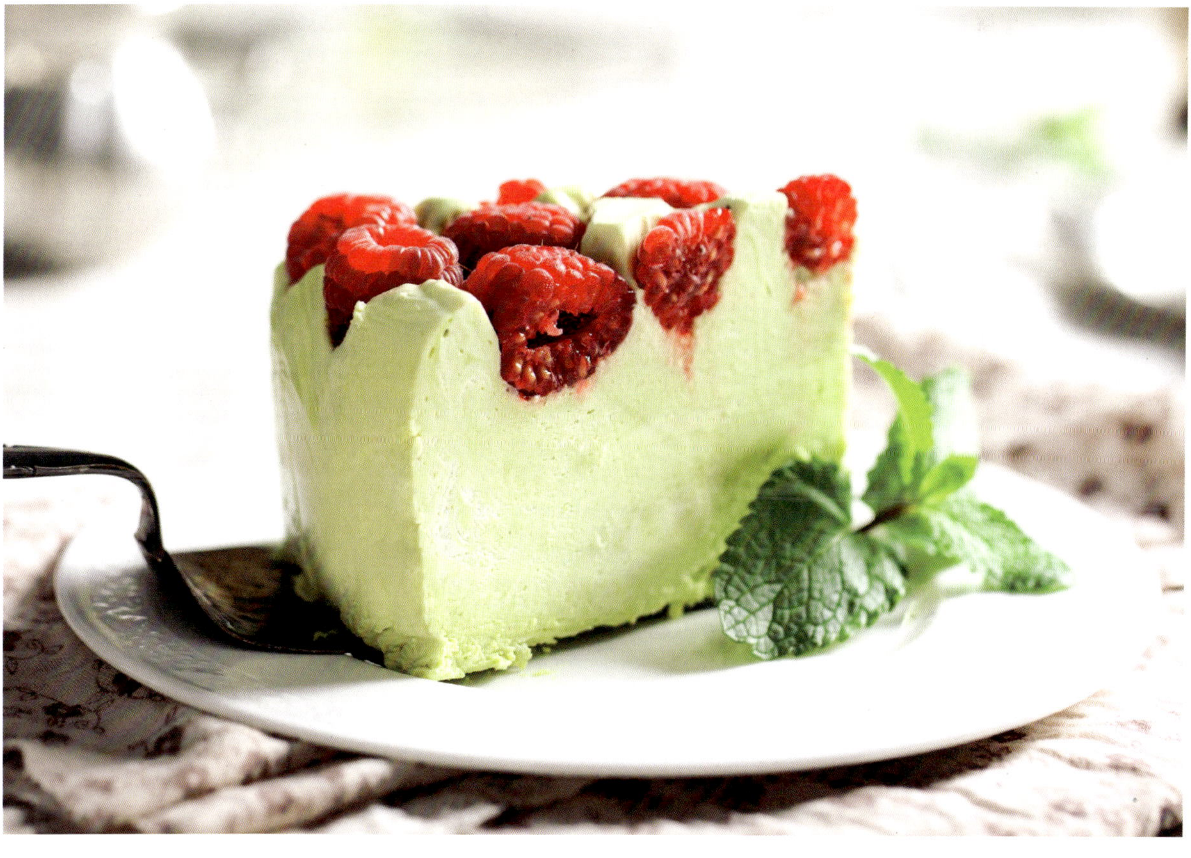

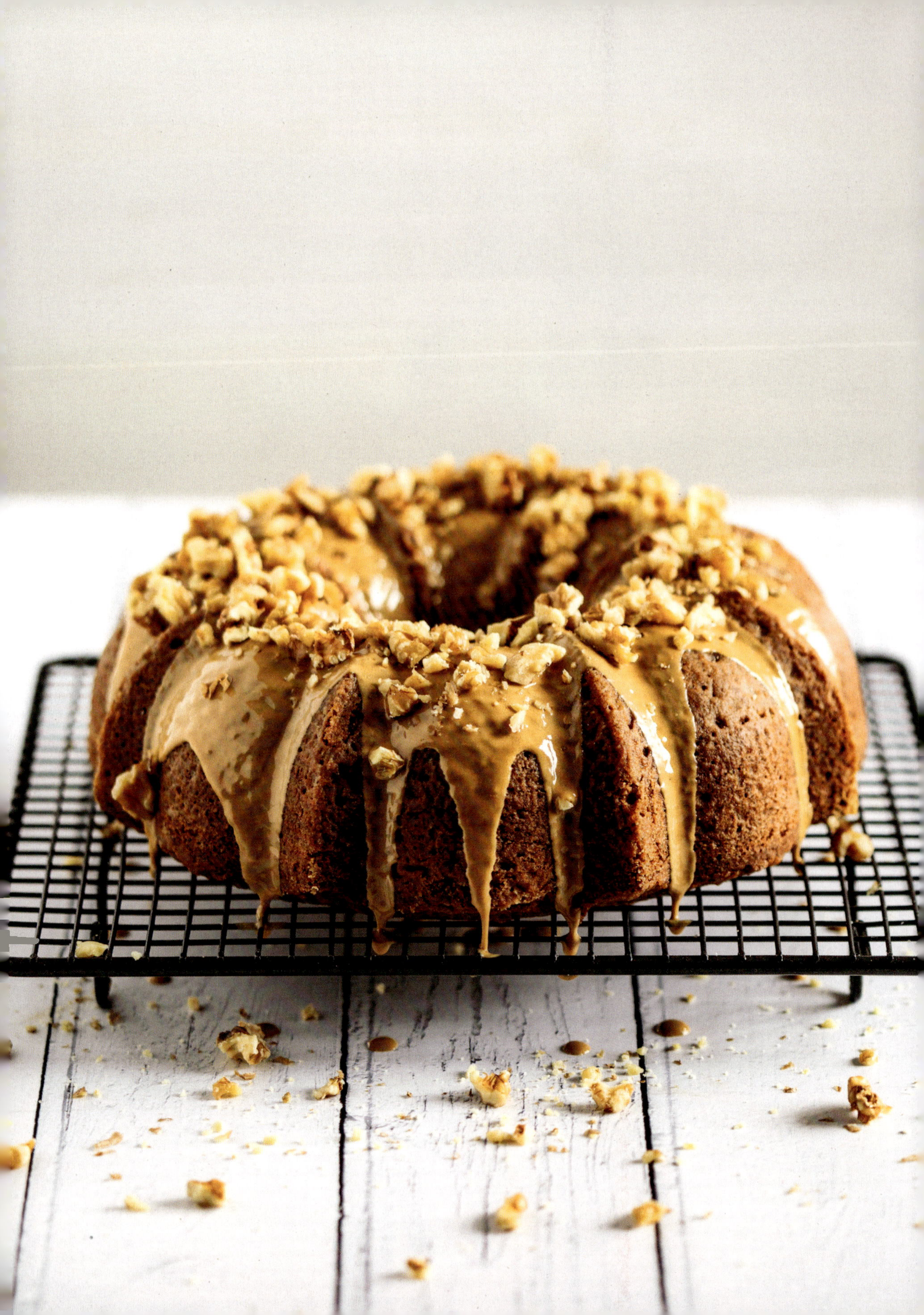

Coffee & Walnut Cake

SERVES 8-10
PREP + COOK TIME: 1 HOUR 20 MIN + COOLING

1¾ cups + 1 tbsp (225g) flour
1 tsp baking powder
⅛ tsp bicarbonate of soda
½ tsp salt
¾ cup (100g) walnuts, chopped + extra for topping
1½ tbsps instant coffee granules
1 tbsp hot water
3 tbsps milk
1 tsp vanilla essence
255g unsalted butter, cubed and at room temperature
1 cup (225g) caster sugar
4 eggs
Coffee glaze (see next recipe)

Preheat oven to 165°C. Grease a bundt tin and lightly dust with flour. Shake off the excess flour.

Sift flour, baking powder, bicarb and salt into a bowl. Stir in the chopped walnuts. Set aside.

In another bowl dissolve instant coffee granules in the hot water. Stir in the milk and vanilla. Set aside.

Cream the butter and sugar with an electric mixer until light and fluffy. Add eggs, one at a time, beating between each addition.

Fold one-third of the flour mixture into the creamed butter mixture then add half of the coffee solution. Fold in another third of the flour mixture, followed by the remaining coffee solution. Lastly fold in the remaining third of the flour mixture until just incorporated.

Pour batter into the prepared tin and bake in the oven for 50-60 minutes or until a skewer inserted into the centre of the cake comes out clean.

Remove from the oven and leave to cool in the tin for 10-15 minutes before turning out onto a wire rack to cool completely.

When the cake is completely cool, pour over the coffee glaze. Scatter with more chopped walnuts and allow glaze to set before serving.

Coffee Glaze

SERVES 8-10
PREP + COOK TIME: 10 MINS
GLUTEN FREE

1 tbsp unsalted butter
⅔ cup (100g) icing sugar
1 tbsp instant coffee granules
1 tbsp hot water

Mix together the butter and icing sugar with an electric mixer until the mixture resembles breadcrumbs.

In a small bowl, dissolve the coffee granules in the hot water.

Stir the coffee solution into the icing sugar a little at a time until you get a pouring consistency.

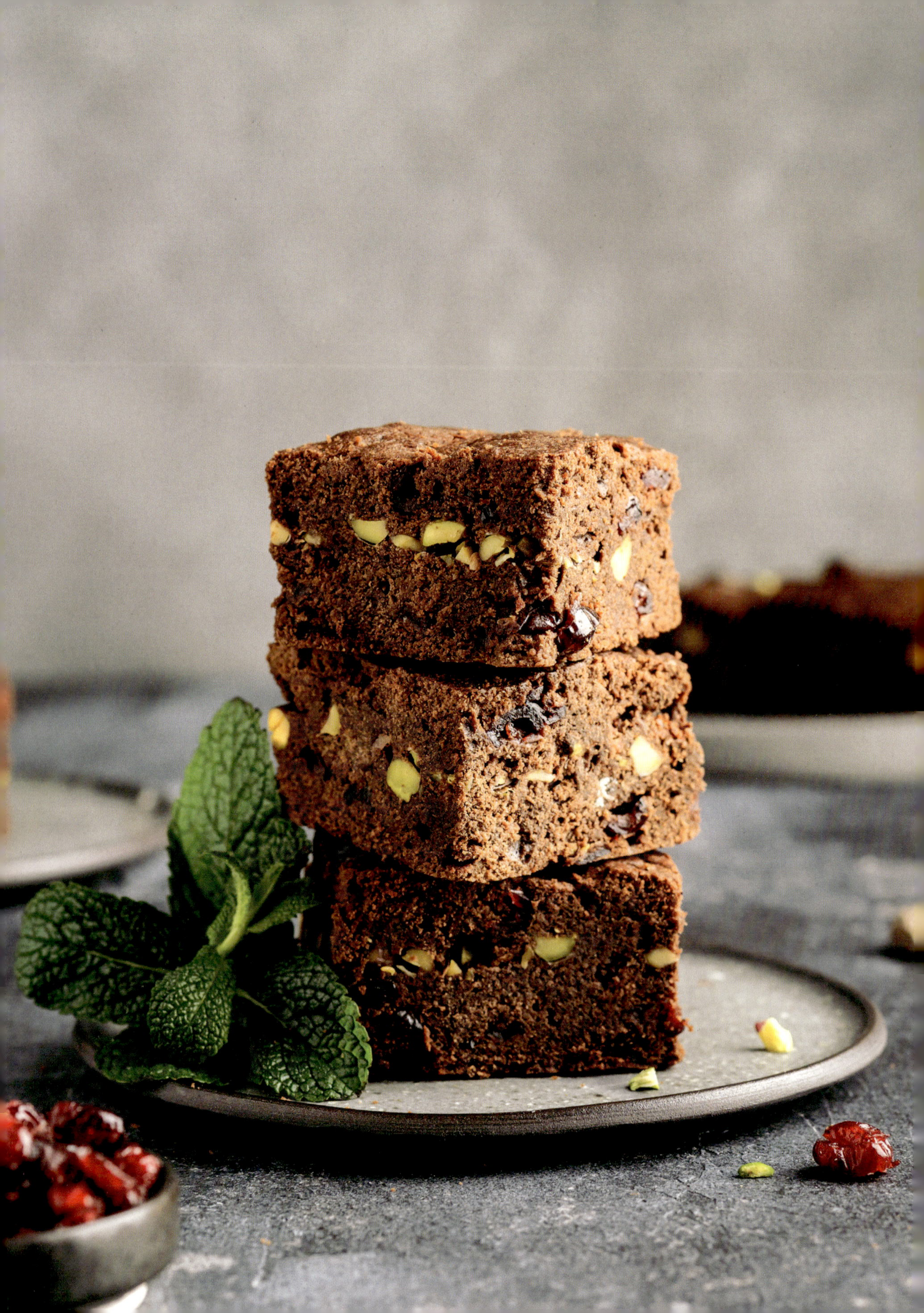

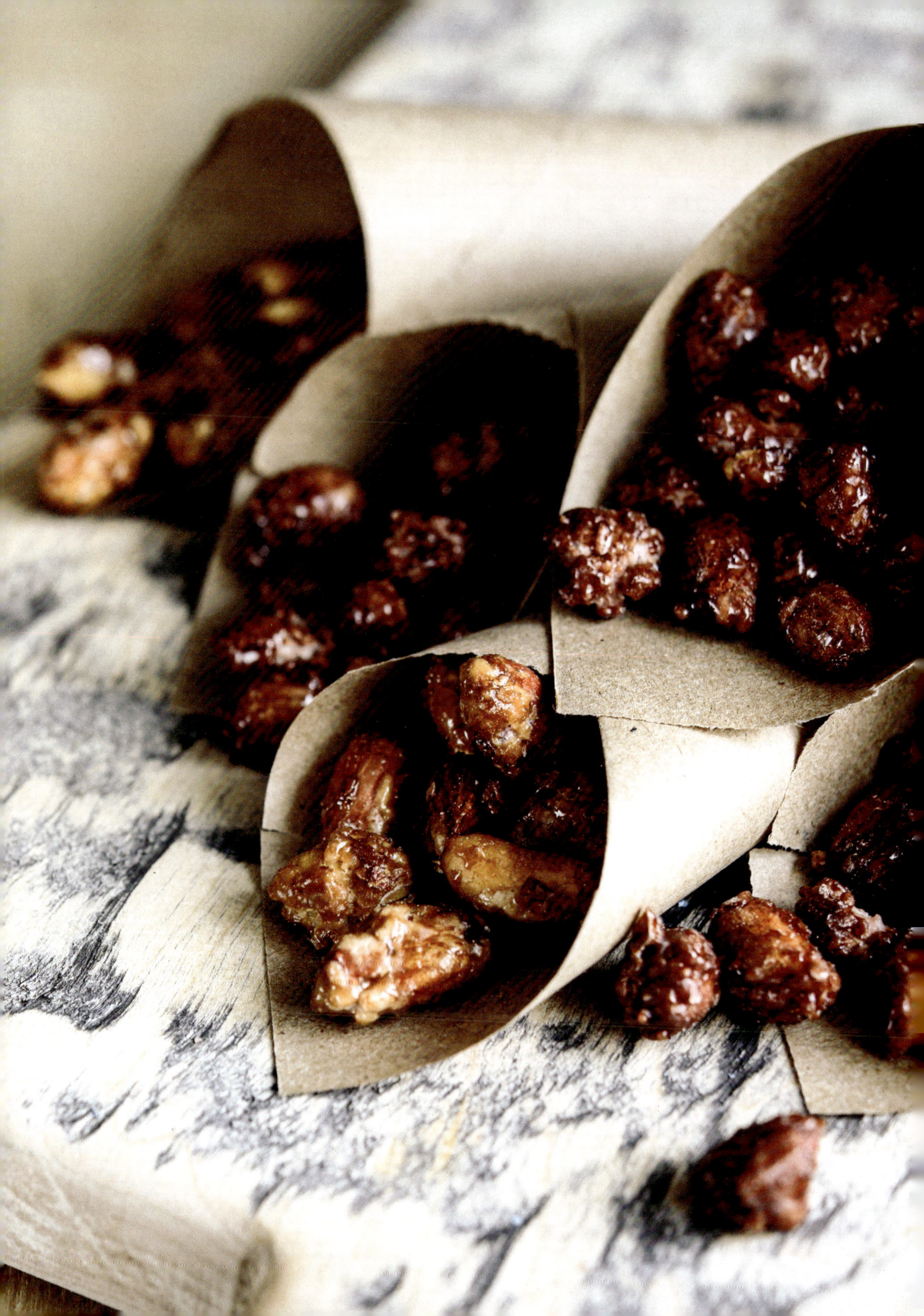

Pistachio & Cranberry Chocolate Brownies

MAKES 12
PREP + COOK TIME: 45 MINS

200g unsalted butter, chopped
250g dark chocolate, roughly chopped
5 eggs, lightly beaten
1 cup + 2 tbsps (250g) caster sugar
1⅓ cups (375g) plain flour
⅓ cup (35g) cocoa powder
½ cup (80g) dried cranberries, chopped
½ cup (60g) pistachios, roughly chopped

Preheat oven to 200°C. Line the base and sides of an 18 x 28cm tin with greaseproof paper, leaving paper overhanging the long sides of the tin for easy removal once cooked.

Melt butter and chocolate in a saucepan over low heat. Set aside and allow to cool slightly. Whisk in eggs until combined, and add sugar, flour and cocoa powder. Stir to combine before mixing in cranberries and pistachios.

Pour mixture into prepared tin and bake for 20-25 minutes until edges are dry and centre is just set. Leave to cool in the tin for 15 minutes before gently lifting out using greaseproof paper.

Cut into squares and either serve immediately for a soft and fudgy texture, or cool on a wire rack before serving for a firmer texture.

Caramelised Peanuts

SERVES 4
PREP + COOK TIME: 1 HOUR 15 MINS
GLUTEN FREE • DAIRY FREE

1 cup (220g) sugar
½ cup (125ml) water
2 cups (250g) raw peanuts, skin on

Preheat oven to 150°C. In a medium saucepan, combine sugar and water and place over medium heat. Stir until sugar dissolves. Add peanuts and cook, stirring constantly, for about 30 minutes until the peanuts are completely coated and no sugar syrup remains. Pour peanuts onto an ungreased baking tray and bake for 30 minutes, stirring every 10 minutes. Allow to cool for 10 minutes before serving.

Granola Cups

MAKES 8
PREP + COOK TIME: 40 MINS + COOLING

1 ripe banana
¼ cup (80g) maple syrup
¼ cup (30g) almonds, chopped
1 tsp vanilla extract
1½ cups (130g) rolled oats
1 tsp cinnamon
Pinch of salt
1½ cups (375ml) Greek yoghurt
⅓ cup (30g) blueberries

Preheat oven to 180°C. In a large bowl, mash banana with a fork. Add maple syrup, almonds, vanilla, oats, cinnamon and salt. Stir to combine. Press mixture into the bottom and sides of eight greased muffin cups. Transfer to the oven and bake for 30 minutes. Allow to cool in the tins for 10 minutes before transferring to a wire rack to cool completely. Fill with Greek yoghurt and blueberries, to serve.

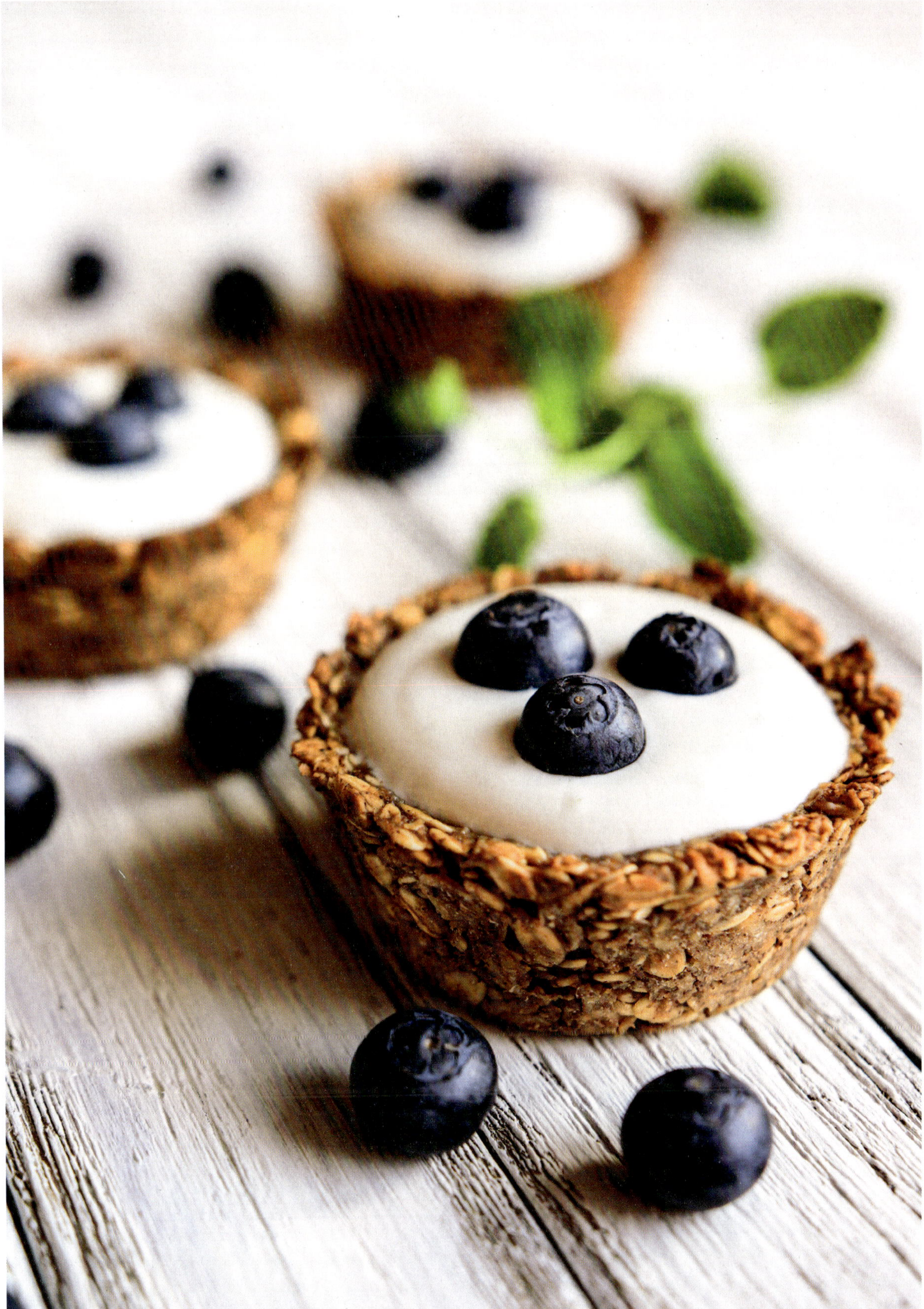

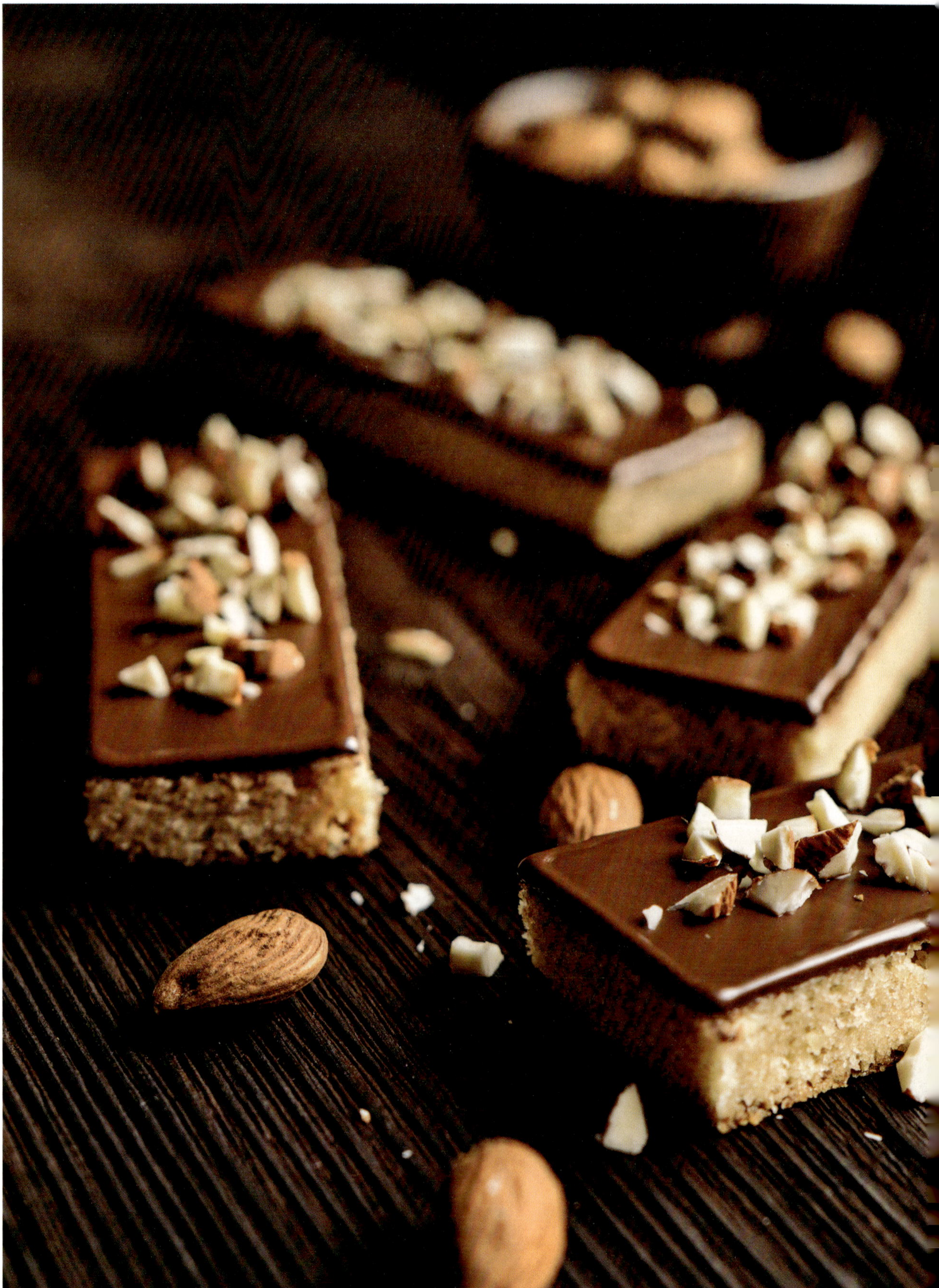

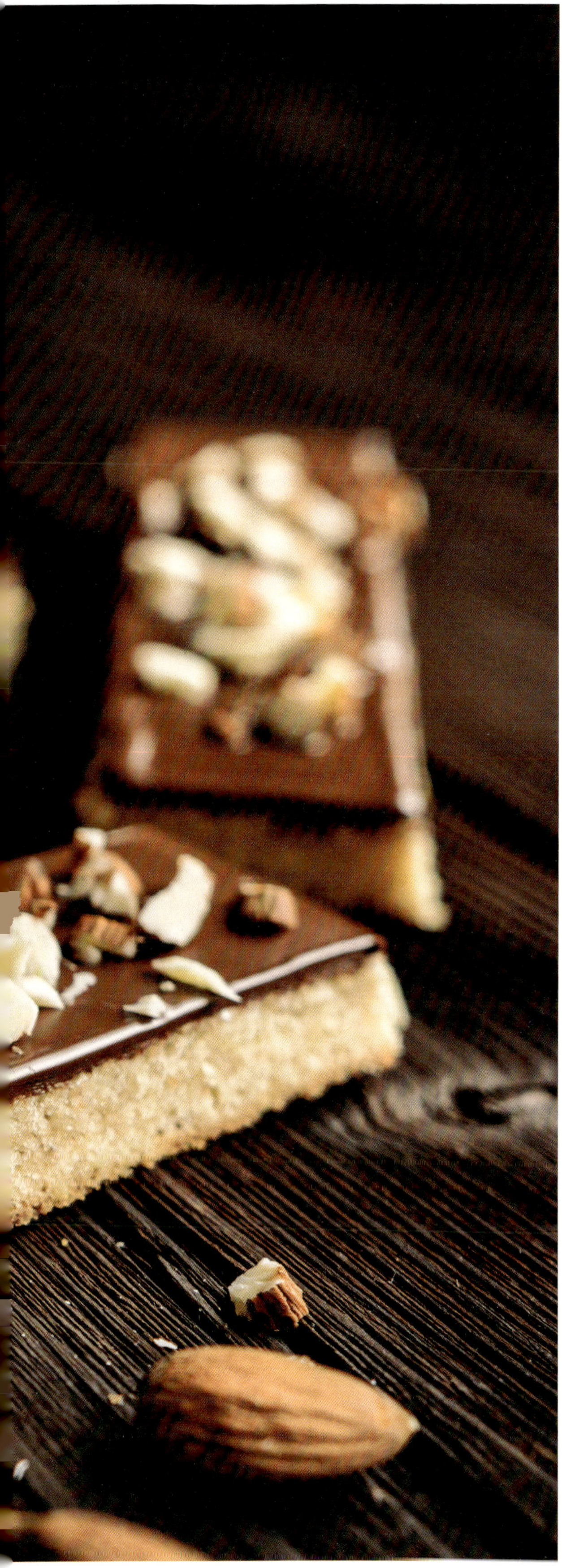

Chocolate Almond Shortbread Bars

MAKES 9
PREP + COOK TIME: 1 HOUR 15 MINS

ALMOND SHORTBREAD

225g unsalted butter
1 cup (220g) sugar
1 tsp vanilla extract
½ tsp almond extract
2 cups (250g) plain flour
½ tsp salt

CHOCOLATE TOPPING

1 cup (250ml) thickened cream
450g dark chocolate, chopped
1 tsp salt
Chopped almonds to serve

Preheat oven to 180°C. Line the bottom and sides of a 22 x 33cm tin with greaseproof paper.

In the bowl of an electric stand mixer or with a hand-held mixer, cream butter and sugar together until light and fluffy. Add vanilla and almond extracts and mix.

Mix in flour and salt on low speed, increase speed to medium and mix until well combined and crumbs form.

Press dough evenly into prepared tin to form the bottom layer and bake for 15 minutes. Remove from oven and cool.

Melt chocolate and cream together in a heatproof bowl set over a pan of simmering water. Add salt and mix until smooth.

Pour chocolate mixture over cooled shortbread layer and sprinkle chopped almonds on top. Refrigerate until set (approximately 1 hour) then cut into bars.

Sesame Tahini Cookies

MAKES 16
PREP + COOK TIME: 25 MINS
GLUTEN FREE • DAIRY FREE

½ cup (80g) sesame seeds
1½ cups (180g) almond meal
½ tsp bicarbonate of soda
¼ tsp salt
⅓ cup (115g) honey
⅓ cup (75g) tahini
1 tsp vanilla extract

Preheat the oven to 175°C and line two baking trays with greaseproof paper.

Place the sesame seeds in a shallow dish.

In a small bowl, whisk the almond meal with the bicarb and salt.

In a large bowl, mix the honey with the tahini and vanilla extract. Add the almond meal mixture to the wet ingredients and stir to incorporate.

Scoop the dough into 3cm balls. Roll the balls in the sesame seeds. Place the balls on the baking trays about 5cm apart. Flatten into rounds.

Bake the cookies for about 8 minutes, until the bottoms are golden.

Transfer to a wire rack to cool before serving.

Peanut Butter Chocolate Slice

MAKES 16
PREP + COOK TIME: 15 MINS + 1 HOUR 30 MINS CHILLING

BASE
1 cup (100g) crushed plain biscuits
115g butter, melted
¼ tsp salt
¾ cup (190g) smooth peanut butter
½ cup (80g) icing sugar

CHOCOLATE TOPPING
1 cup (155g) dark chocolate chips
2 tbsps smooth peanut butter

Grease and line a 20 x 20cm tin with greaseproof paper and set aside.

In a medium-sized bowl mix together crushed biscuits, melted butter, salt, peanut butter and icing sugar until combined. Press into the prepared pan and set aside.

Melt the chocolate chips and peanut butter for the topping in a heatproof bowl in the microwave on medium for 30-second bursts, mixing in between. Alternatively place chocolate and peanut butter in a heatproof bowl set over a saucepan of simmering water and stir with a metal spoon until melted and glossy.

Pour topping over the base and smooth out using a spatula. Refrigerate until set, about 1½ hours.

Remove from fridge and allow to come to room temperature. Cut into squares and serve.

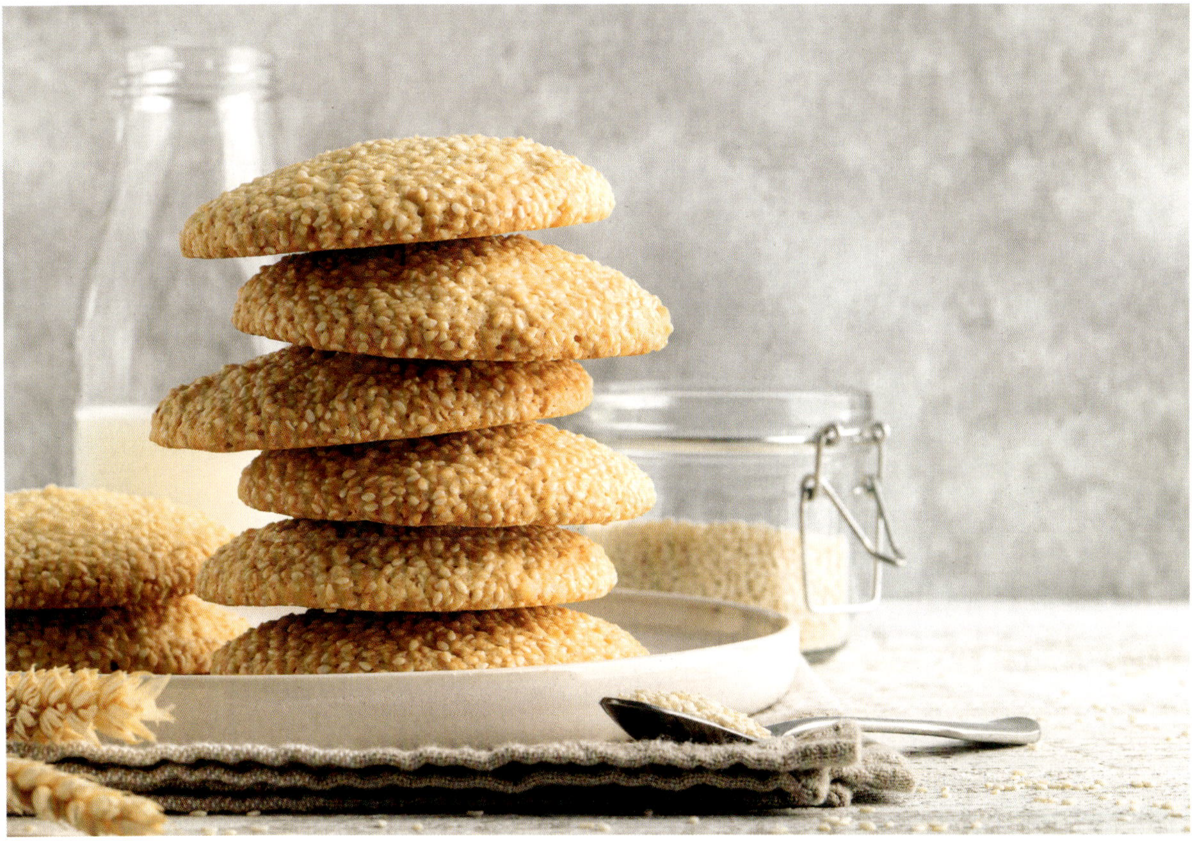

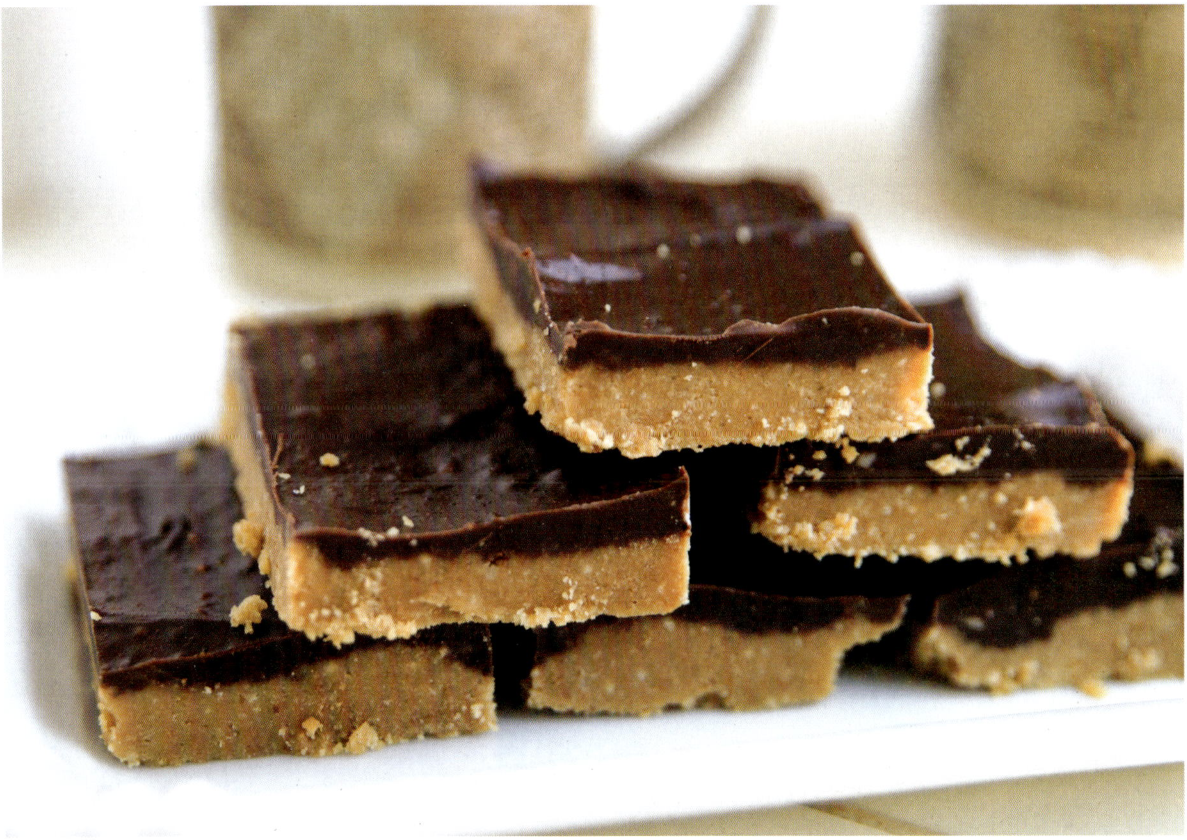

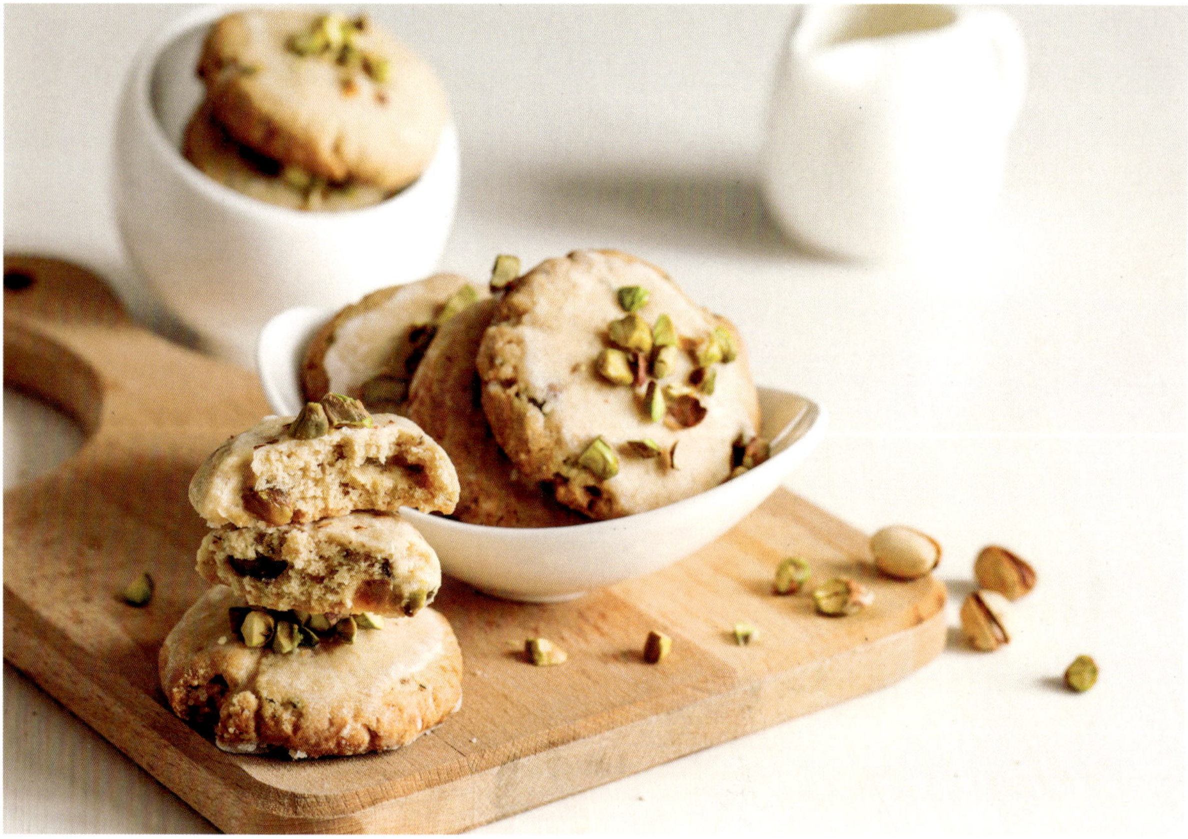

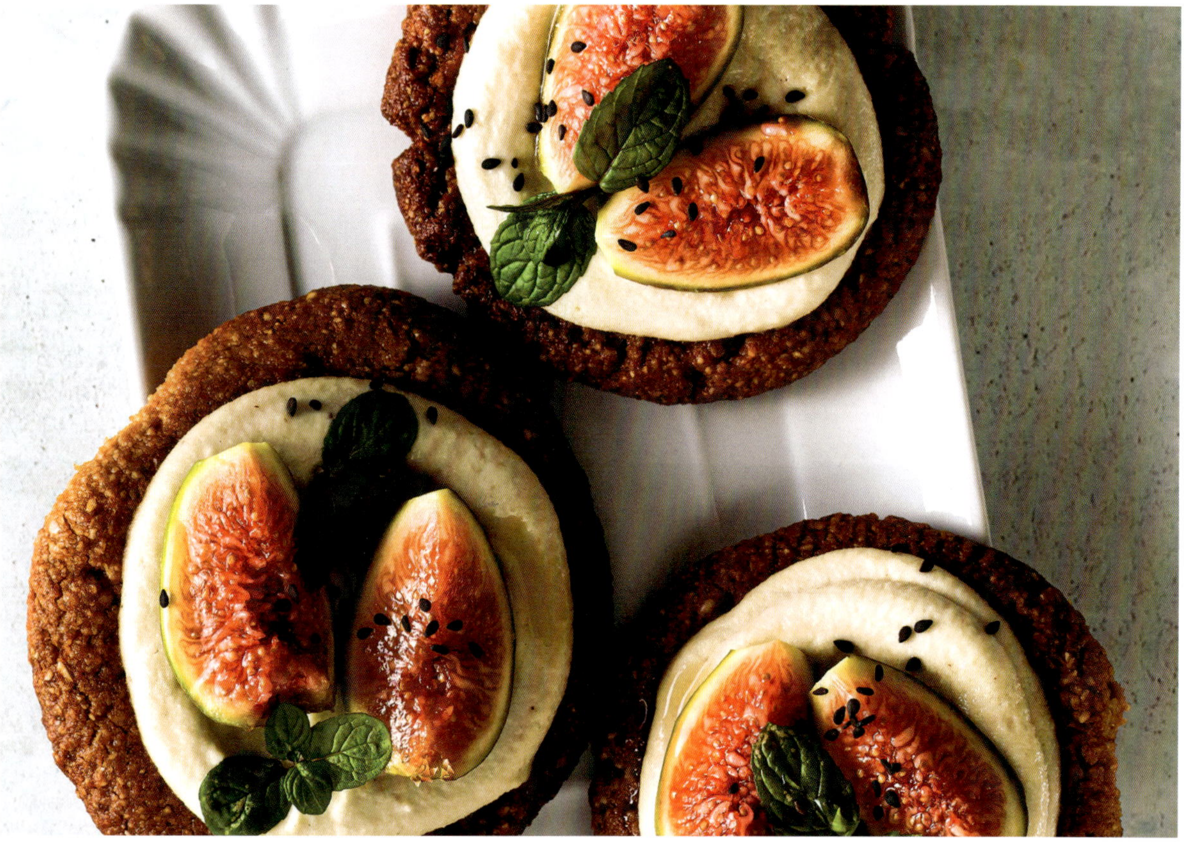

Pistachio Biscuits

MAKES 20
PREP + COOK TIME: 30 MINS + 2 HOURS CHILLING

225g unsalted butter, room temperature
½ cup (110g) sugar
1 tsp vanilla extract
1¾ cups (215g) plain flour
¼ cup (40g) cornflour
1 cup (125g) pistachios, roughly chopped

Cream the butter and the sugar with an electric mixer until light and fluffy. Beat in the vanilla.

In a separate bowl whisk together the flour and cornflour. Add to the butter and sugar and beat to form a dough. Stir in the pistachios.

Cover and refrigerate the dough for at least 2 hours.

Preheat oven to 175°C. Line a baking tray with greaseproof paper.

Roll the dough into 3cm balls and place on prepared baking tray about 5cm apart. Flatten the balls slightly with your fingers.

Bake for about 10 minutes until light golden brown.

Cool for 2 minutes on the baking tray before transferring to a wire rack to cool completely.

Tahini Cookies

MAKES 8
PREP + COOK TIME: 30 MINS
DAIRY FREE

½ cup (115g) tahini, room temperature
½ cup (110g) packed brown sugar
½ tsp vanilla extract
⅓ cup (40g) plain flour
½ tsp bicarbonate of soda
⅛ tsp salt
1 tbsp water

TOPPINGS
Cashew cream (see recipe page 142)
4 figs, quartered
Mint sprigs
1 tbsp black sesame seeds

Preheat oven to 175°C. Line two baking trays with greaseproof paper.

Add tahini, brown sugar and vanilla to a mixing bowl. Cream together with an electric hand mixer until smooth. Add flour, bicarb and salt. Mix until the mixture forms a crumbly dough Add water and mix well.

Scoop the mixture with a tablespoon and roll into balls. Place on the prepared baking trays leaving at least 5cm between each one.

Bake for 7-9 minutes, or until the edges are slightly golden. It is okay if they look underdone in the middle. Remove from oven and allow the cookies to set on the baking trays for at least 5 minutes before very gently transferring to a wire rack to cool completely.

Top with cashew cream, fig quarters, mint sprigs and black sesame seeds, to serve.

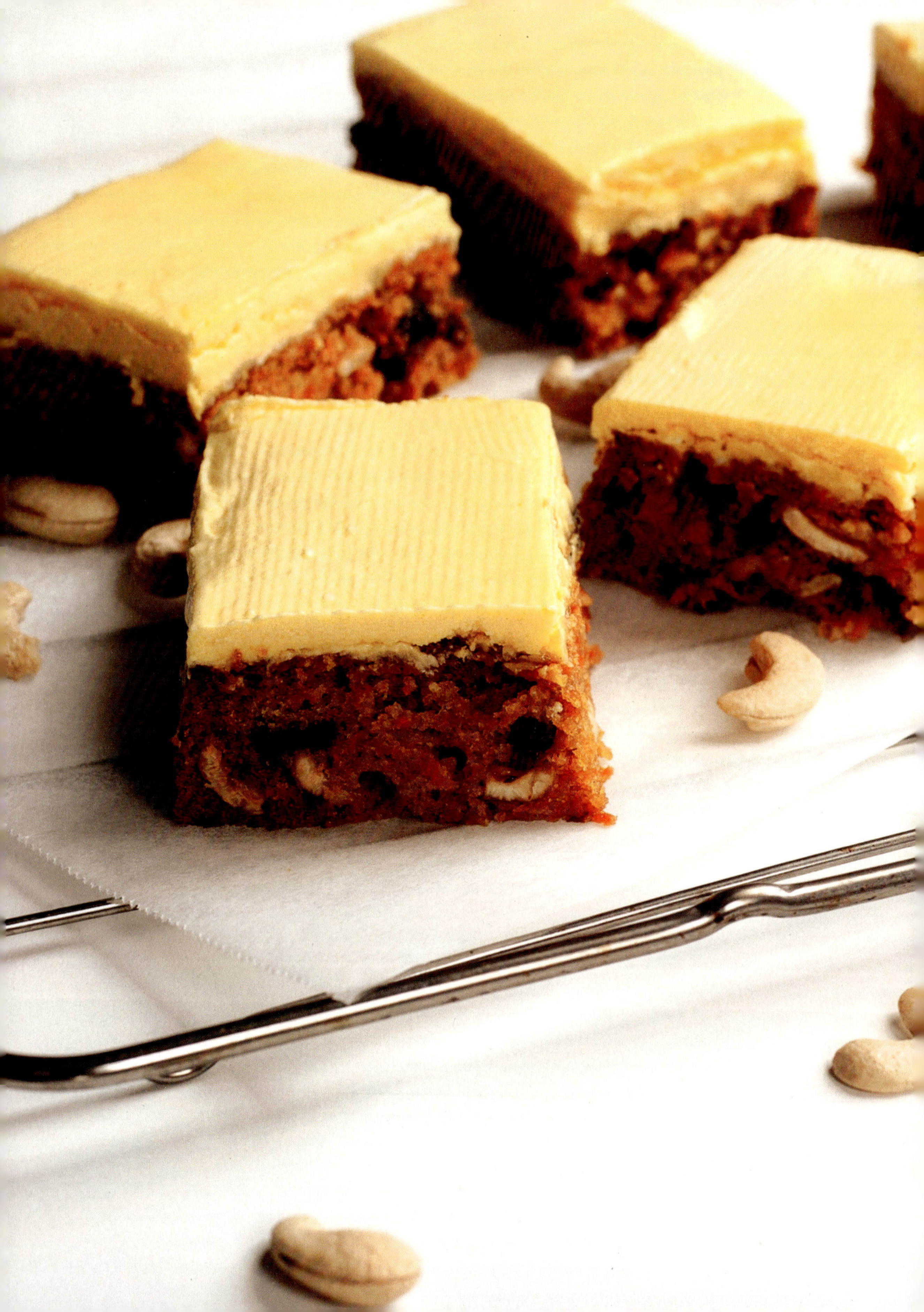

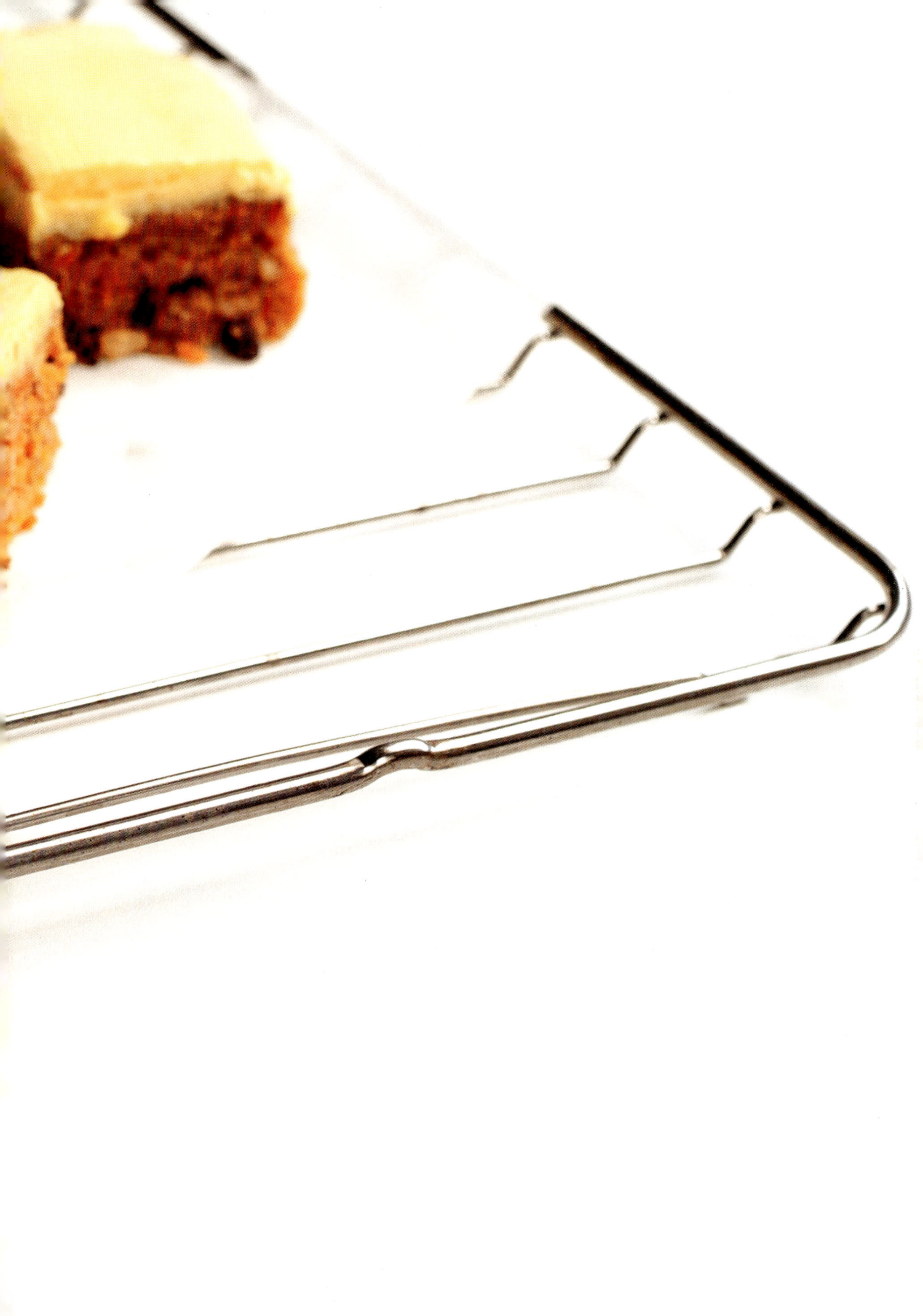

Raw Vegan Carrot Cake

SERVES 16
PREP + COOK TIME: 30 MINS + 3 HOURS FREEZING
GLUTEN FREE • DAIRY FREE

CAKE

2 cups (350g) Medjool dates, pitted
2½ cups (310g) raw walnuts
2 tsps vanilla extract
¼ tsp salt
1¼ tsps cinnamon
¾ tsp ground ginger
Pinch of nutmeg
2 cups (220g) finely grated carrots
½ cup (50g) coconut flour
¼ cup (40g) raisins

TOPPING

Cashew cream (see next recipe)
2 tsps orange zest

Line an 18 x 23cm springform tin with greaseproof paper.

Place dates in a food processor and pulse until finely chopped. Transfer to a bowl and set aside. Add walnuts, vanilla, salt and spices to the food processor. Blend into a semi-fine meal. Add reserved date mixture and grated carrots, pulse until a loose dough forms and carrots are just incorporated. Transfer mixture to a large mixing bowl. Add coconut flour and raisins; mix gently to combine. Add cake mixture to the tin and spread it out evenly across the tin, pressing down to pack mixture into an even layer.

To make the topping, follow the cashew cream recipe, then add orange zest and stir to combine. Pour the cashew cream icing on top of the cake and tap out any air bubbles. Place on a baking tray and freeze for 3-4 hours until the frosting is semi-firm to the touch.

To serve, let the cake thaw for 30 minutes at room temperature and cut into squares.

Cashew Cream

MAKES 2½ CUPS
PREP + COOK TIME: 10 MINS + 2 HOURS SOAKING
GLUTEN FREE • DAIRY FREE

2 cups (250g) raw cashews, soaked for 2 hours
5 Medjool dates
2 tsps vanilla extract
½ cup (125ml) coconut cream
Water as needed

Combine cashews, dates and vanilla in a food processor. Add coconut cream and blend until creamy smooth, scraping down the sides as necessary. Add water a tbsp at a time until desired consistency is reached.

Serve or chill until ready to use.

Peanut Brittle

MAKES APPROX 20 PIECES
PREP + COOK TIME: 35 MINS
GLUTEN FREE

1 cup (125g) unsalted, roasted peanuts
2½ cups (550g) sugar
½ cup (125ml) water
50g butter

Line an 18 x 28cm slice tin with foil. Scatter nuts over the base of the tin.

Combine sugar and water in a small saucepan. Place over medium heat and stir until sugar dissolves, then bring to the boil. Gently boil for 25 minutes, or until a rich golden colour. Remove pan from heat and stir in the butter until just combined. Pour the mixture over the peanuts, then set aside to cool until the toffee sets.

Break into pieces to serve.

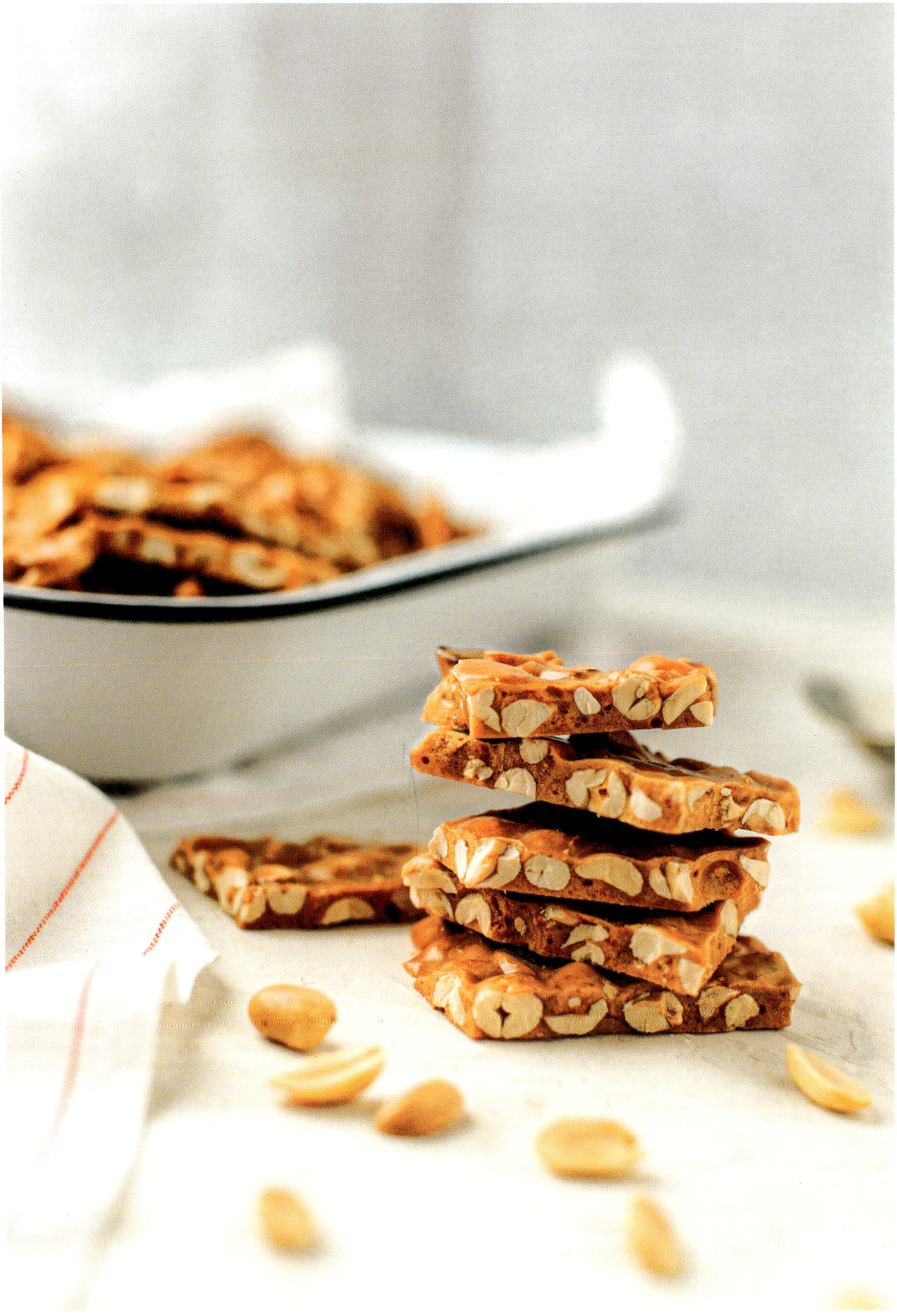

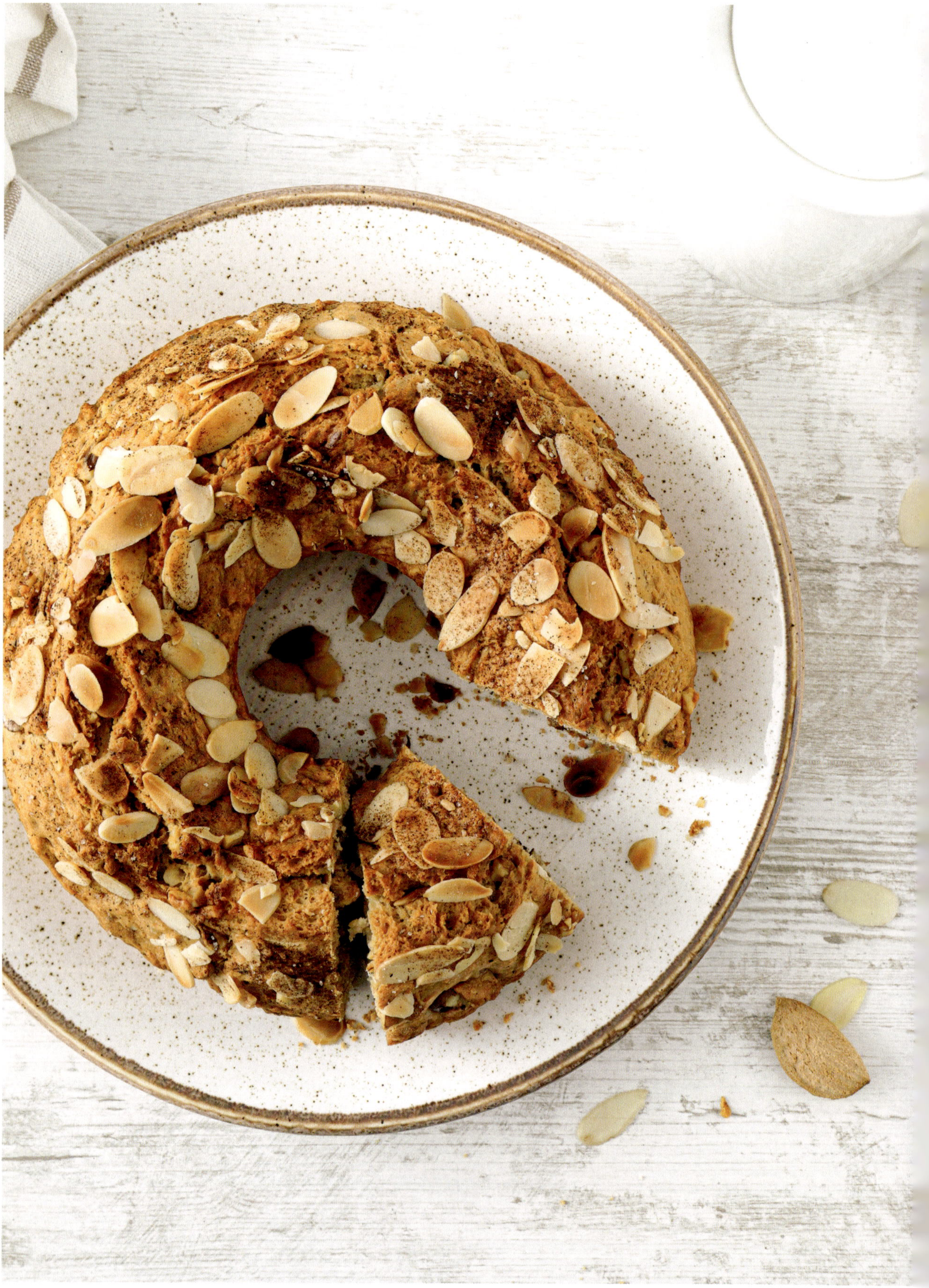

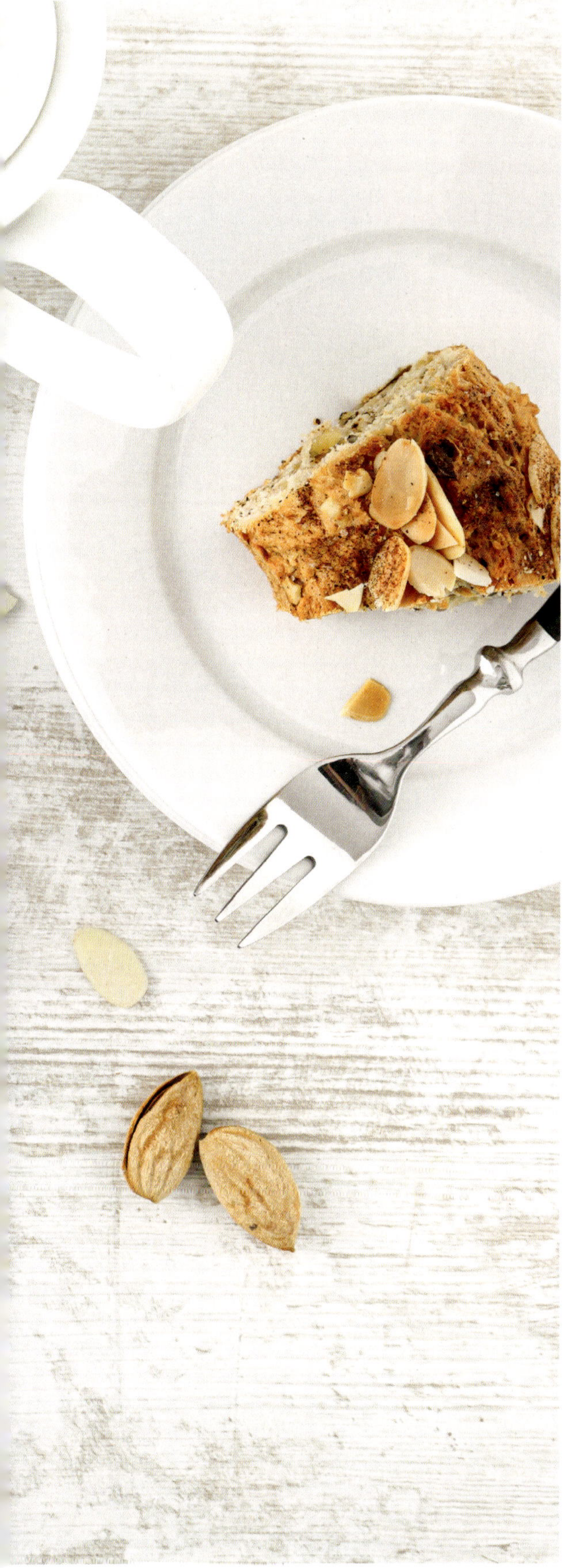

French Apple & Almond Cake

SERVES 10
PREP + COOK TIME: 1 HOUR 30 MINS

3 apples, peeled, cored and thinly sliced
1 egg + 2 egg yolks
1 cup (220g) + 2 tbsps sugar
115g unsalted butter, softened
1 tsp vanilla bean paste
¾ cup (90g) plain flour
¾ cup (90g) almond meal
2 tsps baking powder
½ tsp salt
¼ cup (60ml) milk
1½ tbsps flaked almonds

Preheat oven to 180°C. Butter and flour a 20cm ring cake tin.

In a bowl, microwave apples on high until softened, about 2 minutes. Let cool and strain any excess liquid.

Using an electric mixer beat egg and 2 tablespoons of sugar at medium speed until pale in colour, about 2 minutes. Stir in melted butter and vanilla paste.

In a medium bowl whisk together flour, almond meal, baking powder, salt and remaining 1 cup of sugar. Gradually add flour mixture and milk to egg mixture, beating until just combined.

In a large bowl, whisk together 1 cup of batter and egg yolks. Stir in apples until combined.

Spread egg yolk batter into prepared pan and top with remaining batter, smoothing with a spatula.

Bake in bottom of the oven for 30 minutes. Raise tin to the middle of the oven, and bake for 35 minutes more, loosely covering with foil to prevent excess browning, if necessary.

Let cool in the tin for 15 minutes. Remove from tin and sprinkle with flaked almonds to serve.

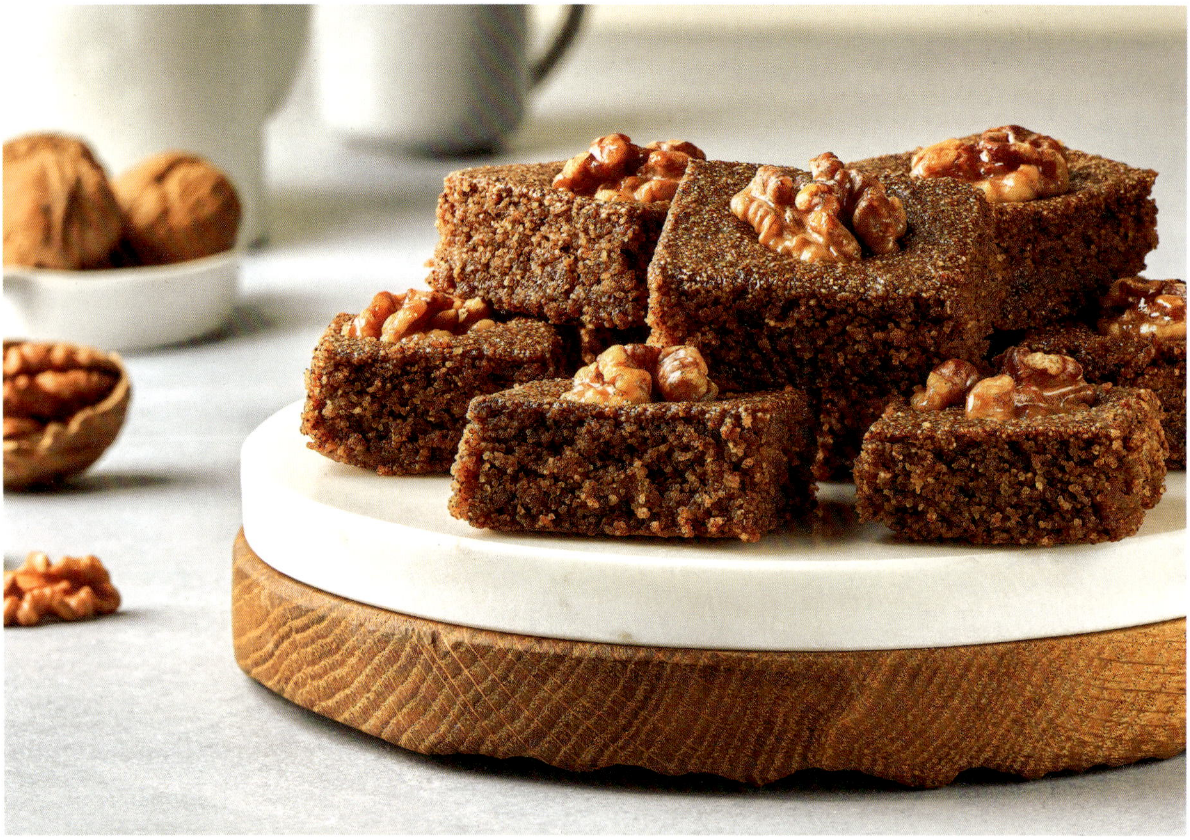

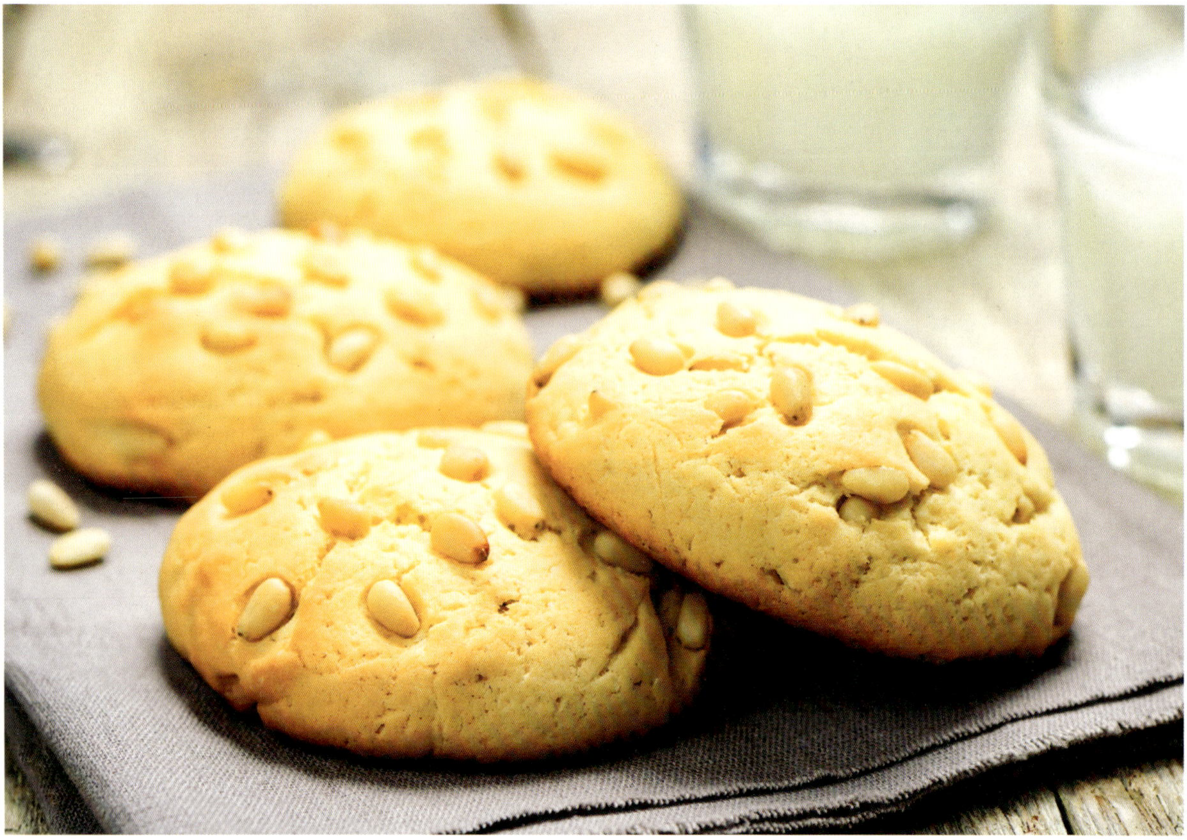

Walnut Semolina Cake

SERVES 9
PREP + COOK TIME: 1 HOUR 30 MINS

1½ cups walnut halves + extra for topping
1 cup (175g) semolina flour
1½ tsps baking powder
½ tsp salt
¾ tbsp unsalted butter, softened
½ cup (180g) honey
¼ cup (55g) sugar
3 eggs
½ tsp vanilla extract

Preheat the oven to 175°C. Butter a 20cm square cake tin and line the bottom with greaseproof paper. Flour the tin, tapping out any excess.

Spread the walnut halves on a baking tray and roast them in the oven for 9 minutes. Let them cool completely.

In a food processor, process the walnuts with the semolina flour until finely ground. Add the baking powder and salt and process until combined.

In a large bowl, using an electric mixer, beat the butter with the honey and sugar at medium speed until fluffy, about 3 minutes.

Add the eggs one at a time, beating well between additions, then add the vanilla extract. On low speed beat in the semolina flour mixture.

Pour the batter into the prepared tin, distribute walnut halves evenly and slightly press into batter. Bake on the middle rack of the oven for 1 hour or until a toothpick inserted into the centre comes out clean.

Let the cake cool in the pan for 10 minutes, and then turn it out onto a wire rack to cool completely. Cut into even squares and serve.

Pine Nut Cookies

MAKES 10
PREP + COOK TIME: 30 MINS
GLUTEN FREE • DAIRY FREE

2 cups (240g) almond meal
½ cup (110g) sugar
½ cup (80g) icing sugar
1 tsp almond extract (optional)
3 egg whites
½ cup (70g) pine nuts

Preheat oven to 180°C with the rack in the lower-middle position. Line a baking tray with greaseproof paper.

In a medium bowl combine almond meal, sugar, icing sugar, almond extract (if using) and egg whites to form a slightly sticky dough.

Place pine nuts in a shallow dish. Using wet hands roll 1 tablespoon of dough into a ball, press one side in pine nuts to coat and place on the baking tray. Press lightly to flatten and repeat with the remaining dough. Make sure cookies are evenly spaced with room between each one.

Bake cookies until light golden brown, 25-30 minutes. Check regularly so they don't overcook Allow to cool completely before serving.

6

Fruity

Plum & Cinnamon Doughnuts

MAKES 10
PREP + COOK TIME: 1 HOUR + 2 HOURS PROVING

1½ cups (375ml) milk + more for brushing
85g butter
4½ tsps (2 packets) active dry yeast
⅓ cup (80ml) lukewarm water
2 eggs, beaten
¼ cup (55g) sugar
2 tsps cinnamon
5 cups (625g) plain flour
1 cup (325g) plum jam
Icing sugar for dusting

Warm the milk and butter in a pan over medium heat until butter melts. Set aside to cool.

Sprinkle yeast over the warm water, whisk, then set aside for 5 minutes until foamy.

In a stand mixer, using the paddle attachment to combine the milk mixture and yeast mixture. Add the eggs, sugar, cinnamon and the flour a little at a time. Beat to incorporate. Change to the dough hook attachment and beat until the dough is smooth and pulls away from the bowl.

Transfer to an oiled bowl, cover and let it rise for 1 hour to double in size. Punch down the dough, cover, and let it rise for 1 more hour.

Roll dough to 1cm thickness on a lightly floured surface. Cut out rounds using a 7cm round cutter. Place half of the dough rounds on a baking tray lined with greaseproof paper and drop teaspoons plum jam in the centre. Brush edges with milk and place another round of dough over and press to seal tightly. Cover with a tea towel and set aside for 30 minutes.

Bake in a preheated oven at 190°C for 12-15 minutes until golden brown. Dust with icing sugar to serve.

Vegan Banana Bread

SERVES 10
PREP + COOK TIME: 1 HOUR 10 MINS
DAIRY FREE

4 medium, ripe bananas
½ cup (100g) light brown sugar
¼ cup (60ml) light olive oil
¼ cup (60ml) almond milk
2 tsps vanilla extract
2 cups (250g) plain flour
½ cup (60g) walnuts, chopped
1 tsp cinnamon
1 tsp bicarbonate of soda
½ tsp salt

Preheat the oven to 175°C. Grease and lightly flour a 20 x 10 x 7cm loaf tin and set aside.

Mash bananas in a large bowl. Add sugar, oil, almond milk and vanilla. Whisk to combine. Add flour, walnuts, cinnamon, bicarb and salt. Stir to incorporate. Pour batter into prepared tin.

Bake for 45 minutes, then cover with foil and bake for 10-15 minutes longer, until a skewer inserted in the centre comes out clean.

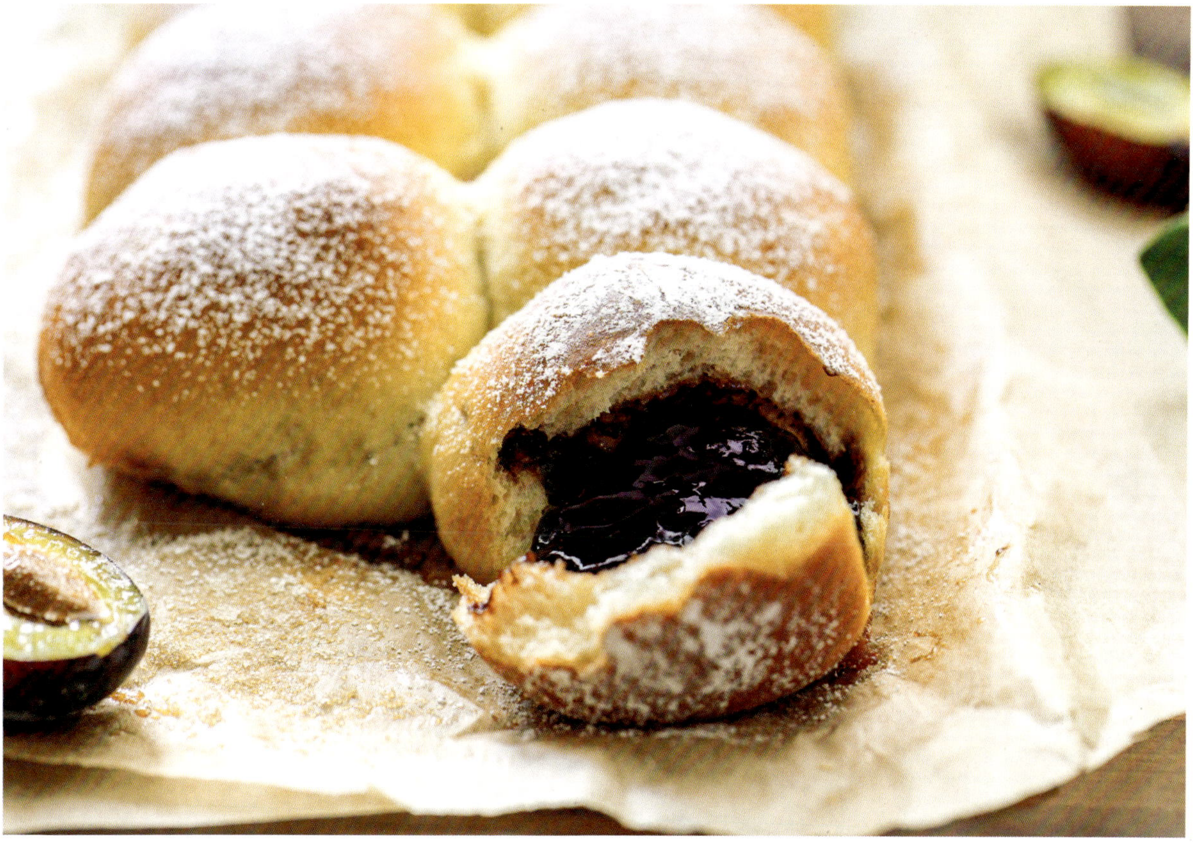

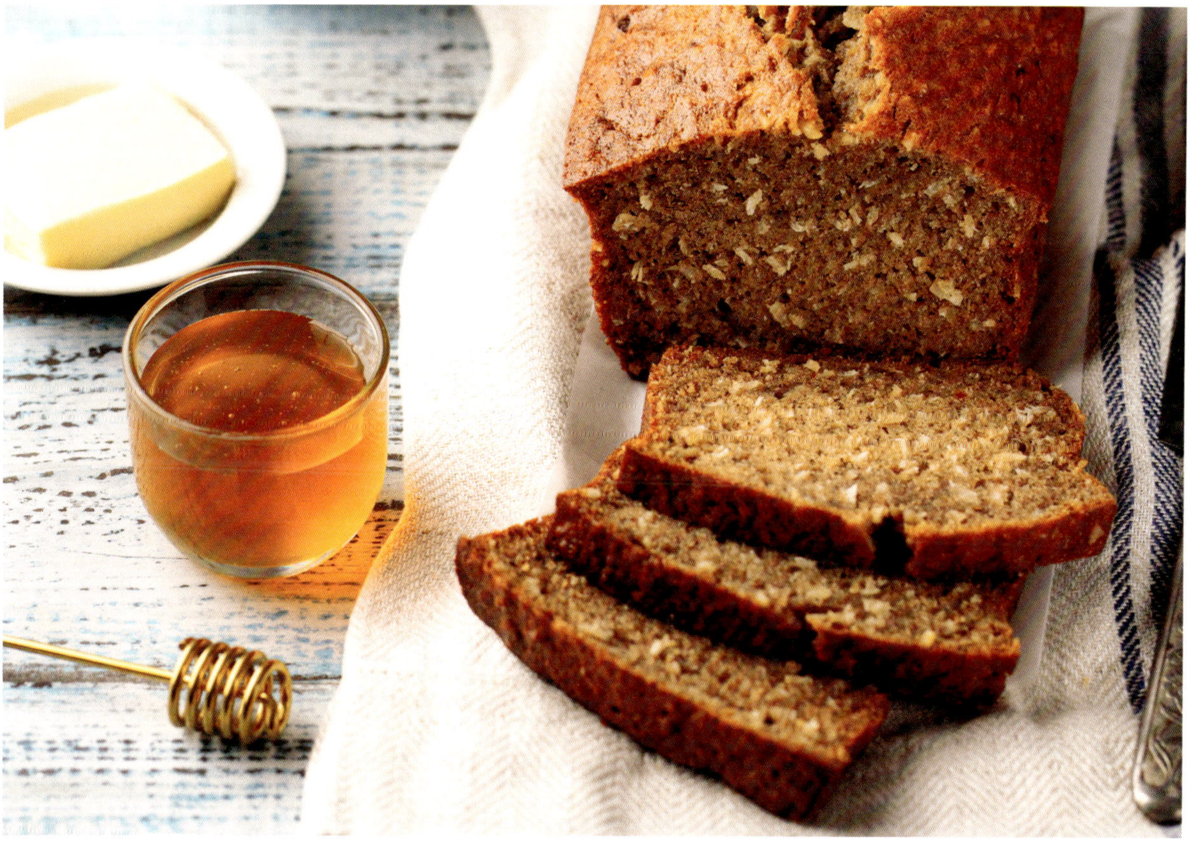

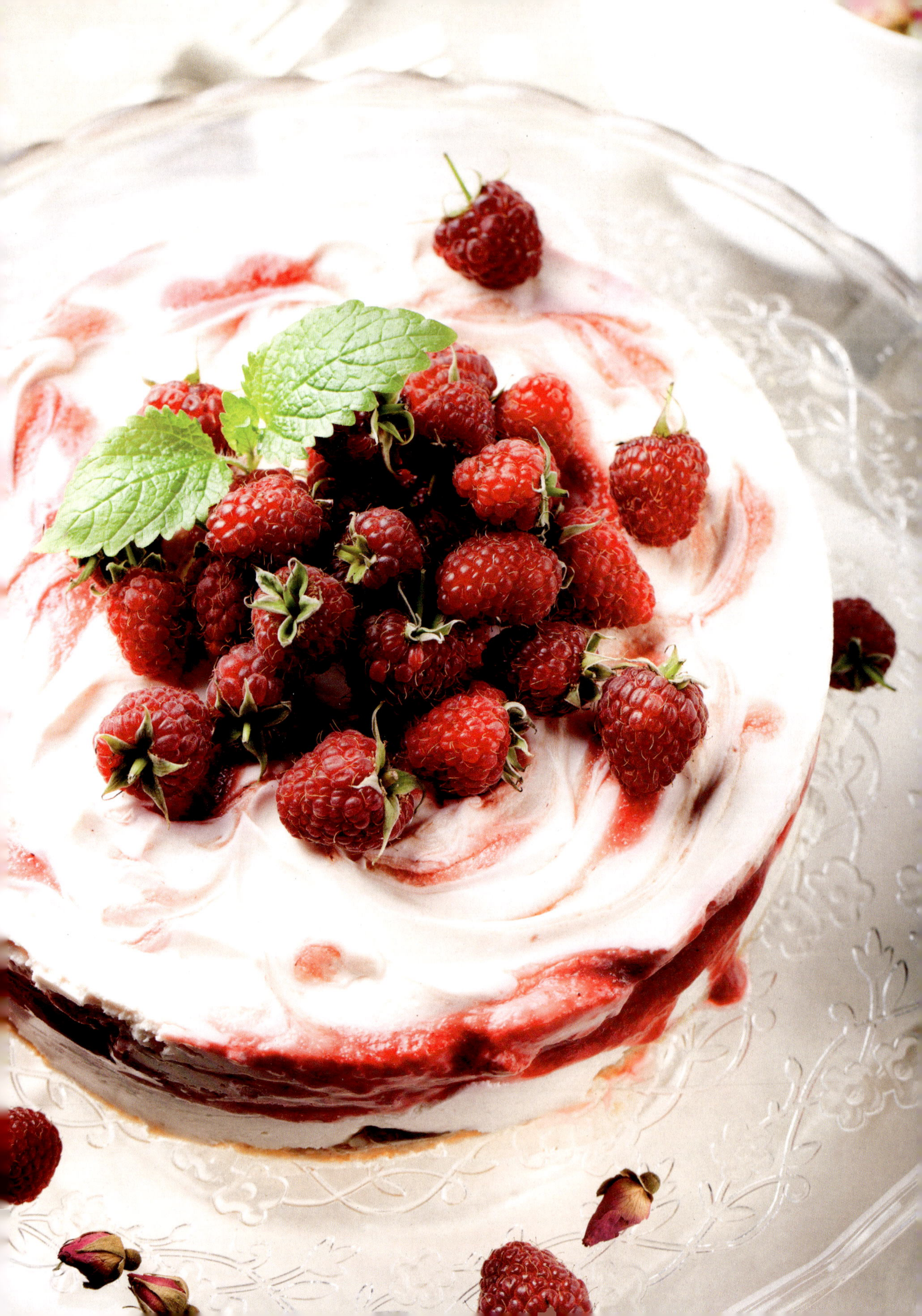

Raspberry & White Chocolate Cheesecake

SERVES 12
PREP + COOK TIME: 40 MINS + 8 HOURS CHILLING

CRUST

250g digestive or ginger biscuits

115g butter, melted

FILLING

1 cup (170g) white chocolate chips

½ cup (125ml) thickened cream

700g full-fat cream cheese, room temperature

1½ cups (235g) icing sugar

1 tsp vanilla extract

1½ cups (185g) fresh raspberries

Raspberry sauce and rosewater cream (see following recipes)

TO SERVE

1 cup (125g) fresh raspberries

Line a 22cm springform tin with greaseproof paper.

Blitz the biscuits in a food processor until they resemble fine breadcrumbs. Add the melted butter and pulse to combine. Press into the bottom of the prepared tin and set aside.

In a medium bowl, stir together white chocolate and ¼ cup cream. Microwave on high for 40 seconds, then stir until completely smooth. Place in the fridge to cool to room temperature.

In a large bowl, beat cream cheese with an electric mixer until smooth. Add sugar, vanilla and remaining ¼ cup cream and beat on high until light and fluffy. Add cooled white chocolate and beat to incorporate.

Place 1½ cups fresh raspberries into the bottom of the crust and pour the cheesecake filling over the top, smoothing with a spatula.

Top with raspberry sauce. Chill for least 8 hours or overnight. Dollop the rosewater cream over the raspberry sauce and gently swirl to combine. Top with fresh raspberries to serve.

Raspberry Sauce

SERVES 12
PREP + COOK TIME: 10 MINS + COOLING
GLUTEN FREE • DAIRY FREE

2½ cups (310g) frozen raspberries, thawed

½ cup (100g) sugar

2 tbsps water

1 tbsp cornflour

Add the raspberries and sugar to a small pan. Bring to a simmer over medium heat and cook for 2-3 minutes. Mash with a potato masher. Combine water and cornflour and stir into sauce to thicken. Set aside to cool completely then refrigerate until ready to use.

Rosewater Cream

SERVES 12
PREP + COOK TIME: 10 MINS
GLUTEN FREE

1¼ cups (310ml) thickened cream

1 tbsp icing sugar

1 tsp rosewater

Beat cream, icing sugar and rosewater in a small bowl with an electric mixer until soft peaks form. Refrigerate until ready to use.

White Chocolate & Apricot Squares

MAKES 20

PREP + COOK TIME: 20 MINS + CHILLING

1 cup (190g) dried apricots, soaked in water for 2-3 hours + ¾ cup (140g) dried apricots, chopped

¼ cup (60ml) coconut oil

2 tbsps lemon juice

2 tbsps maple syrup

⅔ cup (80g) roasted cashews, chopped

1¼ cups (110g) rolled oats

¾ cup (65g) shredded coconut

4 tbsps coconut flour

1½ cups (235g) white chocolate chips

3 tsps olive oil

Line a 20 x 30cm rectangular cake tin with greaseproof paper.

Drain the soaked apricots and place in a food processor with coconut oil, lemon juice and maple syrup. Blend into a thick paste.

Combine the chopped cashews, rolled oats, shredded coconut, chopped dried apricots and coconut flour in a bowl. Add apricot paste and stir well to combine.

Press the mixture down firmly into prepared pan.

Melt white chocolate and olive oil in a heatproof bowl over a pan of simmering water.

Pour melted chocolate over apricot slice.

Chill for 1-2 hours until chocolate is set and slice is firm. Cut into squares to serve.

Apple Fritter Loaf

SERVES 12

PREP + COOK TIME: 1 HOUR 10 MINS

APPLE CINNAMON MIXTURE

1 large apple, cored and diced

1 tbsp white sugar

1 tsp cinnamon

CINNAMON SUGAR MIXTURE

¼ cup (50g) packed light brown sugar

1 tsp cinnamon

BREAD

1 large egg

⅓ cup (70g) white sugar

¼ cup (60ml) vegetable oil

¼ cup (60ml) sour cream

1 tsp vanilla extract

1 cup (125g) plain flour

1 tsp bicarbonate of soda

½ tsp salt, or to taste

GLAZE

1 cup (155g) icing sugar

2-3 tbsps milk

Preheat oven to 180°C. Grease and flour a 20 x 10cm loaf tin and set aside.

In a small bowl, add ingredients for the apple cinnamon mixture. In another small bowl combine brown sugar and cinnamon.

For the bread, whisk egg and sugar until smooth. Add oil, sour cream and vanilla and whisk. Add flour, bicarb and salt and stir until just combined. Sprinkle half the cinnamon mixture over half the apples and fold them through the batter. Pour batter into the prepared tin. Evenly sprinkle the remaining apples on top followed by the remaining cinnamon sugar.

Bake loaf for 40-45 minutes. Allow tin to cool before turning out onto a wire rack. In a small bowl, add icing sugar and slowly drizzle in milk, whisking until smooth. Evenly drizzle glaze over bread before slicing and serving.

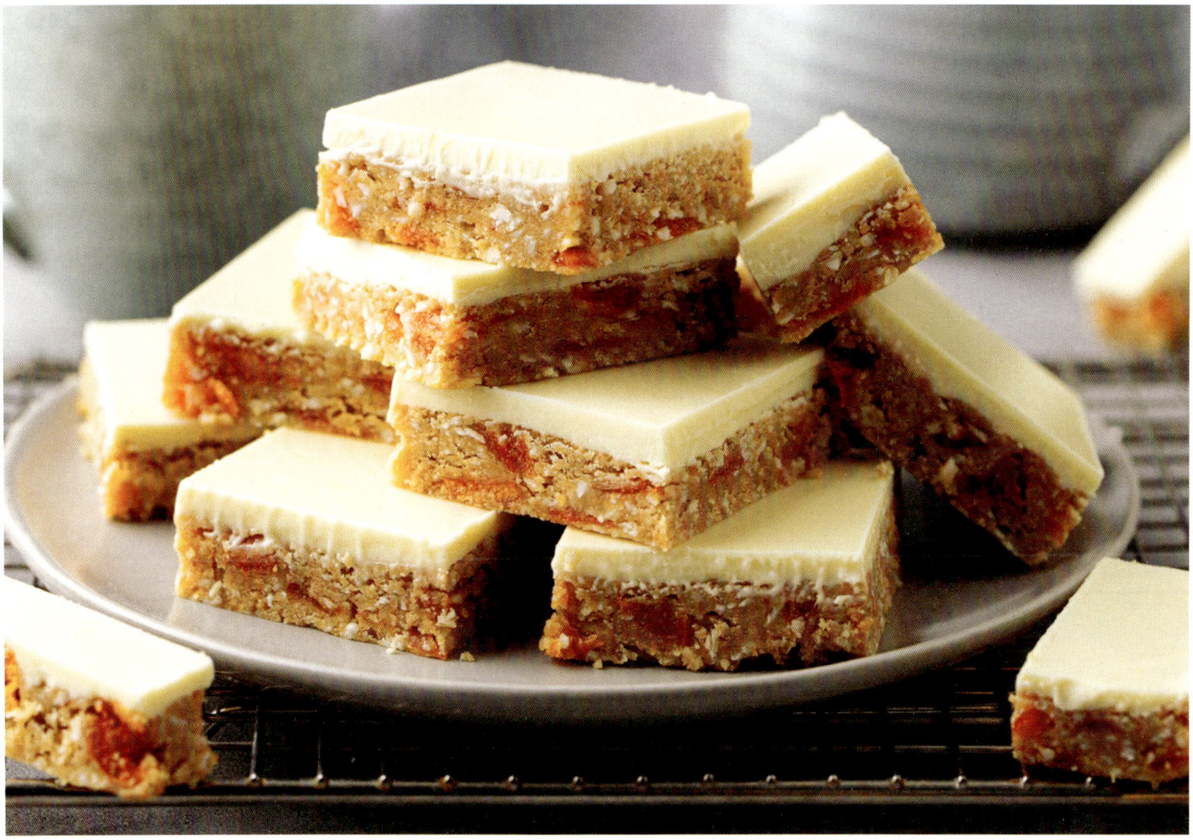

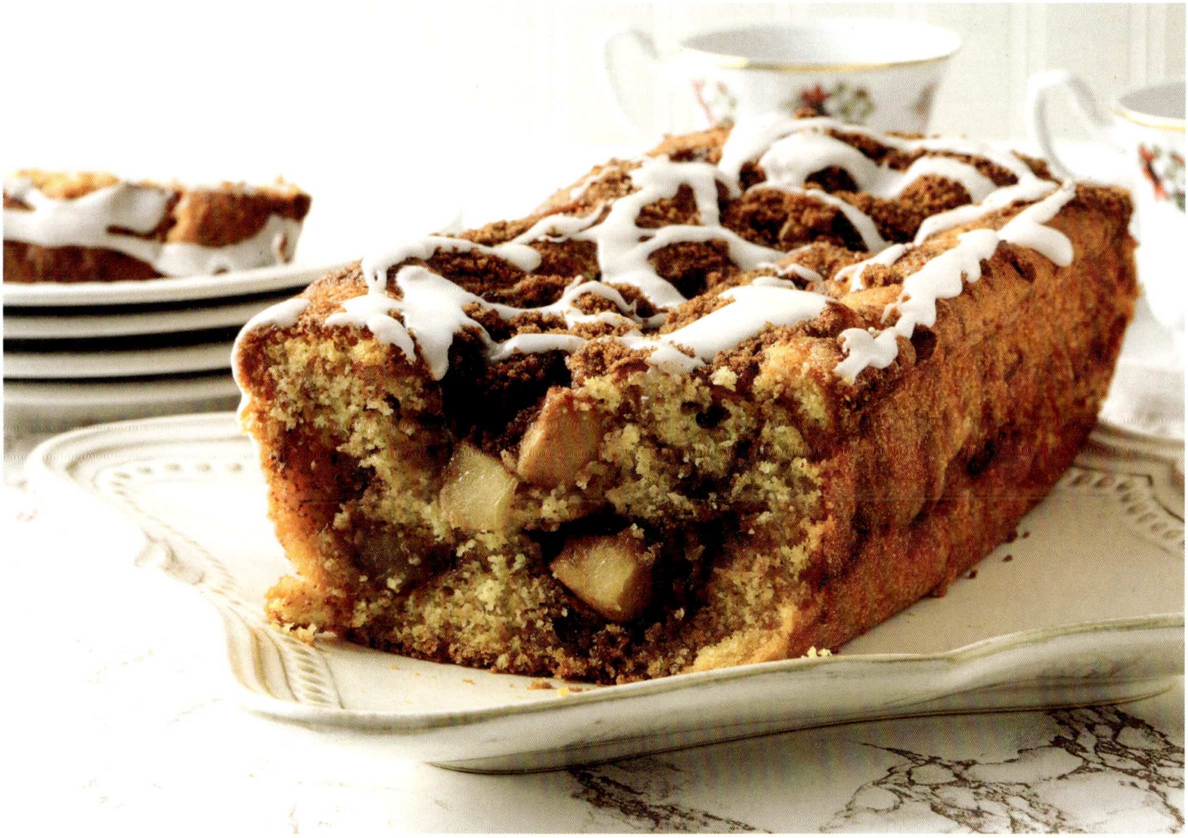

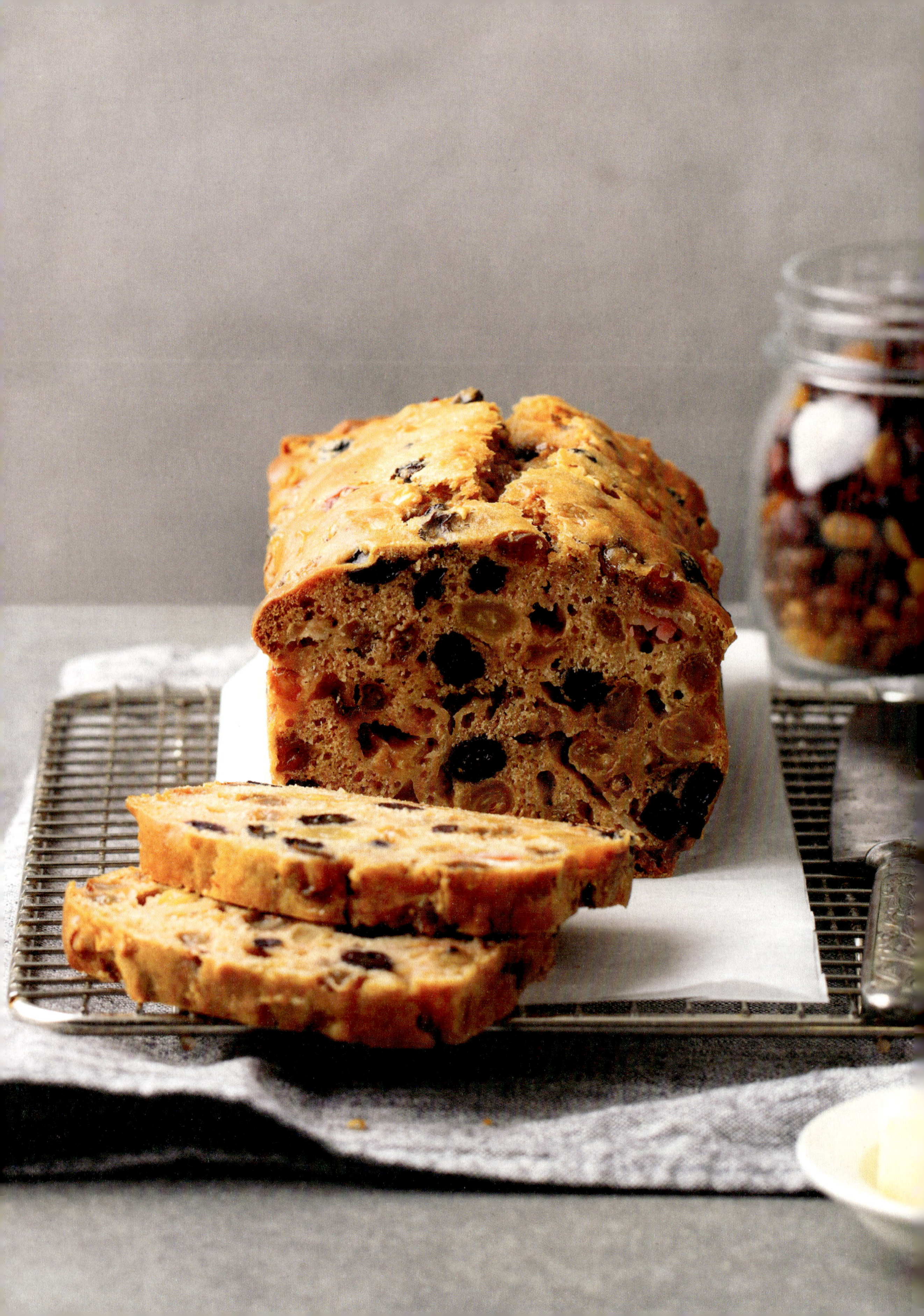

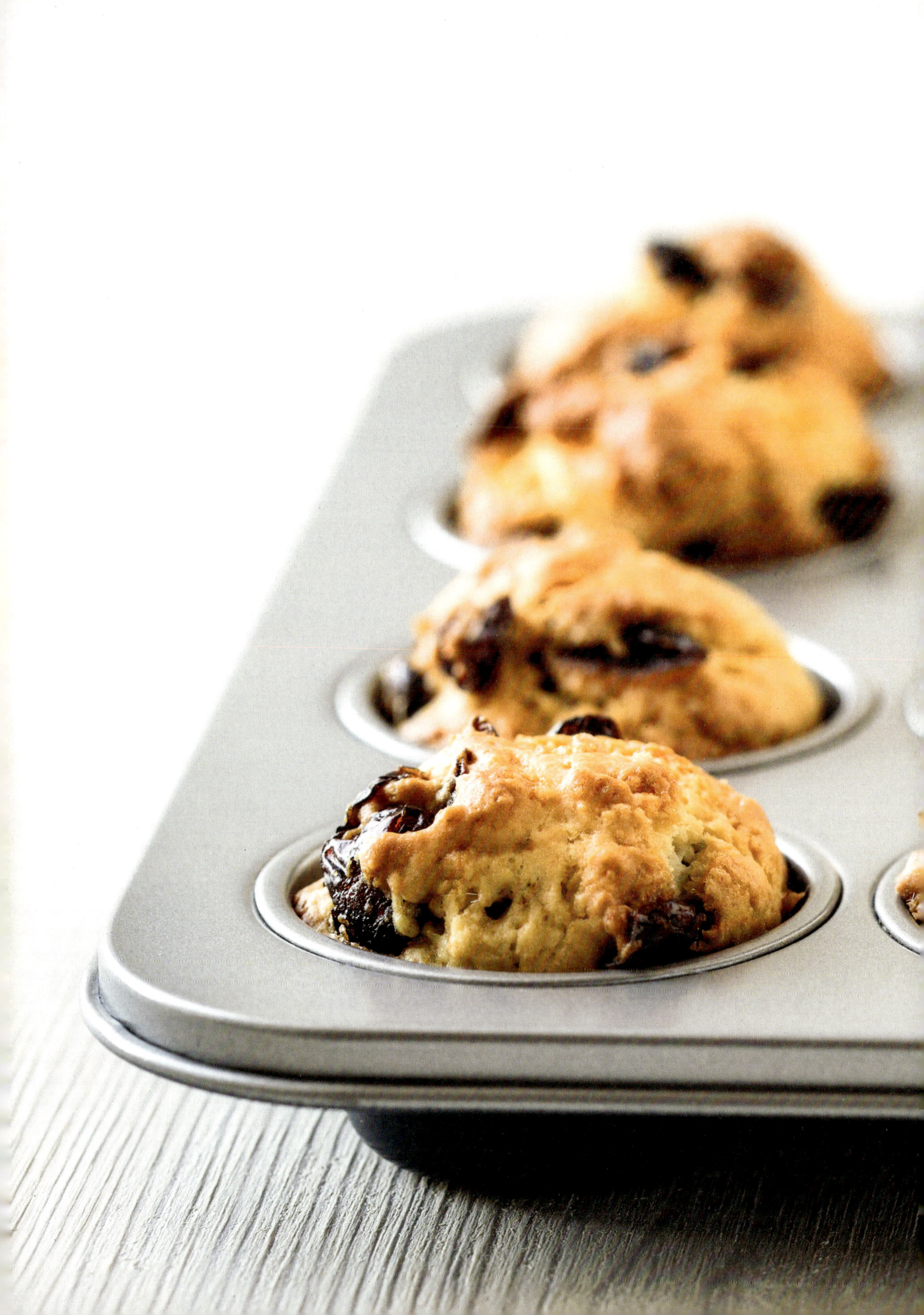

Bara Brith

SERVES 12
PREP + COOK TIME: 1 HOUR 40 MINS + OVERNIGHT SOAKING

- 1 cup (150g) raisins
- 1 cup (150g) sultanas
- ¾ cup (120g) currants
- ⅔ cup (50g) candied peel
- 1⅓ cups (330ml) very strong black tea, hot
- 4 tbsps unsalted butter, softened
- 1 cup (220g) packed dark brown sugar
- 1 large egg, lightly beaten
- 3 cups (375g) plain flour
- 3¾ tsps baking powder
- 1 tsp salt
- 2½ tsps mixed spice

Place raisins, sultanas, currants and candied peel in a bowl. Pour the hot tea over the fruit, stir, cover and let sit overnight.

Preheat the oven to 160°C. Grease a 1kg loaf tin.

Cream the butter and sugar with an electric mixer until light and fluffy. Add the egg and beat to combine. Add flour, baking powder, salt and mixed spice and mix to incorporate. Add the soaked fruits and their juices and stir to combine.

Scoop the batter into the greased loaf tin and smooth the top with a spatula.

Bake for 70-85 minutes or until a skewer inserted into the centre comes out clean.

Allow to cool in the tin for 10 minutes before transferring to a wire rack.

To serve, cut into slices and spread with butter.

Cranberry Muffins

MAKES 12
PREP + COOK TIME: 40 MINS

- 1¼ cups (275g) plain flour
- ⅔ cup (125g) brown sugar
- 2 tsps baking powder
- ⅔ cup (150ml) milk
- ⅔ cup (150ml) vegetable oil
- 1 egg
- 1 cup (170g) dried cranberries

Preheat oven to 200°C. Grease a 12-hole muffin tin.

Combine flour, sugar and baking powder in a large bowl. Add milk, oil and egg and stir well to combine. Fold in the cranberries. Spoon mixture into the muffin tin. Bake for 18-20 minutes or until golden brown.

Filo Fruit Cups

MAKES 12
PREP + COOK TIME: 30 MINS

- 1 cup (250g) mascarpone
- 1½ cups (375ml) vanilla yoghurt
- 1 tsp vanilla extract
- 6 sheets filo pastry
- 60g butter, melted
- 2 cups (250g) raspberries
- Icing sugar for dusting

Preheat oven to 175°C. Grease a 12-hole muffin tin.

Beat mascarpone, yoghurt and vanilla until smooth. Refrigerate until ready to use.

Layer three filo sheets, brushing each with melted butter. Cut six 12cm squares out of the pile of buttered filo. Press squares into six holes of the muffin tin. Repeat with the remaining pastry to fill all 12 muffin holes. Bake for 8-10 minutes or until golden brown. When cool, fill with mascarpone mixture and raspberries. Dust with icing sugar.

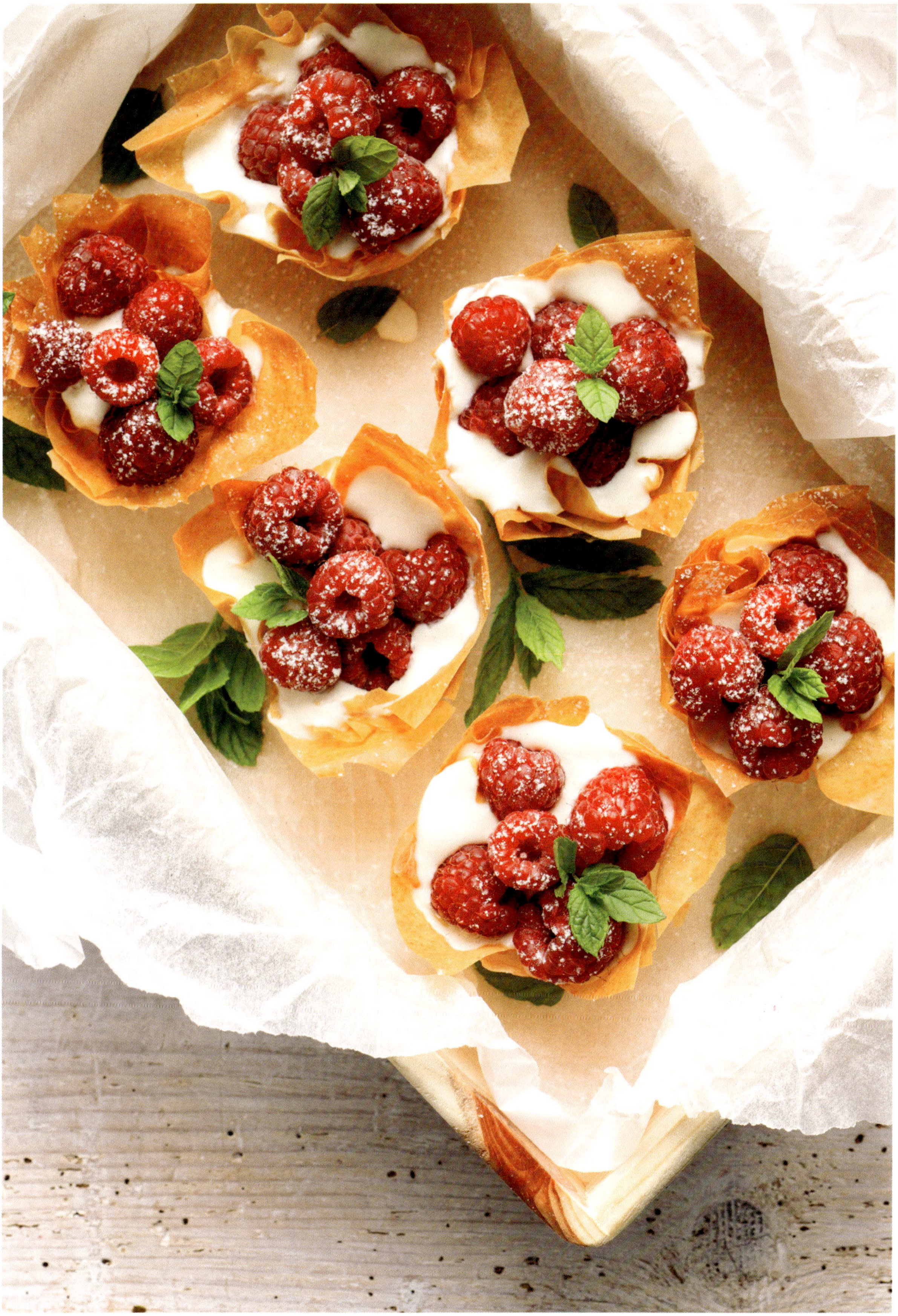

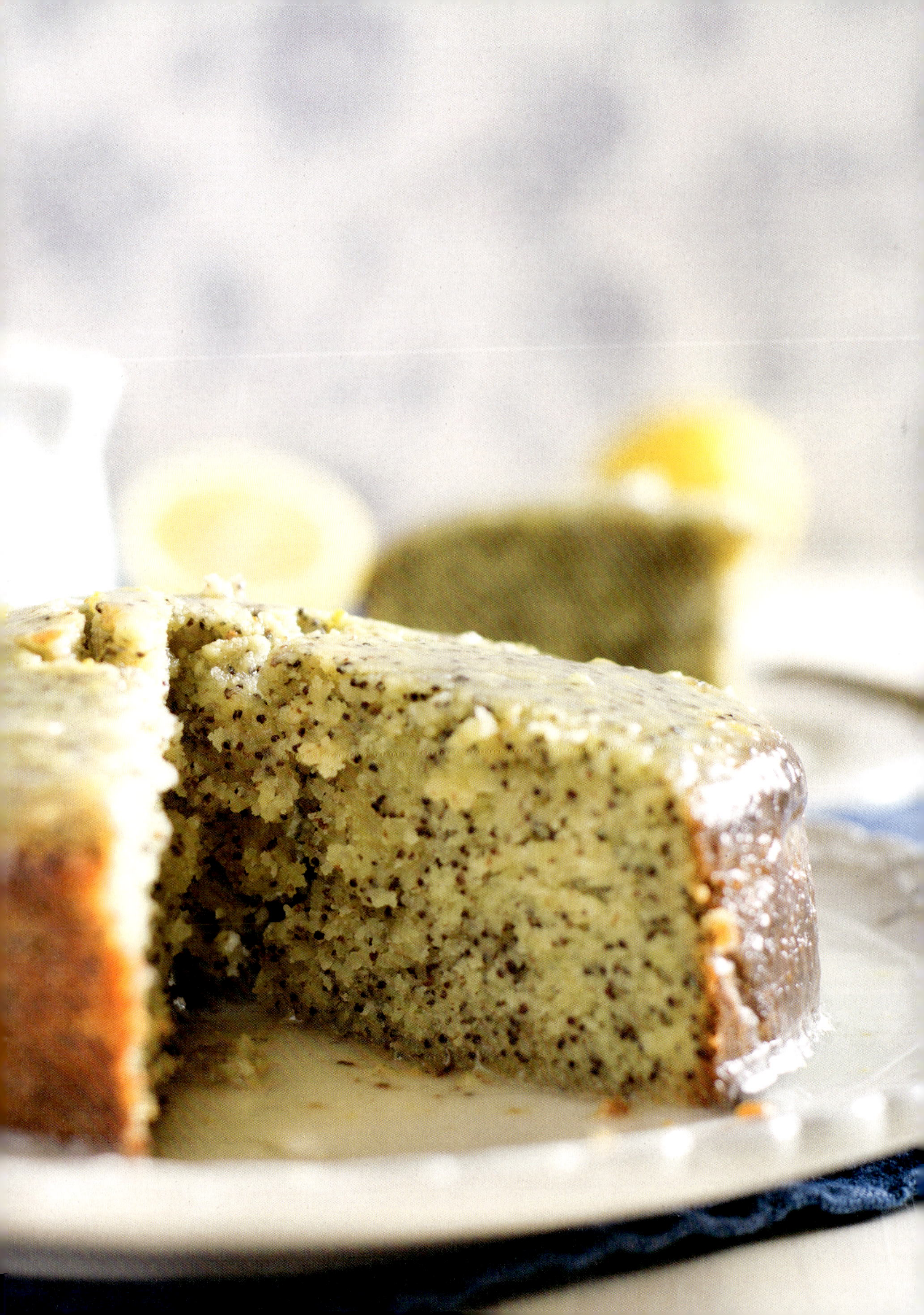

Lemon Poppyseed Cake

SERVES 12
PREP + COOK TIME: 1 HOUR

175g butter, softened
¾ cup (175g) golden caster sugar
1⅔ cups (200g) self-raising flour
4 lemons, zested
3 eggs
2 tbsps poppy seeds
½ cup (125ml) Greek yoghurt
Lemon glaze (see next recipe)

Preheat oven to 160°C. Grease and line a deep 23cm round cake tin with greaseproof paper.

In a large bowl, cream together the butter and sugar with an electric mixer until light and fluffy.

Add the flour, lemon zest, eggs, poppy seeds and yoghurt. Beat to incorporate.

Spoon mixture into the tin and smooth the top with a rubber spatula.

Bake for 40-45 minutes. Cool in the tin for 10 minutes, then turn out onto a wire rack to cool completely.

Pour over the lemon glaze. Leave to set before serving.

Lemon Glaze

MAKES ENOUGH FOR 1 CAKE
PREP + COOK TIME: 5 MINS

1¼ cups (200g) icing sugar
3-4 tbsps lemon juice

Sift the icing sugar into a large bowl. Beat in the lemon juice to make a thin, runny glaze. Add enough lemon juice to reach your desired consistency.

Berry Crumble

SERVES 8
PREP + COOK TIME: 1 HOUR

4 cups (500g) mixed berries
2 cups (400g) pitted cherries
¼ cup (55g) sugar
2 tbsps cornflour
Juice of 1 lemon
¾ cup (90g) plain flour
½ cup (110g) firmly packed light brown sugar
Pinch of salt
5 tbsps butter, diced
½ cup (60g) chopped almonds
¼ cup (20g) shredded coconut
Vanilla ice cream to serve

Preheat oven to 190°C.

Combine the berries, cherries, sugar, cornflour and lemon juice in a large bowl. Stir to coat. Set aside.

In another bowl combine the flour, brown sugar and salt. Add the butter and rub in with your fingertips until the mixture resembles breadcrumbs. Mix in the almonds and coconut.

Transfer the fruit mixture to a 2-litre baking dish. Sprinkle the topping evenly over the fruit. Transfer to the oven and bake for 40-45 minutes, or until the topping is golden brown and the filling is bubbly.

Serve warm or cold with ice cream.

Vanilla Raspberry Cake

SERVES 6
PREP + COOK TIME: 50 MINS

200g unsalted butter
1 cup (200g) caster sugar
4 eggs
1 tbsp vanilla extract
1 lemon, zested and juiced
1⅔ cups (200g) plain flour + 2 tbsps to coat raspberries
2 tsps baking powder
1 tsp salt
1¼ cups (150g) raspberries + extra to decorate
½ cup (70g) icing sugar

ICING
125g butter, softened
1½ cups (235g) icing sugar
1 tbsp milk

Preheat oven to 180°C and grease and line a 500g loaf tin with greaseproof paper.

In a mixing bowl, cream butter and sugar together with an electric whisk. Add eggs one at a time then stir in vanilla extract and lemon zest.

Sift together flour, baking powder and salt. Place raspberries and 2 tablespoons of flour in a bowl and stir with a spoon to combine until raspberries are fully covered with flour. Fold the dry ingredients through the wet ingredients followed by the raspberries. Pour the batter into the lined tin and bake for 35-40 minutes until a skewer inserted in the centre comes out clean.

To make the icing, beat the butter with an electric mixer until pale. Gradually add the icing sugar and milk, beating constantly until combined.

Allow the cake to cool then turn it out of the tin and set aside on a wire rack. Decorate with icing and fresh raspberries.

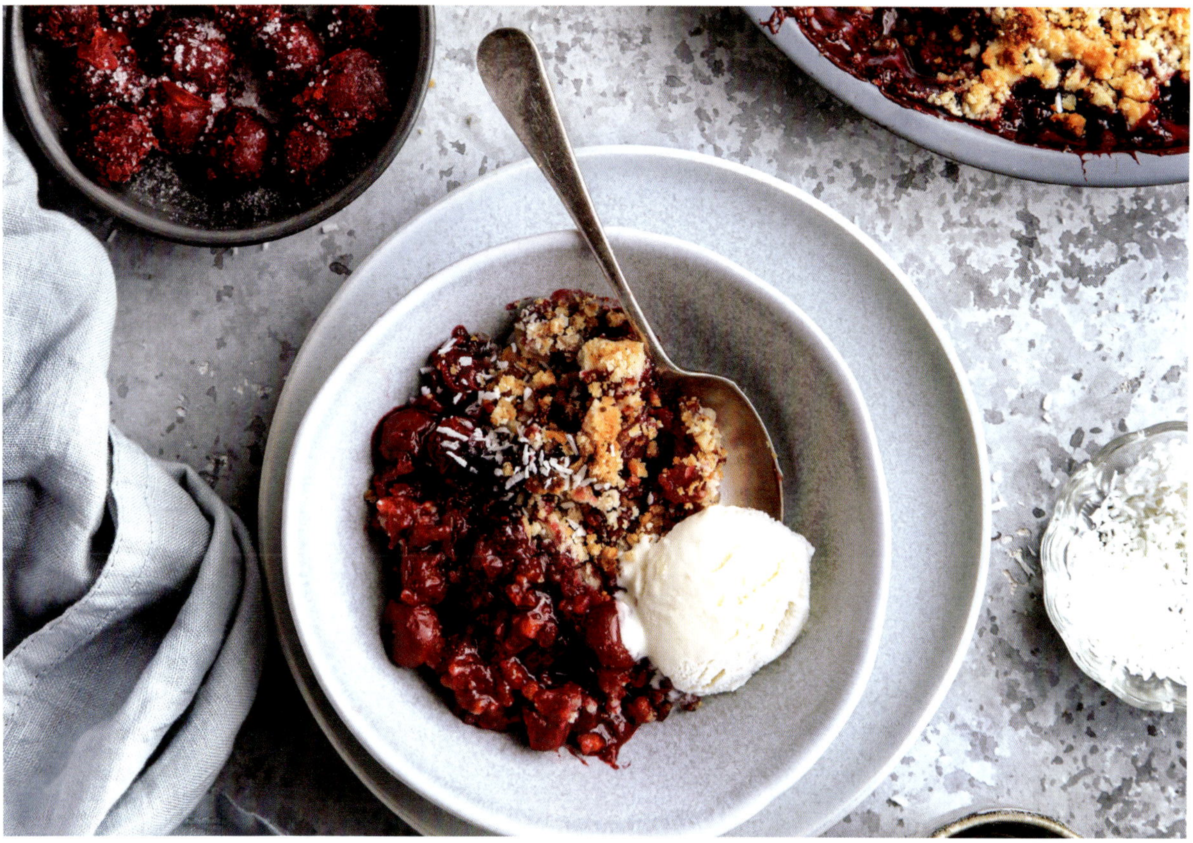

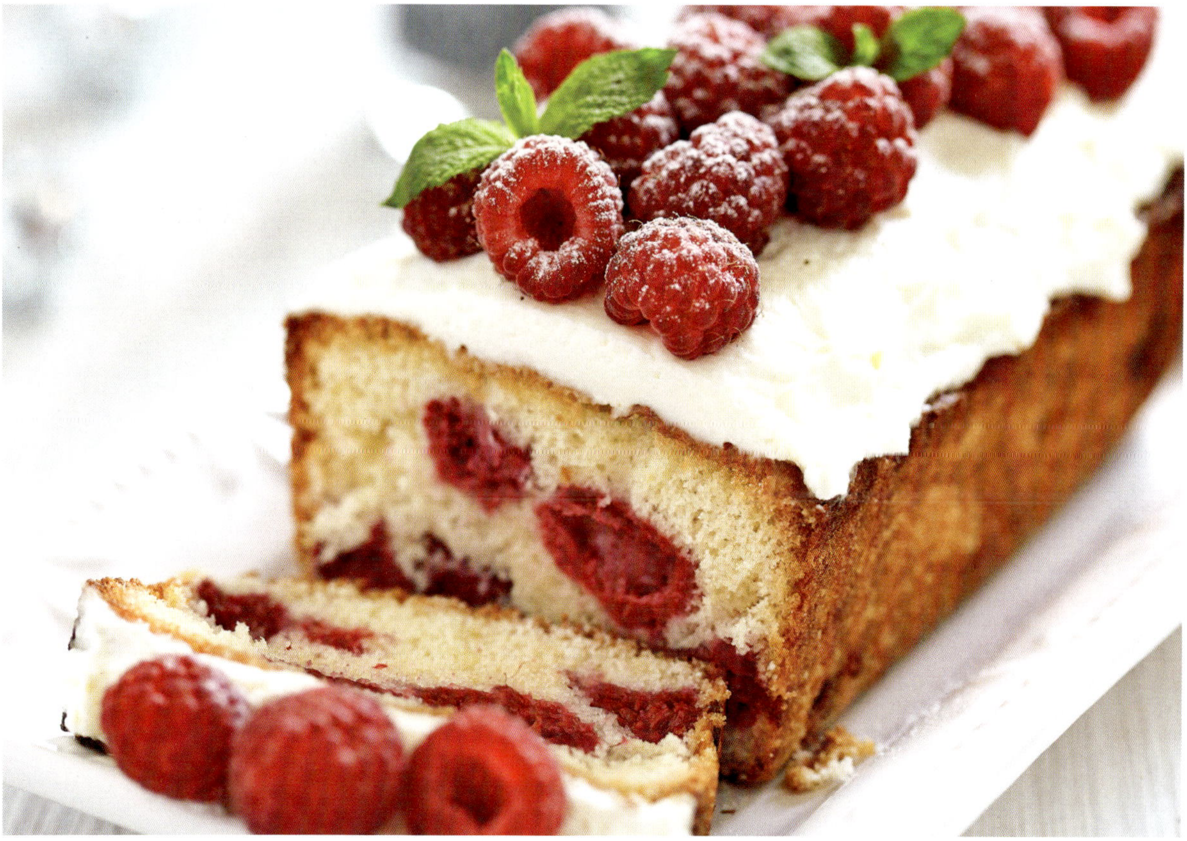

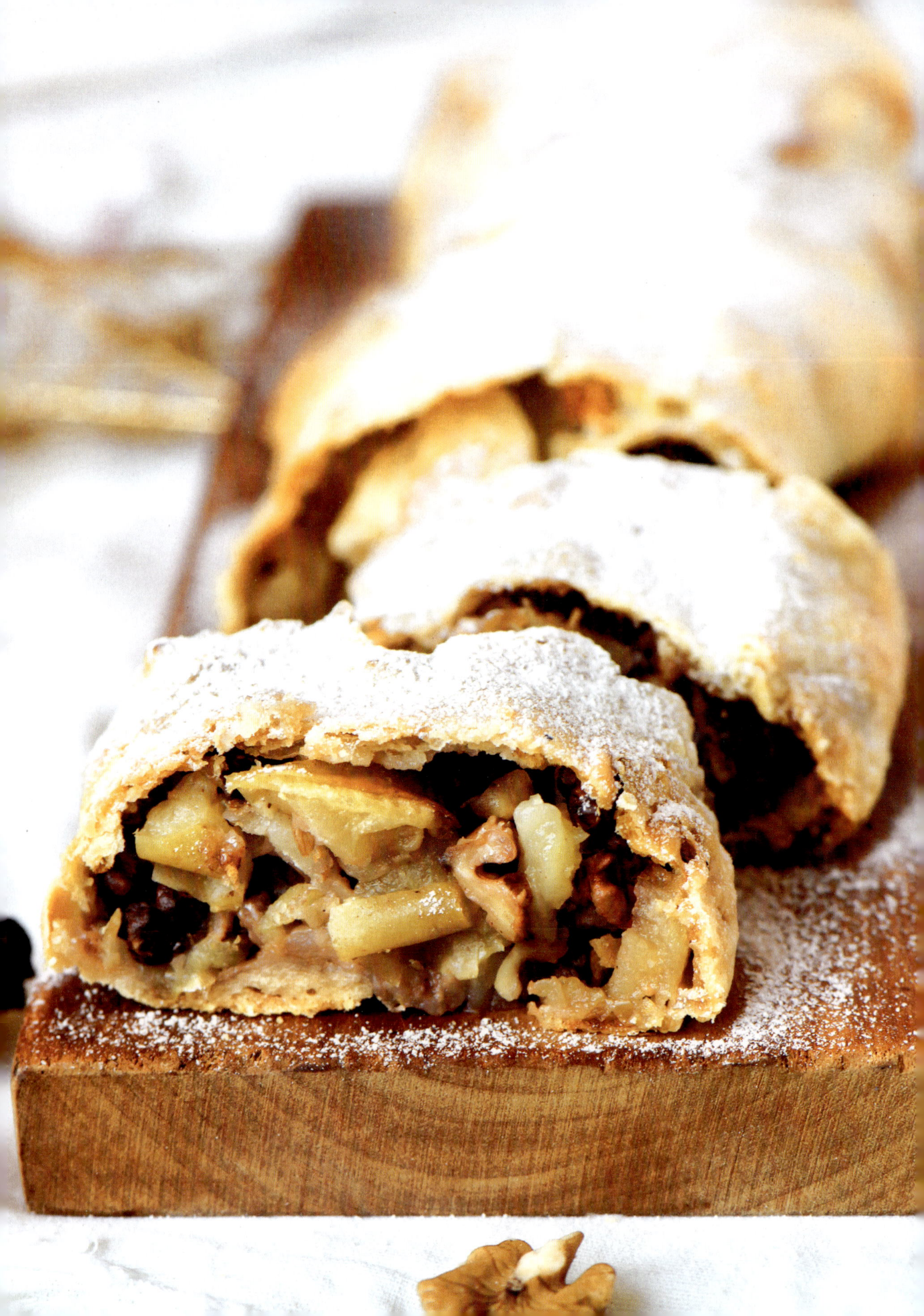

Apple Strudel

SERVES 8
PREP + COOK TIME: 2 HOURS 5 MINS

DOUGH

55g unsalted butter, melted
$1^2/_3$ cups (200g) plain flour
Pinch of salt
$^1/_3$ cup (80ml) lukewarm water

FILLING

4 medium apples, peeled and diced
1 tbsp lemon juice
1 tsp cinnamon
½ cup (110g) sugar
½ cup (80g) golden raisins, plumped in hot water for 10 minutes then drained
$^1/_3$ cup (40g) walnuts, roughly chopped
1 tsp vanilla extract

TO ASSEMBLE

90g unsalted butter, melted
¼ cup (30g) breadcrumbs
Icing sugar for dusting

Combine melted butter, flour salt, and lukewarm water in a bowl and mix until a smooth and elastic dough forms. Transfer to a greased bowl and set aside in a warm place for 60 minutes.

Combine apples with lemon juice, cinnamon, sugar, raisins, walnuts and vanilla. Set aside.

Preheat oven to 180°C. Line a baking tray with greaseproof paper.

Lay a tea towel flat and sprinkle with flour. Roll the dough out as thin as you can, then carefully stretch it to about 45 x 30cm. You should be able to see through the dough to the towel below. Brush with half the melted butter.

Scatter breadcrumbs over the pastry leaving a 5cm border along the long edges of the dough. Cover the breadcrumbs with apple filling.

Fold the crumb free borders over the filling then roll up the strudel from a short side with the help of the towel. Place seam-side down.

Transfer to the baking tray, brush with melted butter and cook for 50 minutes, brushing with butter every 10 minutes.

Dust with icing sugar to serve.

Lemon Loaf

SERVES 8
PREP + COOK TIME: 1 HOUR 15 MINS + COOLING

125g butter
1 cup (220g) sugar
2 eggs
½ cup (125ml) milk
1½ cups (185g) plain flour
1 tsp baking powder
½ tsp salt
Zest of 1 lemon

LEMON GLAZE
½ cup (80g) icing sugar
1-2 tbsps lemon juice
Zest of 1 lemon

Preheat oven to 180°C. Grease and lightly flour a 20 x 10 x 7cm loaf tin and set aside.

In a large bowl, cream butter and sugar with an electric hand mixer until light and fluffy. Add eggs, one at a time, beating after each addition. Add milk and beat to combine.

In a large mixing bowl combine flour, baking powder, salt and lemon zest.

Add wet mixture to dry mixture and stir well to combine.

Pour batter into prepared loaf tin. Bake for 55 minutes or until a skewer inserted in the centre comes out clean.

Remove from oven and cool in pan for 5 minutes. Transfer to a wire rack and allow to cool slightly.

Stir together all the glaze ingredients in a small bowl, adding enough lemon juice to make a pourable glaze. Place a baking tray under the cooling rack to catch any drips and spoon glaze slowly over top of loaf, allowing it to drip down the sides a little. Scatter with lemon zest and allow to cool completely. Decorate as desired, then slice and serve.

Apricot & Almond Galette

SERVES 6
PREP + COOK TIME: 1 HOUR + 1 HOUR CHILLING

DOUGH
½ cup (60g) almond meal
2 cups (250g) plain flour + more as needed
3 tbsps sugar
170g unsalted butter, chilled, cut into cubes
2 tbsps cream cheese
1 egg yolk, beaten
4 tbsps ice water + more as needed

FILLING
680g apricots, halved and pitted
1 tbsp fresh lemon juice
½ cup (110g) sugar
⅓ cup (110g) apricot jam
1 egg beaten with 1 tbsp water
3 tbsps flaked almonds

In a food processor add almond meal, flour and sugar and pulse briefly. Add the butter, cream cheese and egg yolk and pulse to combine.

Stir in the ice water to bring the dough together. Gather the dough into a ball (add a bit more water if needed) and press into a disk. Wrap tightly and refrigerate for at least 1 hour.

Preheat oven to 190°C. Line a baking tray with greaseproof paper. Place the apricots in a bowl and add the lemon juice and sugar. Toss to coat the apricots.

Roll out the dough into a 40cm round. Fold the dough into quarters and unfold it onto the prepared baking tray. Spread the apricot jam over the dough, leaving a border uncovered, then arrange the apricots evenly on top of the jam. Fold the dough edges over the apricots, leaving the galette open in the centre. Brush the dough with the egg wash and sprinkle with the almonds.

Bake the galette for 35-45 minutes. Cool on a wire rack and serve.

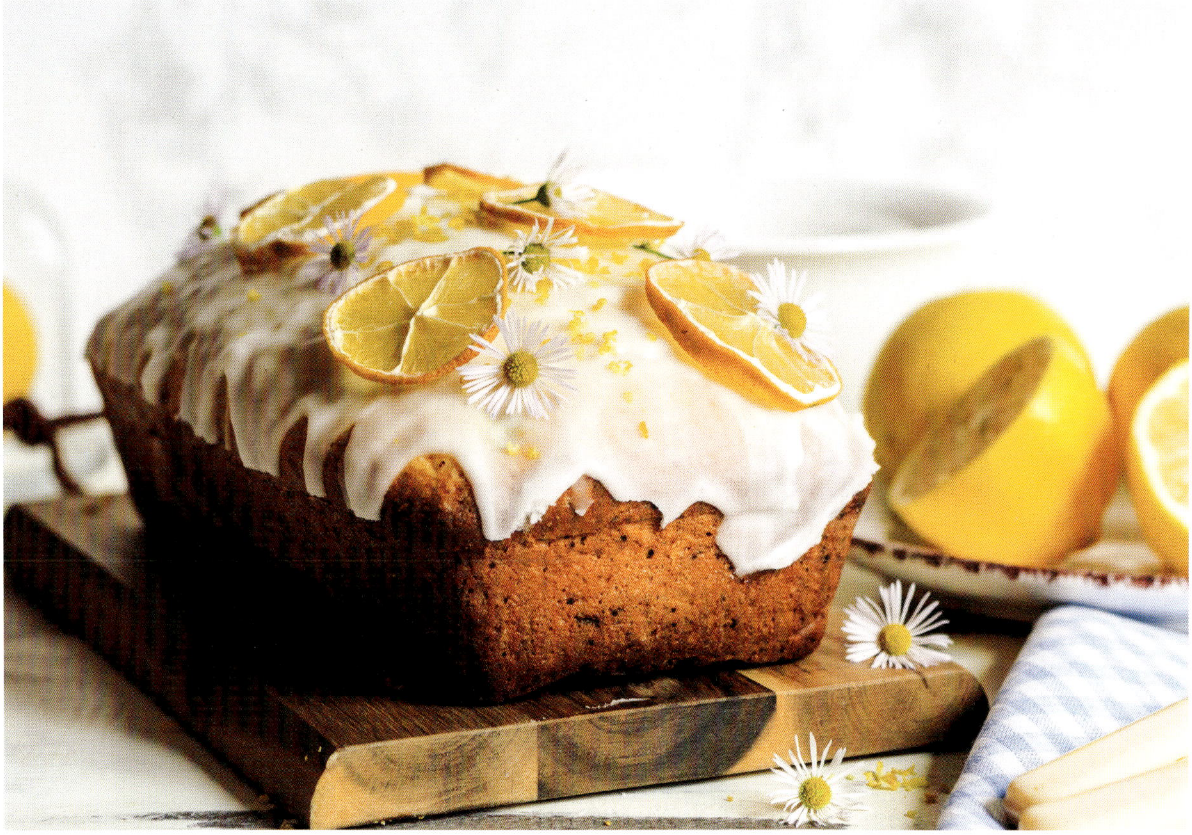

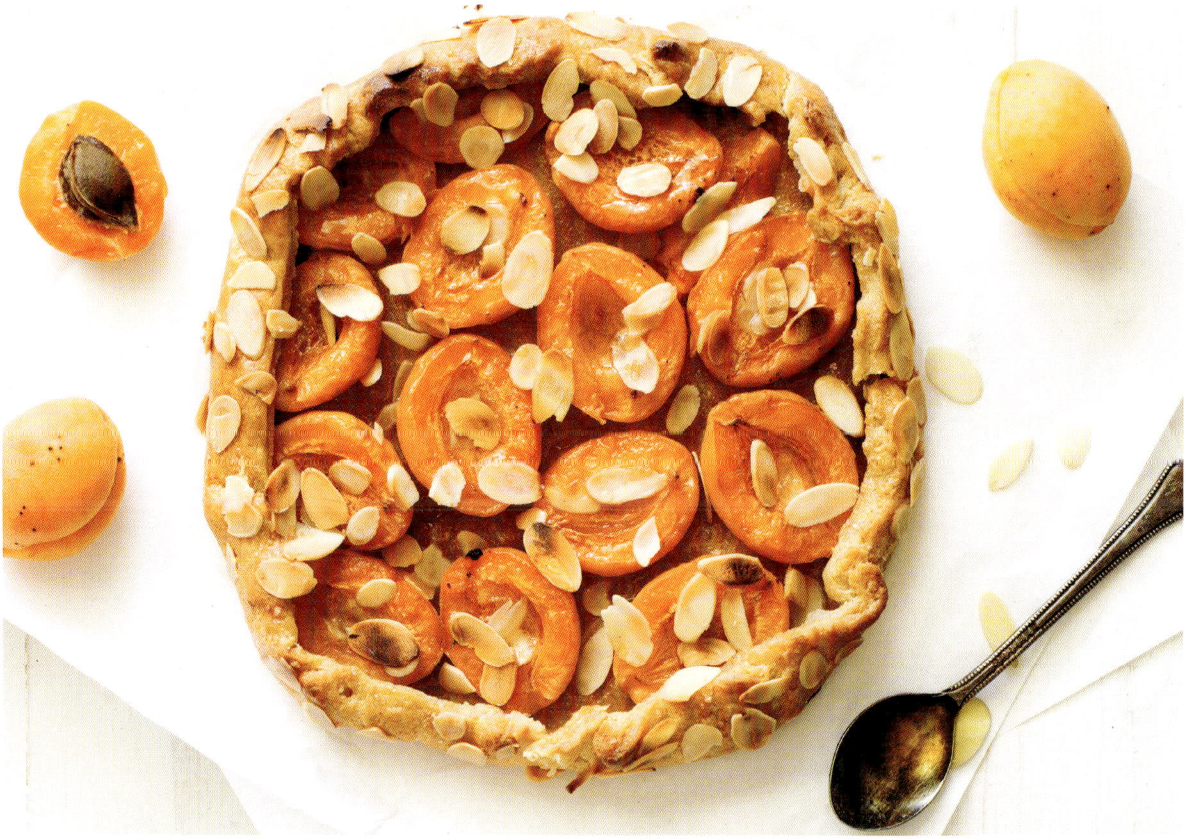

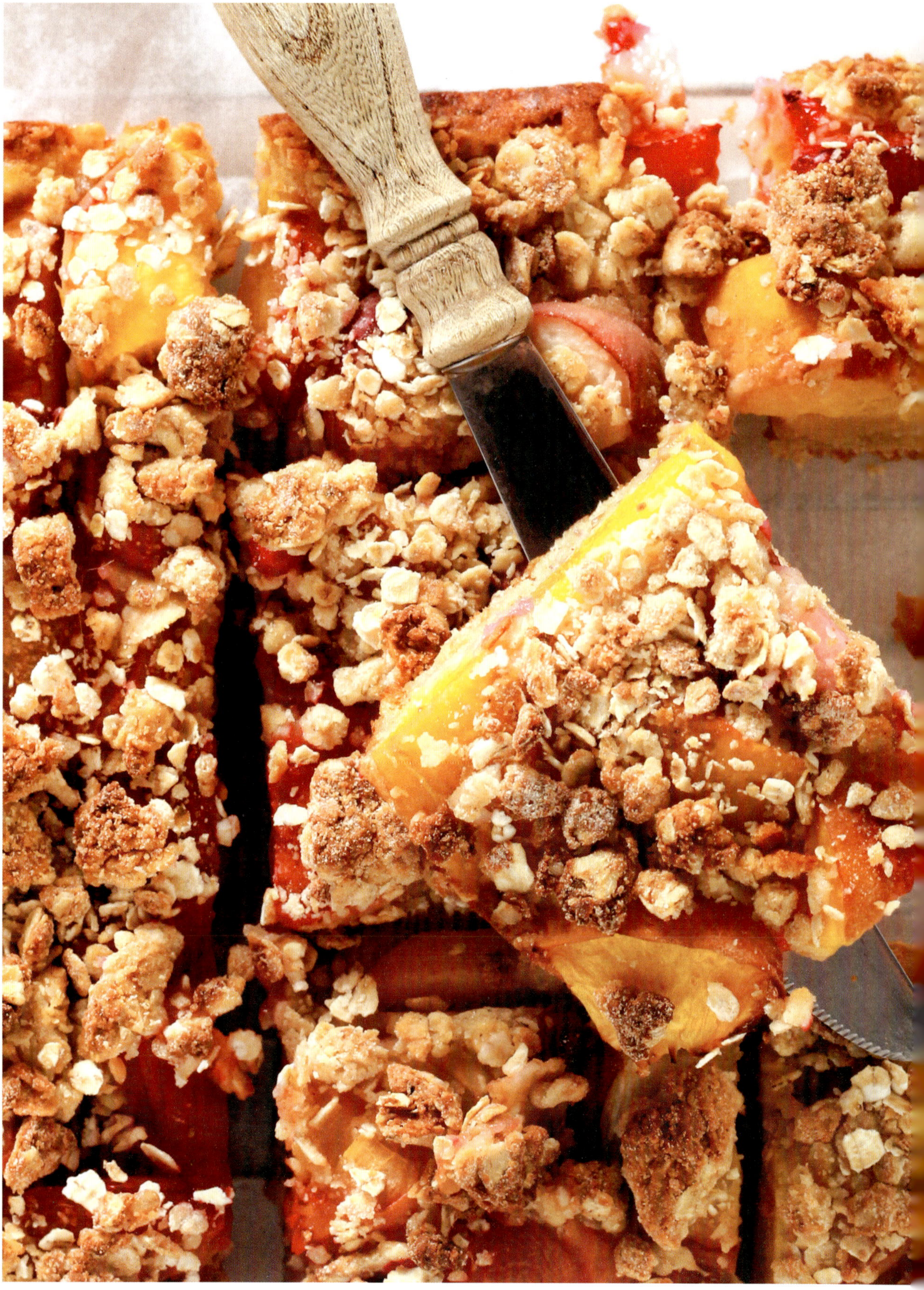

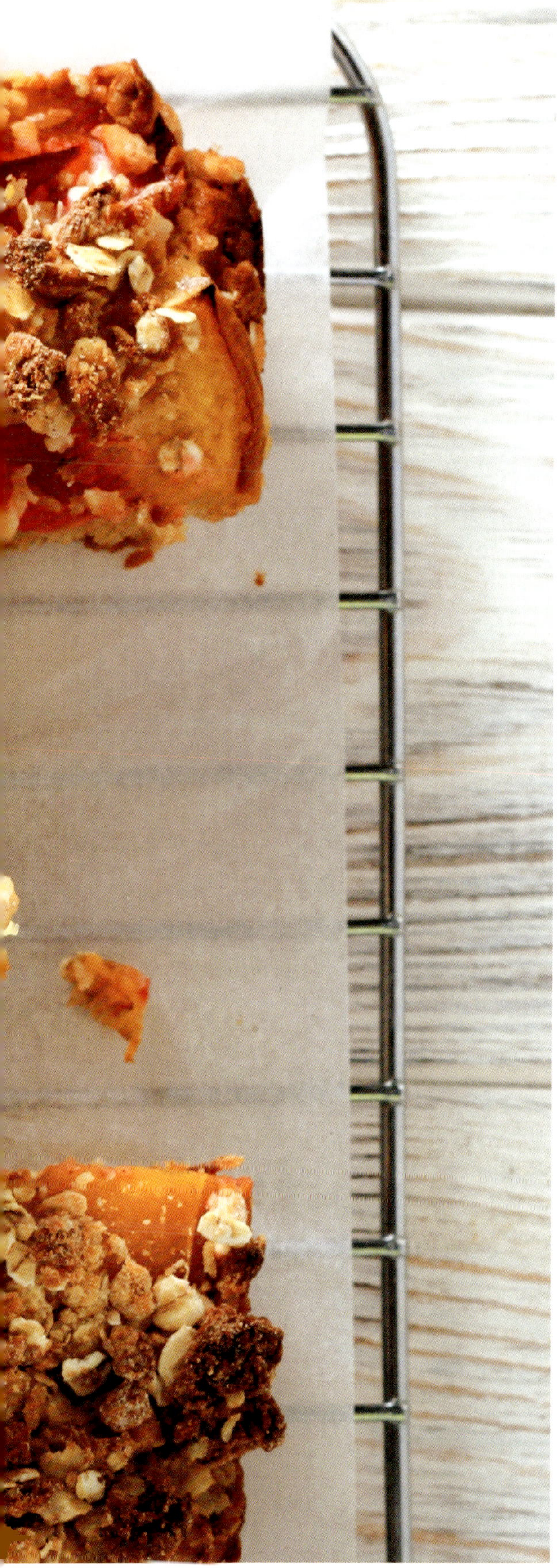

Peach Crumble Slice

SERVES 16-20
PREP + COOK TIME: 1 HOUR

BASE

1 cup (125g) plain flour
90g unsalted butter, melted
1/3 cup (70g) caster sugar

FILLING

1 2/3 cups (250g) peaches, sliced
1 cup (250ml) water
1/4 cup (55g) caster sugar

CRUMBLE

90g unsalted butter, melted
2/3 cup (60g) rolled oats
1/2 cup (60g) plain flour
1/2 cup (100g) brown sugar

Preheat oven to 180°C. Grease and line an 18 x 30cm rectangular slice tin with greaseproof paper.

In a small bowl, combine the plain flour, melted butter and sugar. Stir well to combine, then press the mixture evenly across the base of the prepared pan. Bake for 20 minutes until light golden brown.

Meanwhile combine the fruit, water and sugar in a small saucepan. Bring to the boil then reduce to a simmer. Simmer for 5 minutes, stirring occasionally, until the liquid thickens.

For the crumble, combine the melted butter, oats, flour and brown sugar in a small bowl.

Cover the hot base evenly with the fruit then sprinkle over the crumble mixture.

Return to the oven and bake for 20 minutes, or until the top is golden brown.

Allow to cool slightly before slicing and serving.

Peach Cupcakes

MAKES 12
PREP + COOK TIME: 45 MINS + COOLING

¾ cup (185ml) sour cream or yoghurt
2 large eggs, room temperature
½ cup (125ml) light olive oil, avocado oil or macadamia oil
2 tsps vanilla extract
½ cup (110g) packed brown sugar
½ cup (110g) white sugar
1¾ cups (215g) plain flour
¾ tsp bicarbonate of soda
1¼ tsps baking powder
½ tsp salt
¾ tsp cinnamon
2 peaches, peeled, pitted and finely chopped (about 1½ cups)

ICING
1½ cups (235g) icing sugar
4 tbsps thickened cream
½ tsp almond or vanilla extract

Preheat the oven to 175°C. Line a 12-hole cupcake tin with liners.

In a medium-sized bowl, stir together the sour cream or yoghurt, eggs, oil and vanilla. In a large bowl, whisk together the sugars, flour, bicarb, baking powder, salt and cinnamon. Pour the wet mixture into the dry ingredients and whisk until smooth. Stir in the chopped peaches.

Divide the mixture evenly between the cupcake liners, three-quarters filling each. Bake for 15-18 minutes or until a skewer inserted in the centre comes out clean. Allow cupcakes to cool completely before icing.

Place the icing sugar in a medium bowl. Add the cream a tablespoon at a time until you reach your desired consistency. Mix in almond or vanilla extract. Mix well, then use a teaspoon to drizzle over cupcakes.

Apricot & Raspberry Tart

SERVES 8
PREP + COOK TIME: 50 MINS

320g puff pastry
3 tbsps apricot jam
250g ripe apricots, halved and pitted
1 tbsp butter, melted
1 egg, beaten
¾ cup (85g) raspberries
2 tsps caster sugar
1 tbsp flaked almonds
Mint leaves to garnish (optional)

Preheat the oven to 200°C.

Roll out puff pastry on a baking tray lined with greaseproof paper, then score it lightly around the edges to create a 1.5cm border. Lightly score a diamond pattern over the middle to keep the pastry from rising in the centre during cooking.

Spread the apricot jam inside the border and top with apricots, cut-side down. Brush apricots with melted butter and brush the pastry border with beaten egg, then bake for 15 minutes.

Scatter over raspberries, sugar and flaked almonds. Bake for 5-10 minutes more until the almonds are golden and the pastry has cooked through.

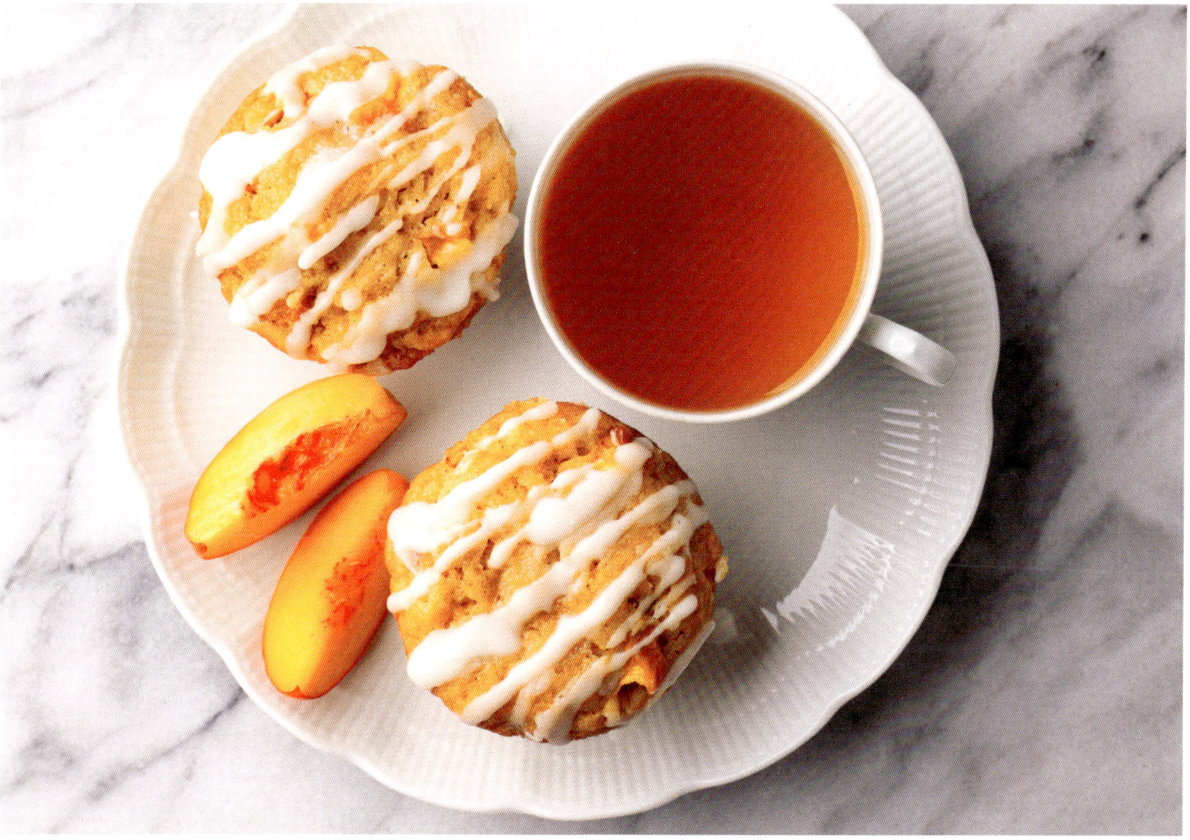

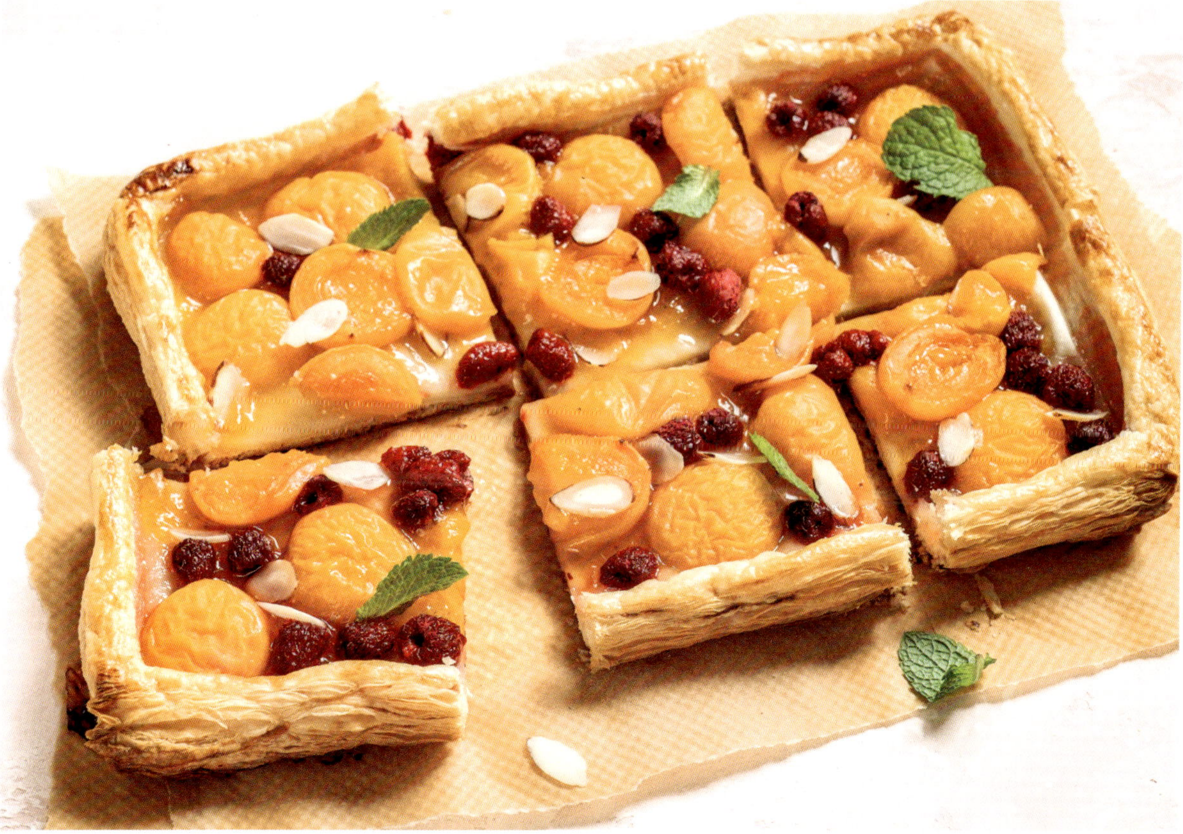

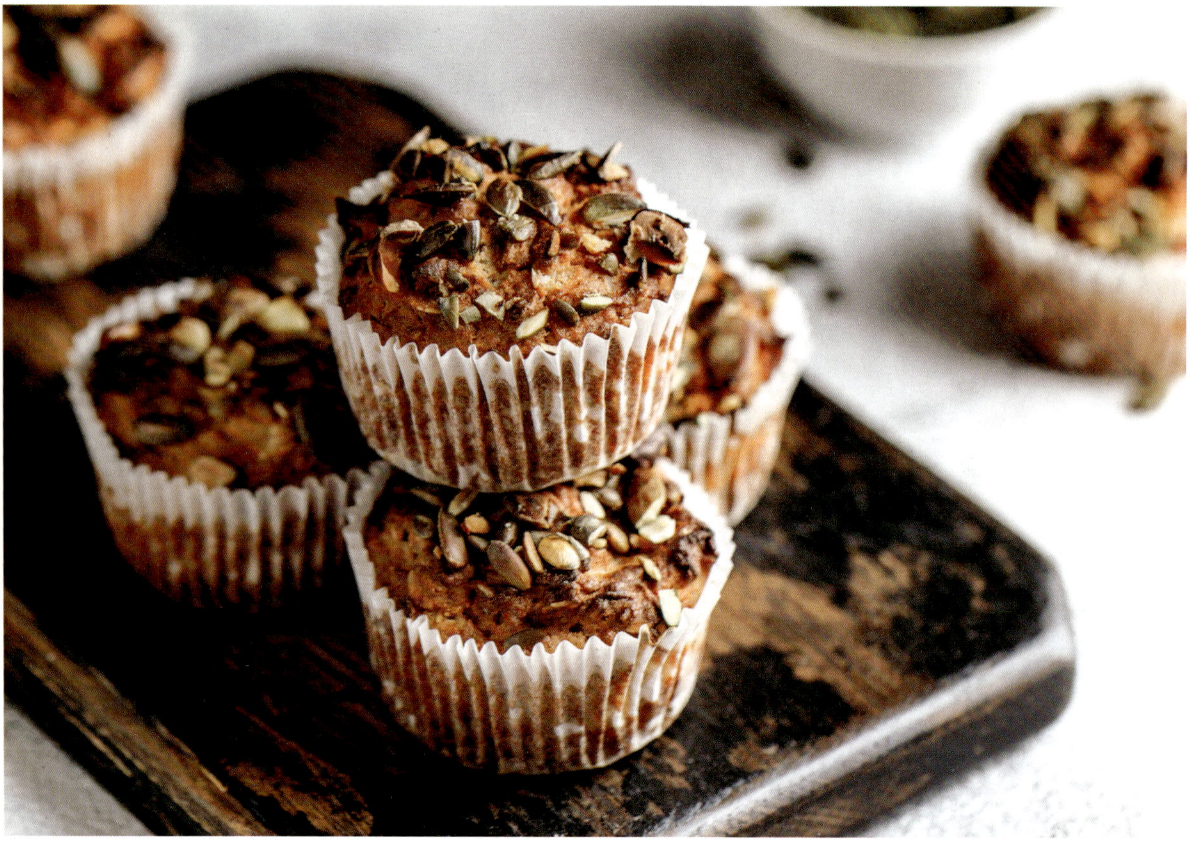

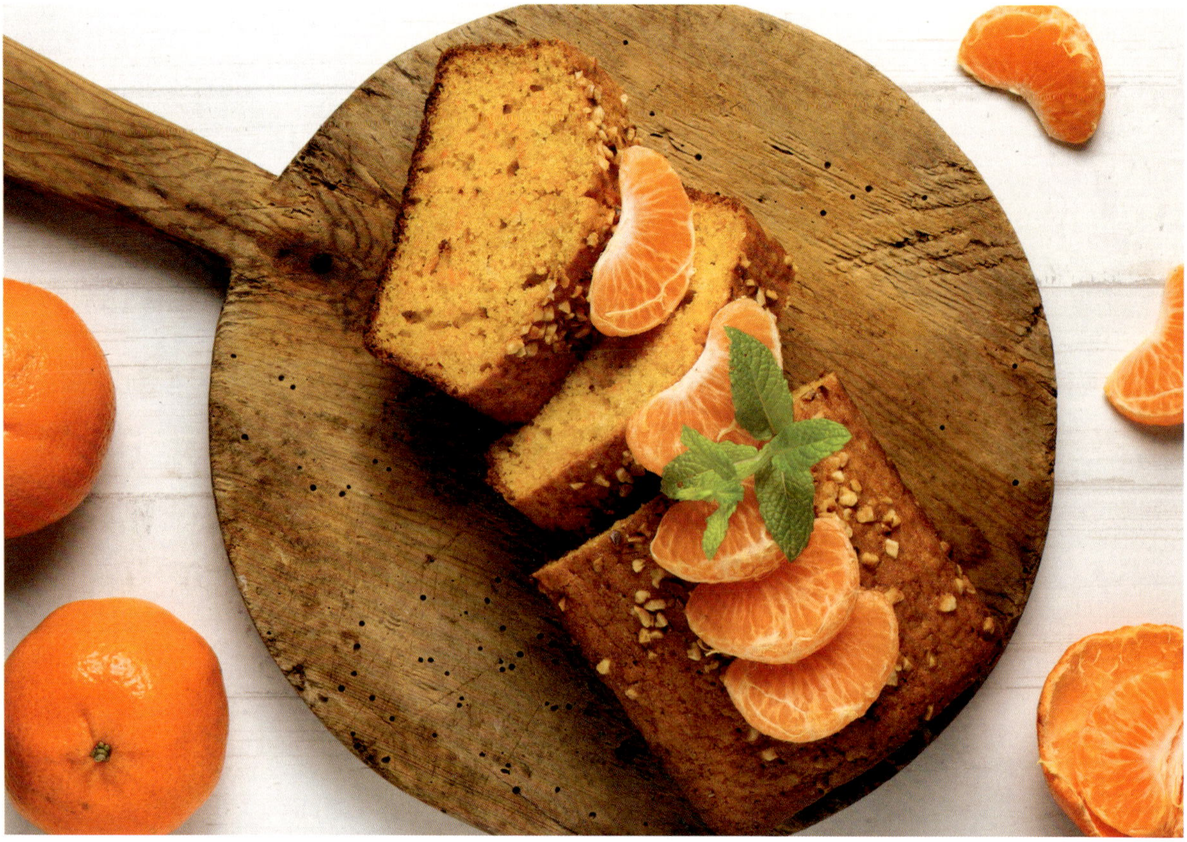

Apple Cinnamon Muffins

MAKES 12
PREP + COOK TIME: 30 MINS

1¾ cups (215g) wholemeal flour
1½ tsps baking powder
1 tsp cinnamon
½ tsp bicarbonate of soda
½ tsp salt
1½ cups (225g) grated apple + 1 cup (120g) diced apple
⅓ cup (80ml) melted coconut oil or olive oil
½ cup (155g) maple syrup
2 eggs
½ cup (125ml) plain yoghurt
1 tsp vanilla extract
1 tbsp raw sugar
¼ cup (30g) pepitas

Preheat the oven to 220°C. Line a 12-hole muffin tin with paper cases.

In a large mixing bowl, combine the flour, baking powder, cinnamon, bicarb and salt. Mix well with a whisk. Add the grated apple and chopped apple. Stir to combine.

In a medium mixing bowl, combine oil and maple syrup and beat together with a whisk. Add eggs and beat well, then add yoghurt and vanilla and mix well.

Pour the wet ingredients into the dry and mix until just combined. Divide the batter evenly between the 12 muffin cases.

Sprinkle the tops of the muffins with raw sugar and pumpkin seeds. Bake muffins for 13-16 minutes, or until the muffins are golden on top and a toothpick inserted into a muffin comes out clean.

Place the muffin tin on a rack to cool.

Carrot & Mandarin Loaf

SERVES 6
PREP + COOK TIME: 1 HOUR 10 MINS

⅓ cup (80ml) sunflower or vegetable oil
2 eggs
3 tbsps sugar
1⅓ cups (350ml) mandarin or orange juice
Zest of 1 mandarin
1⅓ cups (150g) grated carrot
¼ cup (50g) diced mandarin + extra segments to serve
2 cups (250g) wholemeal flour
1 tbsp baking powder
½ cup (60g) blanched almonds, chopped

Preheat oven to 160°C. Grease a 26 x 13cm loaf tin.

Add oil, eggs, sugar, juice and zest to a mixing bowl and whisk to combine.

Add grated carrot and diced mandarin and mix. Add flour and baking powder and mix to combine.

Pour mixture into loaf tin and sprinkle with chopped almonds. Bake for 50 minutes or until a skewer inserted in the centre comes out clean.

Cool completely on a wire rack before serving, topped with extra mandarin segments.

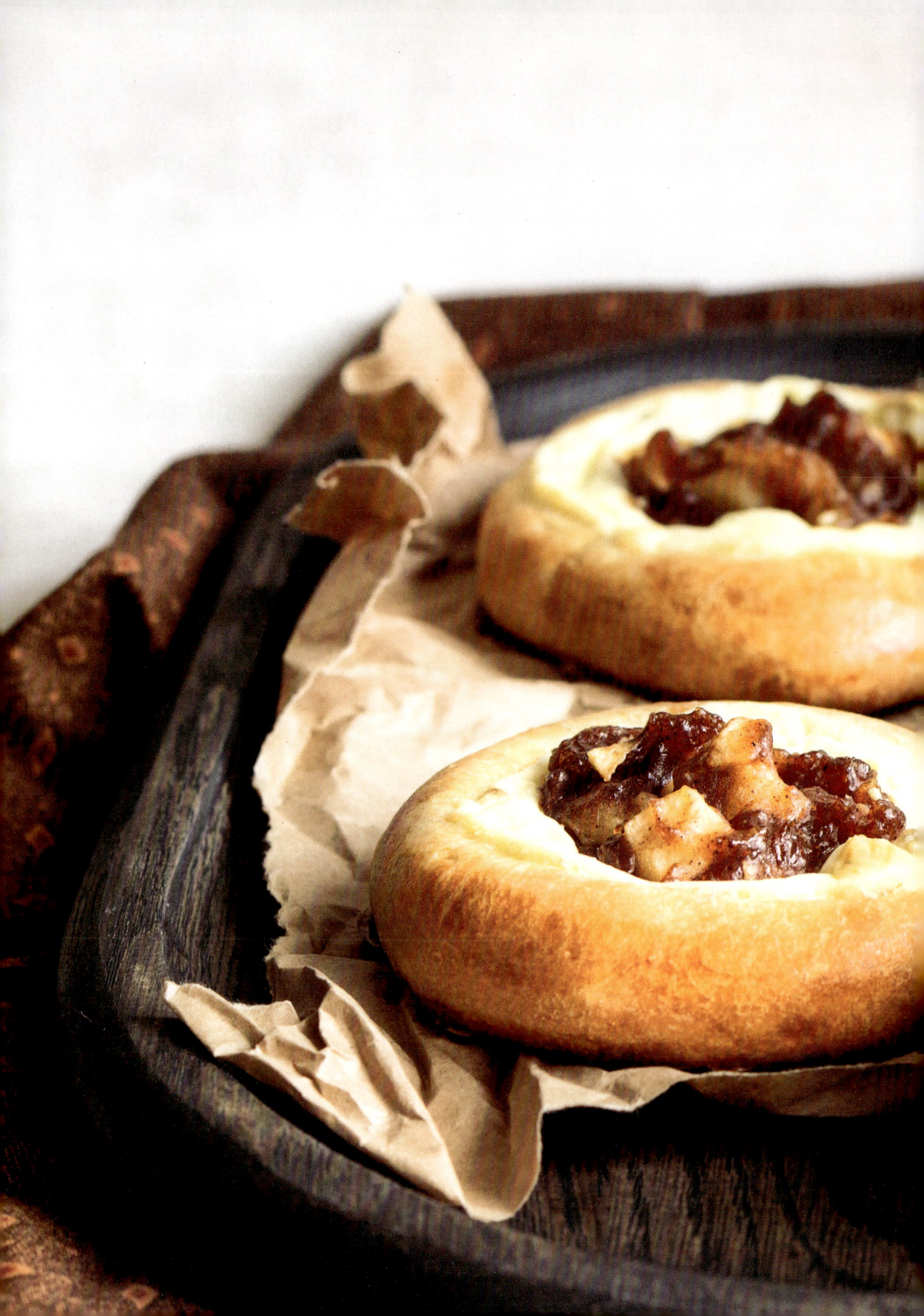

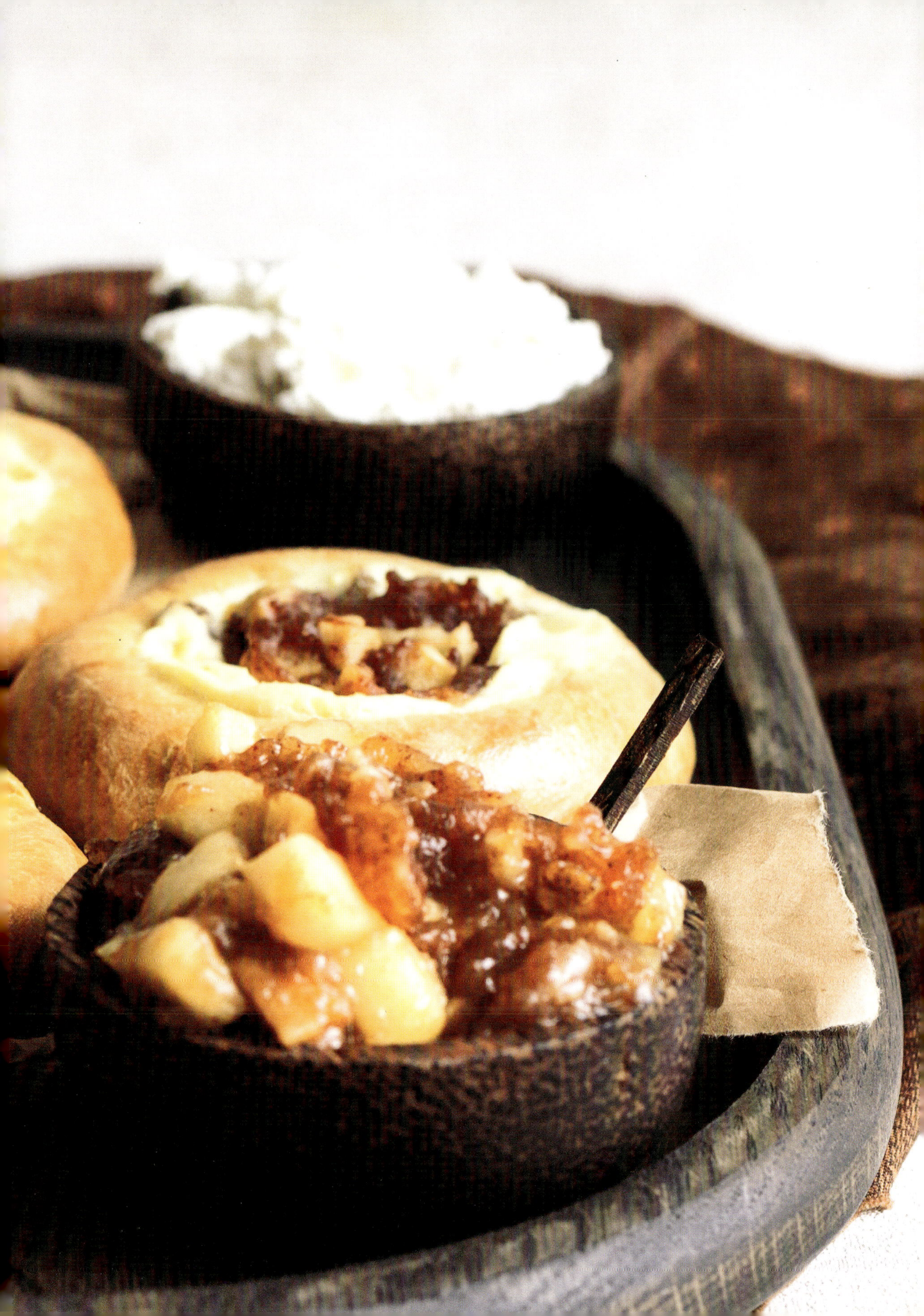

Apple Brioche Buns

MAKES 6
PREP + COOK TIME: 1 HOUR + 1 HOUR 30 MINS PROVING

¼ cup (60ml) whole milk
1 tsp active dry yeast
1 tbsp sugar
1⅓ cups (160g) plain flour
½ tsp salt
1 egg, room temperature
3 tbsps unsalted butter, room temperature
¾ cup (120g) apple strudel filling (see recipe page 165)
1 egg + 1 tbsp milk, beaten together

Heat the milk to 38°C. Whisk in the yeast and the sugar. Set aside for 5 minutes until the mixture begins to foam.

Add the flour, salt, egg and butter to the bowl of a stand mixer fitted with the dough hook. Add the yeast mixture and knead the dough on low speed for 1 minute to allow the ingredients to come together. Increase the speed to medium-high and knead for an additional 15 minutes until the dough cleans the sides and bottom of the bowl.

Cover with a tea towel and leave to rise in a warm spot for 1 hour until doubled in size. Punch down the dough then transfer to a lightly floured surface. Divide dough into six equal pieces and roll each piece into a 10cm diameter ball. Transfer balls to a baking tray lined with greaseproof paper, leaving 5cm between each one. Use the bottom of a bowl or cup that is 7cm in diameter to slightly indent the centre of each bun. Fill each indent with approximately 2 tablespoons of apple filling.

Set the buns aside in a warm place for 30 minutes until doubled in size.

Preheat oven to 175°C.

Brush buns with egg wash and bake for 15-20 minutes until golden on the edges.

Strawberry Clafoutis

SERVES 8
PREP + COOK TIME: 1 HOUR 10 MINS

½ cup (100g) sugar
4 eggs
¾ cup (100g) plain flour
35g butter, melted
½ tsp vanilla extract
1¼ cups (300ml) milk, room temperature
2¼ cups (450g) strawberries, hulled
Icing sugar for dusting

Preheat the oven to 200°C and grease a 23cm square tin.

In a large bowl whisk sugar and eggs until well combined. Fold in flour, melted butter, vanilla and milk. Mix well until smooth.

Halve any large strawberries and place strawberries in tin. Pour batter on top, sprinkle with icing sugar and bake for 20-30 minutes until set and golden.

Dust with more icing sugar to serve.

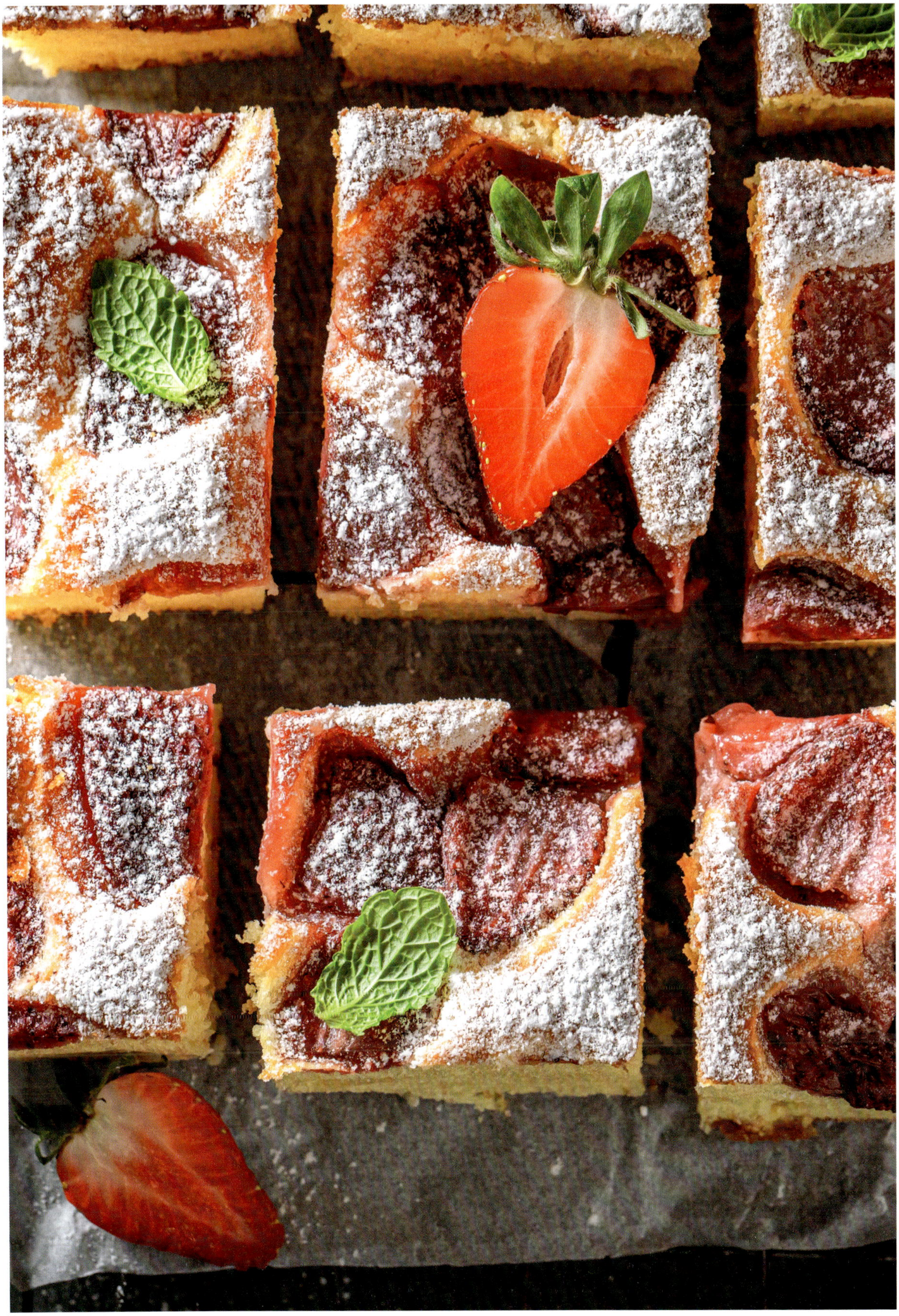

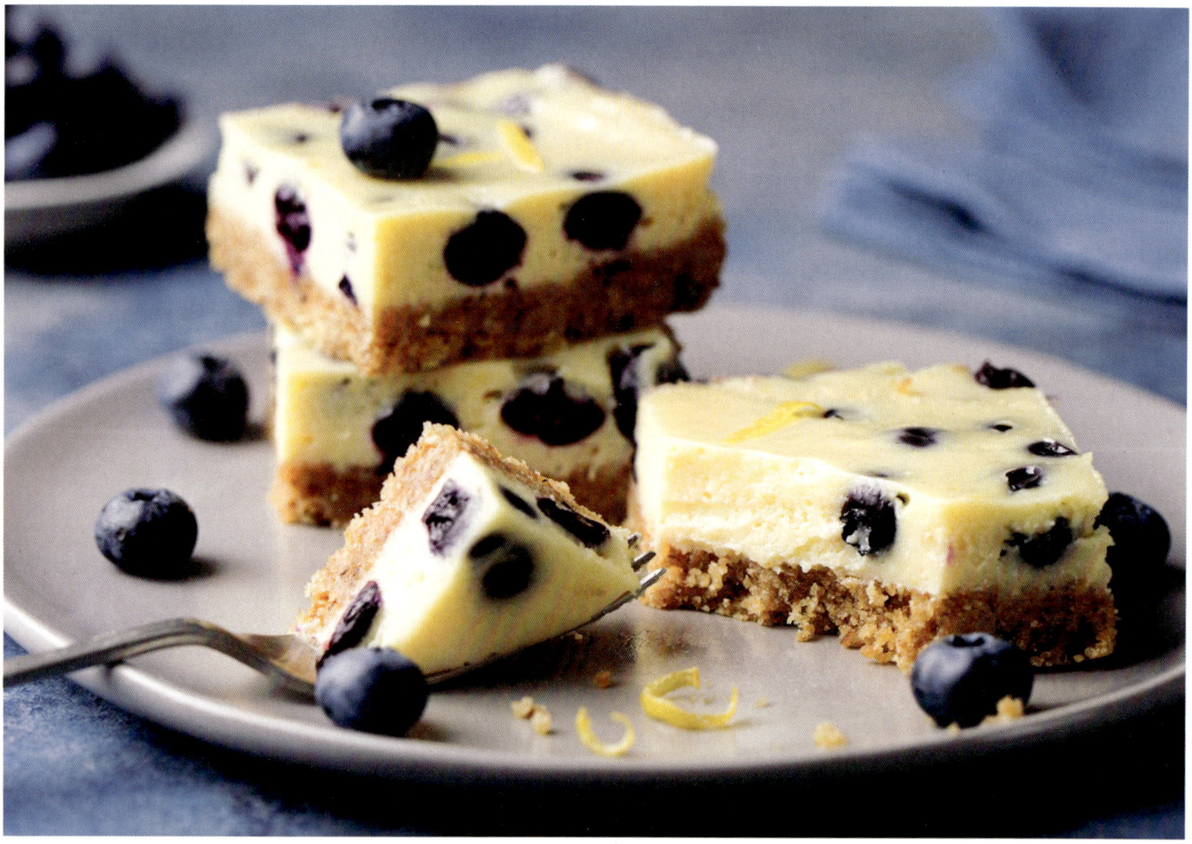

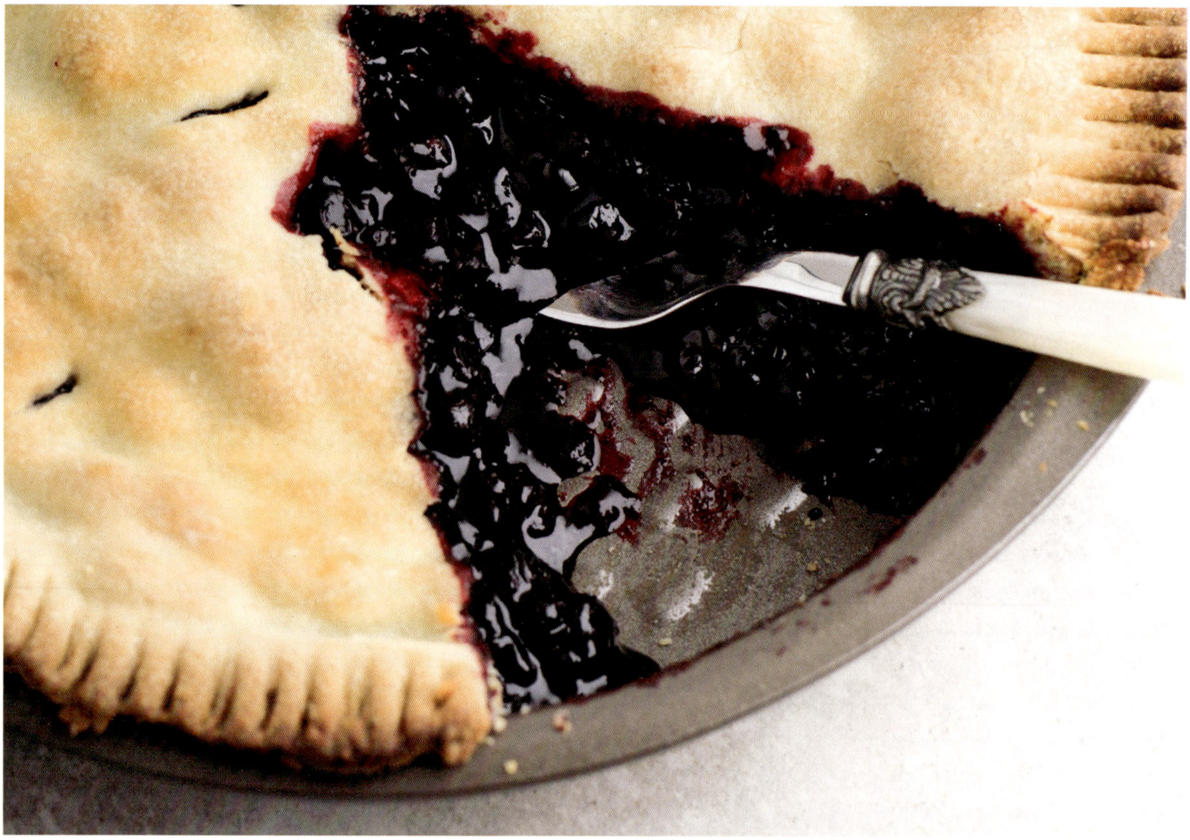

Blueberry Cheesecake Slice

SERVES 16
PREP + COOK TIME: 50 MINS + COOLING AND CHILLING

BASE

150g digestive biscuits

100g unsalted butter, melted

2 tbsps sugar

FILLING

320g cream cheese, softened

1 tbsp plain flour

⅓ cup (80ml) sour cream

1 cup (220g) caster sugar

2 tsps vanilla extract

Zest of 1 lemon

2 eggs, room temperature

2½ cups (250g) blueberries

Preheat oven to 160°C. Grease and line a 20cm square cake tin with greaseproof paper, leaving the edges of the paper overhanging.

Place biscuits in a food processor and process until fine crumbs form. Add butter and sugar and pulse until the mixture resembles wet sand. Pour into tin and press into the base with the back of a spoon.

Beat cream cheese with an electric hand mixer until smooth. Add flour and beat to incorporate. Add sour cream, sugar, vanilla and lemon zest. Beat to combine. Add eggs, one at a time, beating between each addition. Fold in the blueberries. Pour mixture into the tin and smooth the surface.

Bake for 35 minutes until cheesecake is set.

Cool in tin, then refrigerate, covered, for at least 4 hours.

Use paper overhang to lift out of the tin. Cut into squares to serve.

Blueberry Pie

SERVES 8
PREP + COOK TIME: 1 HOUR 10 MINS

6 cups (600g) fresh or frozen blueberries

½ cup (110g) sugar

¼ cup (40g) cornflour

½ tsp cinnamon

1 tsp lemon zest

1 tbsp lemon juice

1 quantity sweet shortcrust pastry (see recipe page 105)

1 egg

1 tbsp milk

Preheat oven to 220°C.

Place the blueberries, sugar, cornflour, cinnamon, lemon zest and lemon juice in a large bowl. Gently stir them so that all of the blueberries are coated with some sugar and flour. Place the mixture into a 22cm pie dish.

On a lightly floured surface, roll out pastry into a circle roughly 25cm wide. Place the pastry onto the blueberries. Use a fork to press pastry edges onto the dish.

Whisk egg and milk together to make an egg wash. Brush pastry with egg wash. Score the pie on the top with several cuts (so steam can escape while cooking).

Place the pie on the middle rack of the oven. Bake for 20 minutes at 220°C then reduce heat to 180°C and bake for 30-35 minutes more or until juices are bubbling and have thickened.

7

Special

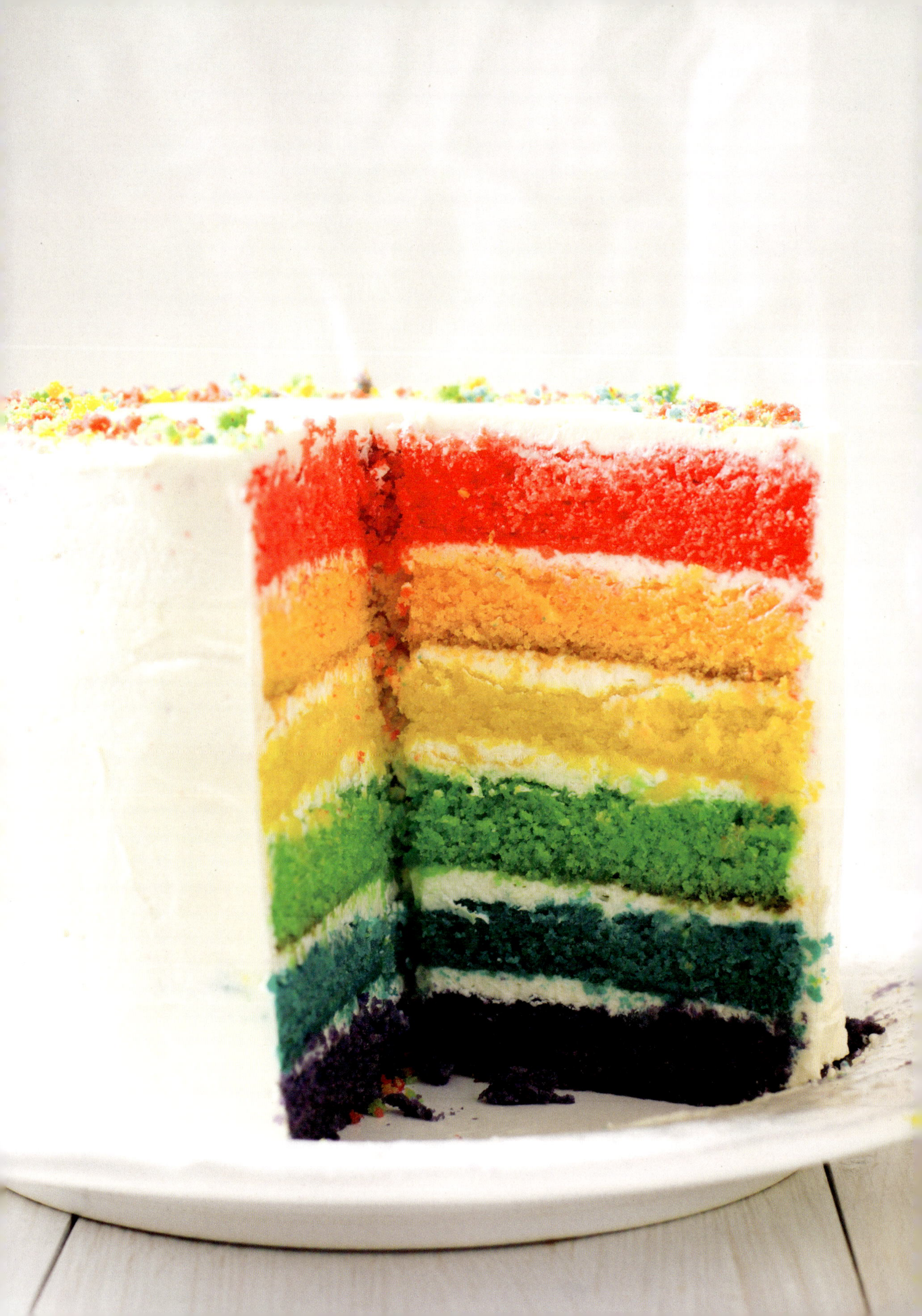

Rainbow Cake

SERVES 18
PREP + COOK TIME: 3 HOURS

THE FOLLOWING MAKES 2 SPONGE CAKES. YOU'LL NEED 3 X THESE INGREDIENTS FOR 6 SPONGES

125g butter, softened

1¾ cups (225g) plain flour

⅔ cup (150g) golden caster sugar

2 medium eggs

2 tbsps millk

1 tsp baking powder

Pinch of salt

1 tsp vanilla extract

Food colouring – red, orange, yellow, green, blue and purple

ICING

1 quantity Cream Cheese Icing (see next recipe)

1 tbsp rainbow sprinkles

Preheat oven to 180°C. Grease two 20cm round sandwich tins and line with baking paper.

Place all the sponge ingredients, apart from the food colouring, into a mixing bowl, then beat with an electric mixer until smooth.

Pour exactly half of the mixture into another mixing bowl. Pick two of your colours and stir a little into each batter. Keep going until you are happy with the colour. The colour of the batter now will be very similar to the finished cake. Scrape the batters into the tins. Smooth with a rubber spatula. Bake on the same oven shelf for 18 minutes until an inserted skewer comes out clean.

Gently turn the cakes out onto a wire rack to cool. Wash the tins and bowls thoroughly, and start again, making fresh batter for two further cakes and this time using another two colours. Repeat the process one more time until you have created all six coloured sponges.

Smear a little icing on your cake stand or plate to stick the first sponge. Start with the purple. Spread with icing all the way to the edge. Repeat, sandwiching on top the blue, green, yellow, orange and red sponges. Spread the remaining icing thickly all over the sides and top of the cake. Decorate with rainbow sprinkles.

Refrigerate until ready to serve.

Cream Cheese Icing

MAKES ENOUGH TO ICE 6 CAKES
PREP + COOK TIME: 3 HOURS
GLUTEN FREE

1 tsp vanilla extract

250g packages cream cheese

120g butter (room temperature)

3 cups (425g) icing sugar

Briefly beat the vanilla, cream cheese and butter with an electric mixer until smooth. Sift in the icing sugar and beat on a slow speed until fully combined. Refrigerate until ready to use.

Pistachio Meringue Roll

SERVES 6
PREP + COOK TIME: 45 MINS
GLUTEN FREE

MERINGUE

4 egg whites

1 cup (200g) caster sugar

¾ cup (100g) pistachios, chopped + ¼ cup (30g) pistachios, chopped for topping

PISTACHIO CREAM

2 cups (500ml) thickened cream

½ cup (125g) pistachio paste (see recipe page 126 for homemade)

1 cup (225g) mascarpone

½ tsp pistachio extract or ¼ tsp almond extract

½ tsp vanilla extract

Preheat the oven to 160°C. Line a 23 x 30cm baking tray with greaseproof paper.

Whisk the egg whites until stiff peaks form. Slowly add the sugar, 1 tablespoon at a time, whisking between each addition until the whites are glossy and thick. Gently fold in the chopped pistachios. Tip the mixture onto the prepared baking tray and spread out in an even layer.

Bake for 25-30 minutes until crisp on the outside. Remove from the oven and leave to cool.

Combine ½ cup of cream and the pistachio paste, and mix with an electric mixer until smooth. Add remaining cream, mascarpone, pistachio or almond extract and vanilla extract and beat until stiff.

Place a large piece of greaseproof paper on the work surface, place the meringue upside-down on top and carefully peel away the greaseproof paper from cooking. Spread the cream evenly over the top of the meringue. Starting at one of the short ends roll up the meringue, using the paper to help fold it over. Scatter with chopped pistachios, before slicing and serving.

Cake Pops

MAKES 24
PREP + COOK TIME: 1 HOUR

1 x 465g sponge cake

225g cream cheese, room temperature

4 tbsps butter

2 cups (310g) icing sugar

1 tbsp milk + more as needed

24 cake pop or lollipop sticks

2 cups (300g) white chocolate chips

Food colouring, as required

Decorative sprinkles

Crumble cake into a large bowl to a breadcrumb consistency.

In a separate bowl, whip the cream cheese, butter, icing sugar and milk together until smooth. Add to the bowl with the cake crumbs and mix until fully incorporated. Add additional milk, as required, until the mixture will hold together when rolled into a ball.

Roll all the mixture into balls and insert sticks. Place in the freezer for 20 minutes.

Melt chocolate in a heatproof bowl over a pan of simmering water on a medium heat. Add a few drops of food colouring and stir until smooth.

Place sprinkles onto baking paper.

Dip the cake pops into the chocolate. Let the excess chocolate drip off. Swirl and tap gently if needed.

Roll the cake pops in sprinkles and other decorations as desired.

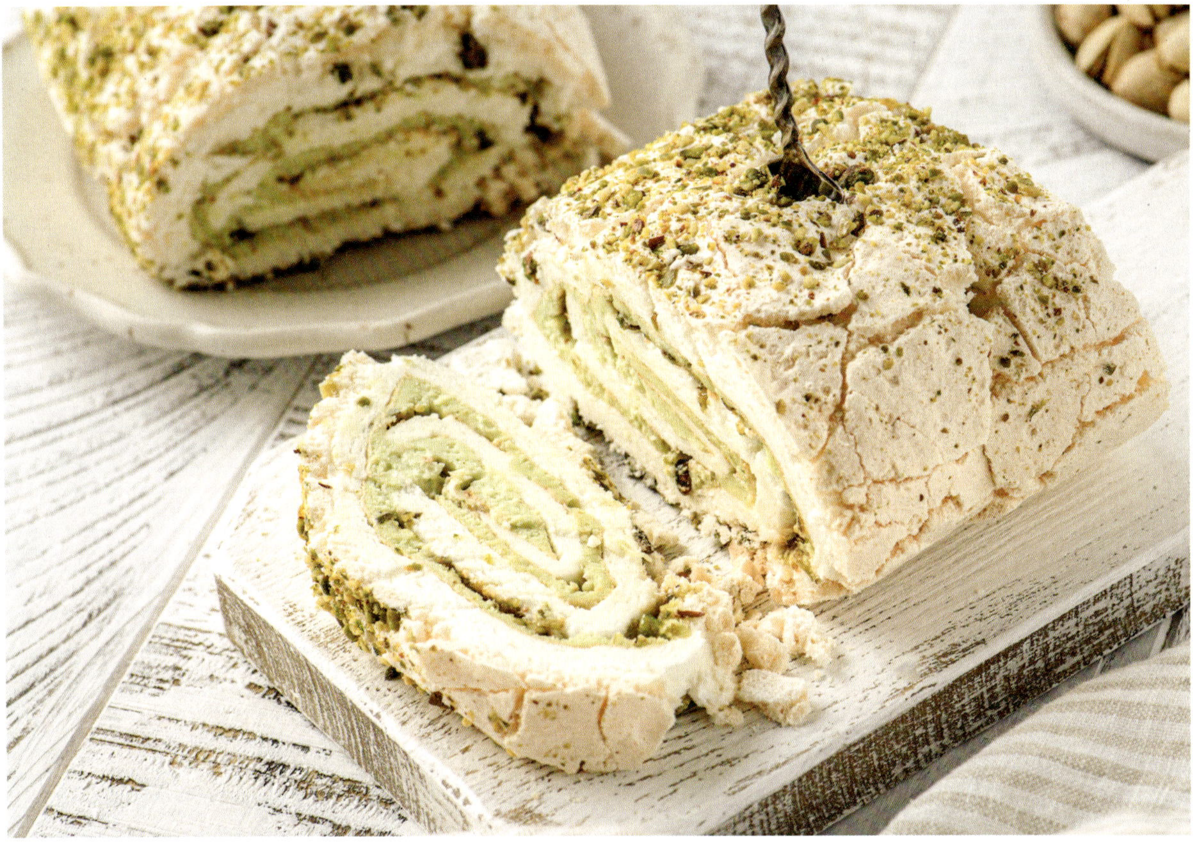

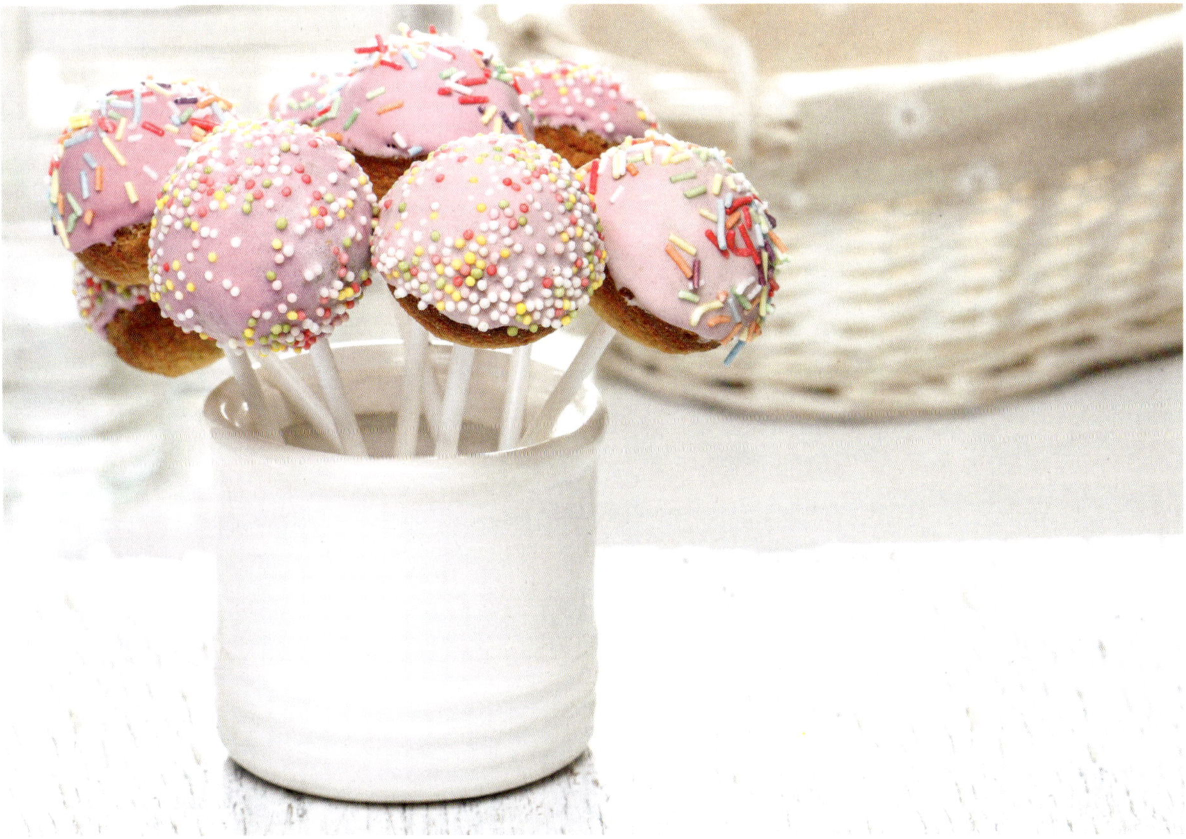

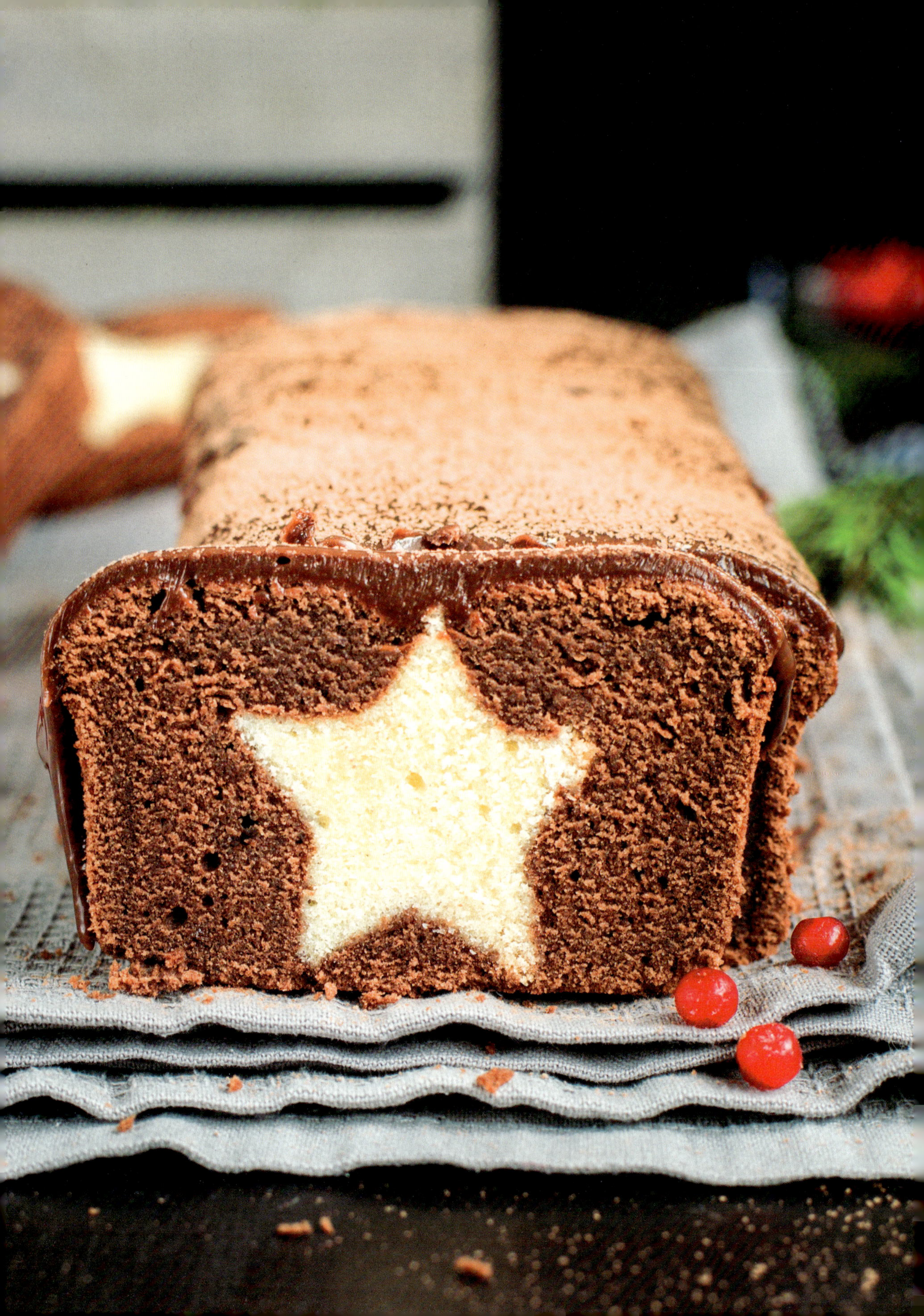

Surprise Star Chocolate Cake

SERVES 10
PREP + COOK TIME: 3 HOURS + COOLING

STAR CAKE

250g butter

1 cup (220g) sugar

1 tsp vanilla extract

4 eggs

2 cups (250g) plain flour, sifted

3 tsps baking powder

⅓ cup (40g) almond meal

Pinch of salt

⅓ cup (90ml) milk

CHOCOLATE CAKE

¼ cup (30g) cocoa powder

¼ cup (60ml) hot water

170g butter

¾ cup (165g) sugar

1 tsp vanilla extract

1 tbsp white vinegar

3 eggs

1½ cups (185g) plain flour, sifted

2 tsps bicarbonate of soda

¼ cup (60ml) buttermilk

ICING

125g dark chocolate, chopped

150g butter, softened

1⅓ cups (205g) icing sugar

1 tsp vanilla extract

¼ cup (30g) cocoa powder

Preheat the oven to 180°C. Line a loaf tin with greaseproof paper.

To make the batter for the star cake, add butter, sugar and vanilla extract into a large mixing bowl. Cream with an electric mixer until light and fluffy. Add eggs one at a time and beat after each addition. Stir in flour, baking powder, almond meal, salt and milk. Mix to combine. Pour batter into prepared loaf tin and bake for 1 hour or until an inserted skewer comes out clean. Allow to cool for 3 hours.

When cool, cut cake into thick slices. Using a star cookie cutter cut out individual stars. Place stars on a plate lined with plastic wrap and freeze for 30 minutes.

Preheat the oven to 180°C. Line a loaf tin with greaseproof paper.

Mix cocoa with hot water then cool for 10 minutes.

Beat the butter, sugar, cocoa mixture, vanilla extract and vinegar with an electric mixer. Add the eggs and beat to combine. Mix in flour, bicarb and buttermilk until incorporated.

Cover the sides and the bottom of the tin with chocolate batter. Fit the stars tightly together in the centre of the tin and cover with remaining batter. Lightly tap the tin so the batter spreads around the stars. Bake for 40-50 minutes or until firm to touch. Allow cake to cool completely before removing from the tin.

Melt chocolate in a heatproof bowl over a saucepan of simmering water. Set aside to cool. Using an electric mixer, beat the butter and sugar until light and fluffy. Add the vanilla extract and melted chocolate. Beat until shiny and smooth.

Spread icing over cake then sift over cocoa powder to finish.

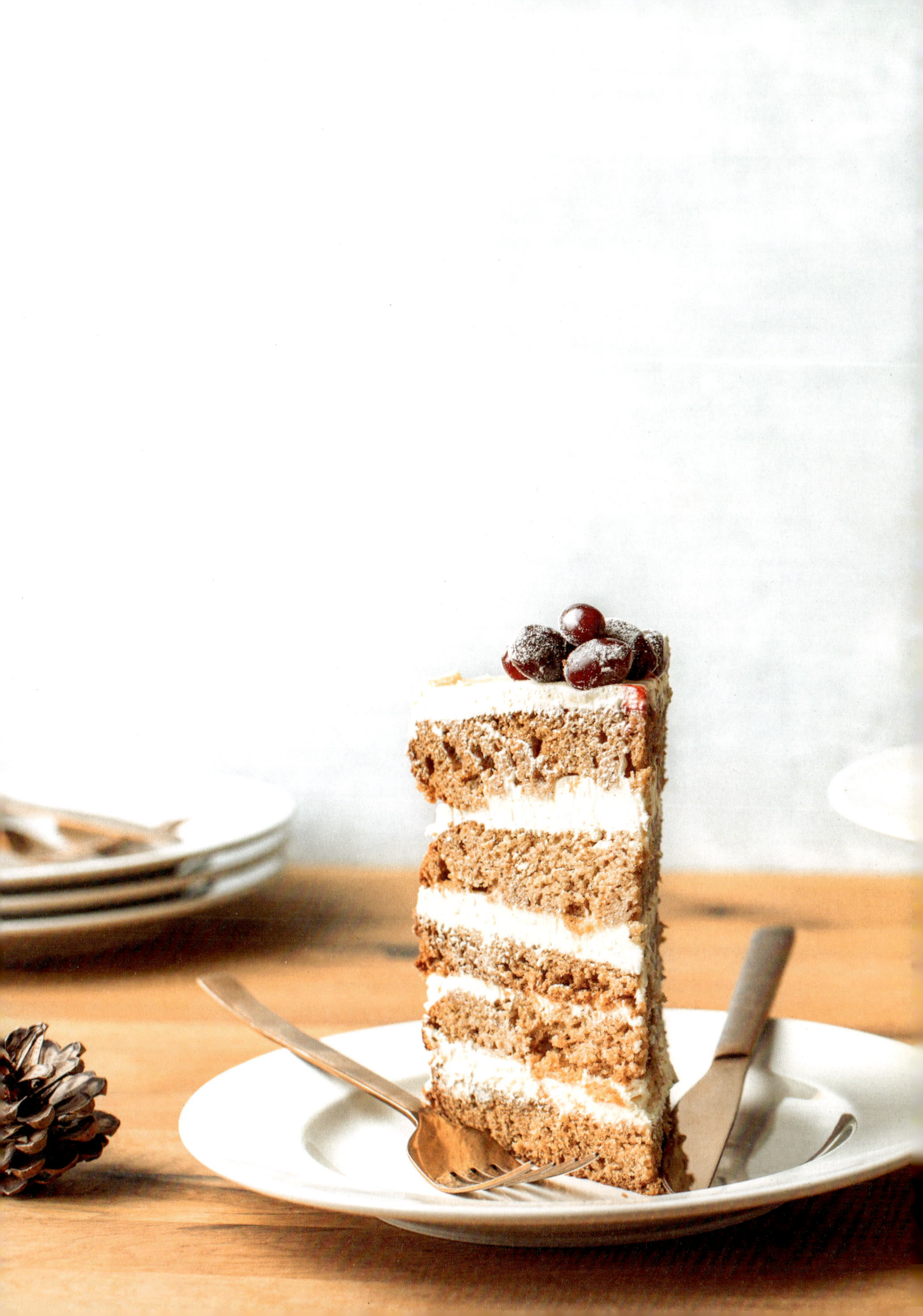

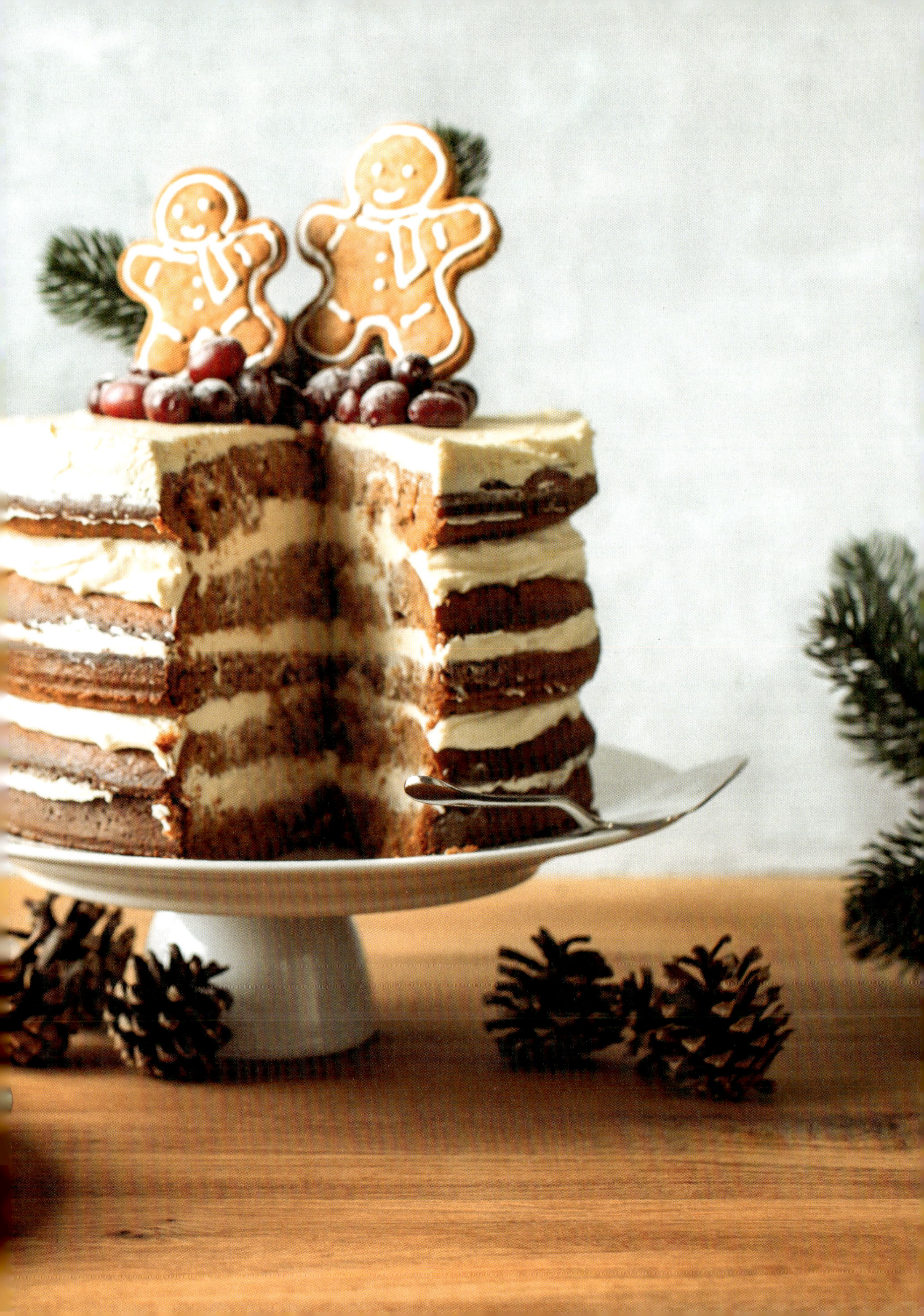

Ginger Layer Cake

SERVES 10
PREP + COOK TIME: 1 HOUR 30 MINS + COOLING

310g butter, diced and softened
1½ cups (330g) caster sugar
¾ cup (260g) golden syrup
5 large eggs
3½ cups (435g) plain flour
2½ tsps baking powder
1¼ tsps bicarbonate of soda
2½ tsps ground ginger
1¼ tsps mixed spice
1⅔ cups (410ml) warm milk
Cinnamon cream (see next recipe)
Gingerbread people and cranberries to decorate (optional)

Preheat oven to 180°C. Grease and line the base and sides of three 20cm cake tins.

Beat together butter, sugar and golden syrup with an electric mixer until pale and creamy. Add eggs one at a time, mixing between each addition. Fold in flour, baking powder, bicarb and spices, alternately with the milk, until the batter is smooth and well combined.

Pour one-fifth of the batter into one of the tins. Divide the remaining batter between the two remaining tins. Transfer to the oven. After 35 minutes check the smallest cake and remove from the oven if golden brown and an inserted skewer comes out clean. Continue cooking the other two cakes for 10-15 minutes until cooked. Allow to cool completely. Cut the larger cakes in half horizontally, to form five layers.

Spread each cake with cinnamon cream and sandwich together. Smooth the cinnamon cream on the top cake with a palette knife and decorate with gingerbread people and cranberries, if desired.

Cinnamon Cream

SERVES 10
PREP + COOK TIME: 10 MINS
GLUTEN FREE

1⅔ cups (400ml) thickened cream
1 cup (260g) mascarpone
⅓ cup (50g) icing sugar mixture, sifted
1½ tsps ground cinnamon

Beat cream until soft peaks form. Add mascarpone, icing sugar and cinnamon and mix well to combine.

Nut Choc Bark

SERVES 8
PREP + COOK TIME: 20 MINS + CHILLING
GLUTEN FREE • DAIRY FREE

300g dark cooking chocolate, roughly chopped
Grated zest of 1 orange
Salt flakes
⅓ cup (40g) + 2 tbsps roughly chopped pistachios
⅓ cup (40g) + 2 tbsps flaked almonds
¼ cup (20g) candied orange peel strips

Melt the chocolate in a large, heatproof bowl over a pan of simmering water. Stir in the orange zest, a pinch of salt flakes and ¼ cup each of pistachios and almonds.

Line a large, flat baking tray with greaseproof paper.

Spread the melted chocolate mixture in a thin even layer over the paper with a flat spatula. Press the candied orange peel and remaining nuts into the top. Sprinkle with salt.

Refrigerate for 2 hours, then break up into bite-size chunks with a knife to serve.

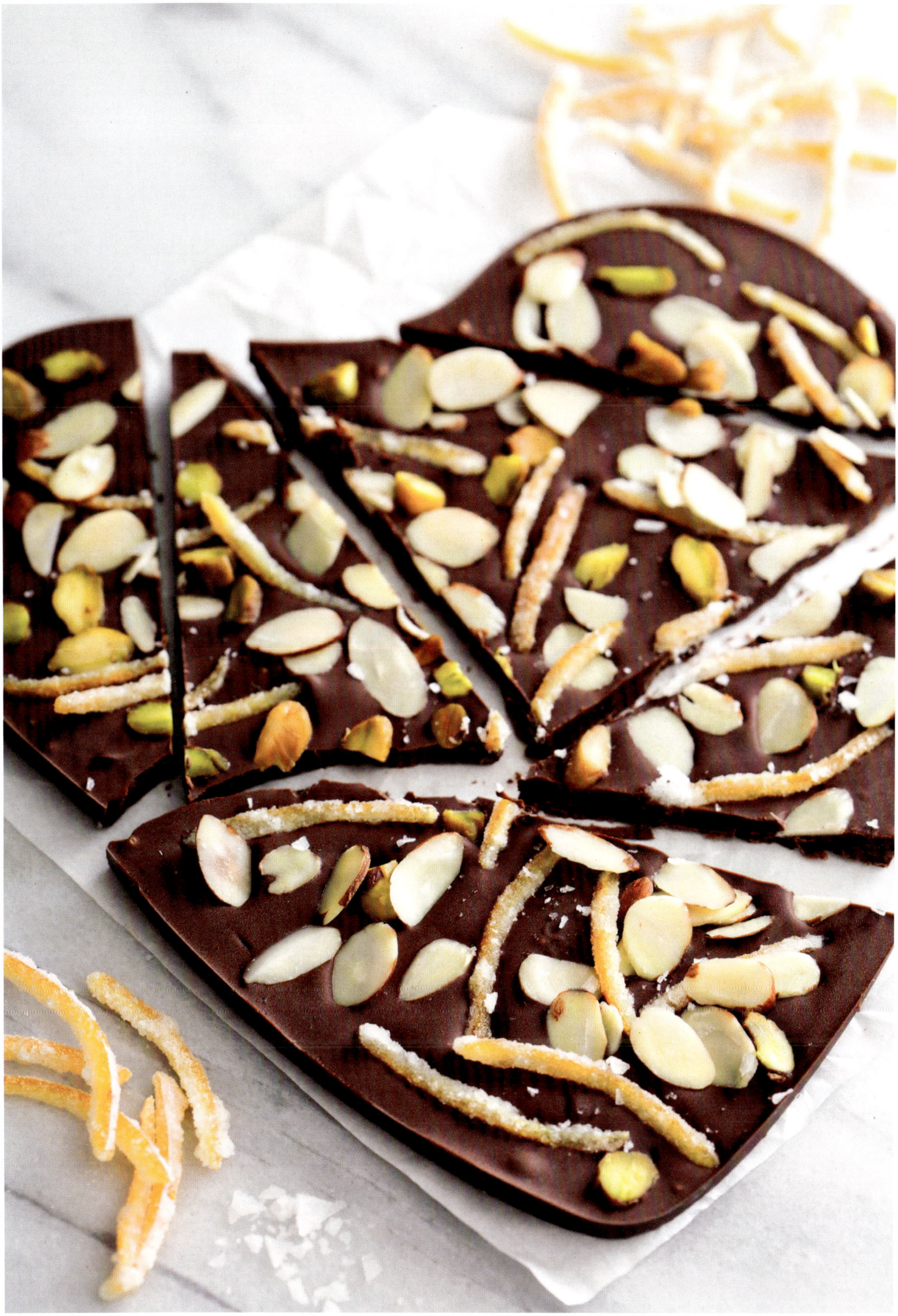

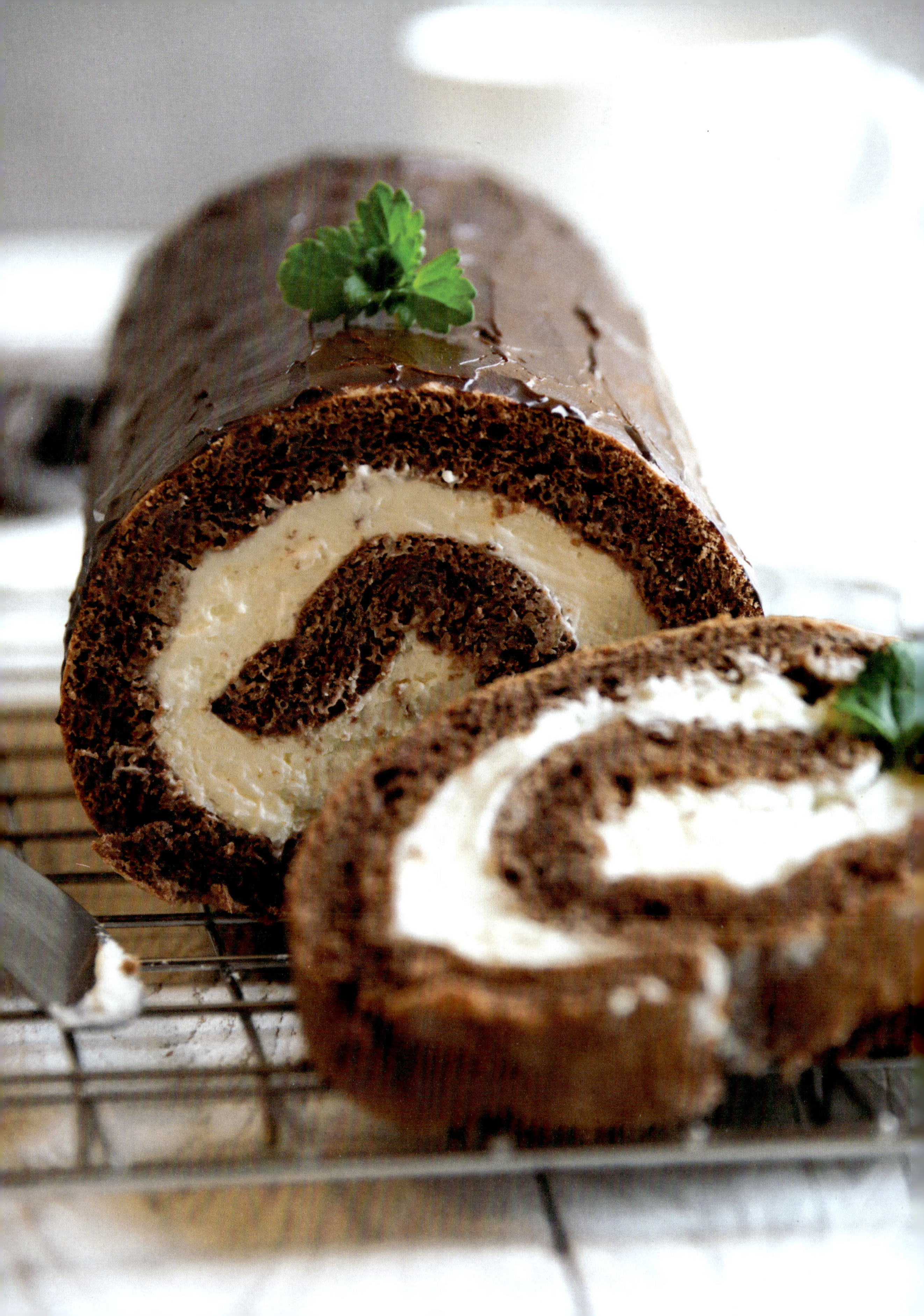

Chocolate Swiss Roll

SERVES 10
PREP + COOK TIME: 45 MINS + COOLING AND CHILLING

4 large eggs, separated
⅔ cup (140g) sugar
1 tsp pure vanilla extract
½ cup (60g) plain flour
5 tbsps cocoa powder
1 tsp baking powder
¼ tsp salt
60g unsalted butter, melted
1 tbsp strong brewed coffee

VANILLA CREAM
1 cup (240ml) thickened cream
3 tbsps icing sugar
1 tsp pure vanilla extract

CHOCOLATE TOPPING
115g dark chocolate, chopped
½ cup (120ml) thickened cream

Preheat oven to 175°C. Grease and line a 31 x 25cm Swiss roll tin with greaseproof paper.

Using an electric hand mixer beat together the egg whites and ⅓ cup sugar until stiff peaks form. In another bowl, beat the egg yolks, remaining sugar and vanilla extract together until pale and creamy.

Sift the flour, 3 tablespoons cocoa powder, baking powder and salt together in a large bowl. Add the melted butter, coffee and egg yolk mixture to the dry ingredients. Beat together to combine. Gently fold in one-third of the egg whites until incorporated. Fold in the remaining egg whites.

Spread batter evenly into prepared pan. Bake for 10 minutes or until the top of the cake gently springs back when touched with your finger. Do not over-bake.

Place a piece of greaseproof paper slightly larger than the cake on a clean work surface. Dust with remaining cocoa powder.

Run a knife around the edges of the cake, then immediately invert it onto the greaseproof paper. Peel off the greaseproof paper that was on the bottom of the cake as it baked. Starting with the narrow end, carefully roll up the cake, using the greaseproof paper to help. Allow the cake to cool completely rolled up in the paper.

Using an electric hand mixer, whisk the cream, sugar and vanilla extract until stiff peaks form.

Slowly and gently unroll the cake. Spread whipped cream evenly on top, leaving about a 1cm border around the cake. Gently roll the cake back up, without the greaseproof paper. Transfer to a wire rack.

Place chopped chocolate in a medium bowl. Heat the cream in a small saucepan until it begins to gently simmer. Pour over chocolate, then let it sit for 2-3 minutes to gently soften the chocolate. Stir until the chocolate is melted and is completely combined with the cream.

Pour ganache all over rolled cake. Spread with a palate knife.

Refrigerate for at least 30-60 minutes before slicing and serving.

Chocolate Orange Macarons

MAKES 22
PREP + COOK TIME: 1 HOUR 15 MINS + COOLING
GLUTEN FREE

MACARONS

3 large egg whites
¼ cup (55g) caster sugar
1⅓ cups (200g) icing sugar, sifted
1 cup (120g) finely ground almond meal
Orange gel food colouring

CHOCOLATE FILLING

1 cup (155g) chocolate chips
1 cup (250ml) thickened cream

Line two baking trays with greaseproof paper.

Beat egg whites in a large bowl with an electric mixer until soft peaks form. Add caster sugar; beat until sugar is dissolved. Fold in sifted icing sugar and almond meal in two batches. Add food colouring until desired colour is reached.

Spoon the mixture into a piping bag fitted with a 2cm round tip. Pipe 4cm rounds about 2cm apart on trays. Tap trays on bench so macarons spread slightly. Set aside for 30 minutes until dry to the touch.

Preheat oven to 150°C.

Bake for 20 minutes, then allow to cool on the trays.

For the filling, pour chocolate chips into a medium bowl. Add cream to small saucepan and heat over medium-high heat until bubbles start to appear around the sides. Pour cream over chocolate chips. Let sit for about 5 minutes, then stir until creamy. Cool the chocolate mixture in the fridge until firm enough to pipe.

Spoon the chocolate filling into a piping bag with a narrow round nozzle. Pipe filling onto flat side of half the macarons. Sandwich together with the remaining halves. Refrigerate until ready to serve.

Raspberry Macarons

MAKES 22
PREP + COOK TIME: 1 HOUR 15 MINS + COOLING
GLUTEN FREE

MACARONS

½ cup (70g) finely ground almond meal
⅓ cup (60g) icing sugar, sifted
¼ cup (30g) freeze-dried raspberry powder
3 large egg whites
½ cup (100g) caster sugar

CINNAMON BUTTERCREAM

225g unsalted butter
55g cream cheese
2 tsps vanilla bean paste
1½ cups (240g) icing sugar
2 tsps cinnamon
¼ tsp salt

Line two baking trays with greaseproof paper.

Sift almond meal, icing sugar and raspberry powder twice through a fine mesh sieve into a bowl. Set aside.

Beat egg whites in a large bowl with an electric mixer until soft peaks form. Add caster sugar; beat until sugar is dissolved. Fold in raspberry mixture in two batches.

Spoon mixture into a piping bag fitted with a 2cm round tip. Pipe 4cm rounds 2cm apart on trays. Tap trays on bench so macarons spread slightly. Set aside for 30 minutes until dry to the touch.

Preheat oven to 150°C.

Bake for 16-18 minutes, then cool on the trays.

Cream butter and cream cheese with an electric mixer until smooth. Add vanilla, icing sugar, cinnamon and salt, and mix until light and fluffy. Spoon into a piping bag with a narrow round nozzle. Pipe filling onto flat side of half the macaron shells. Sandwich together with the remaining halves. Refrigerate until ready to serve.

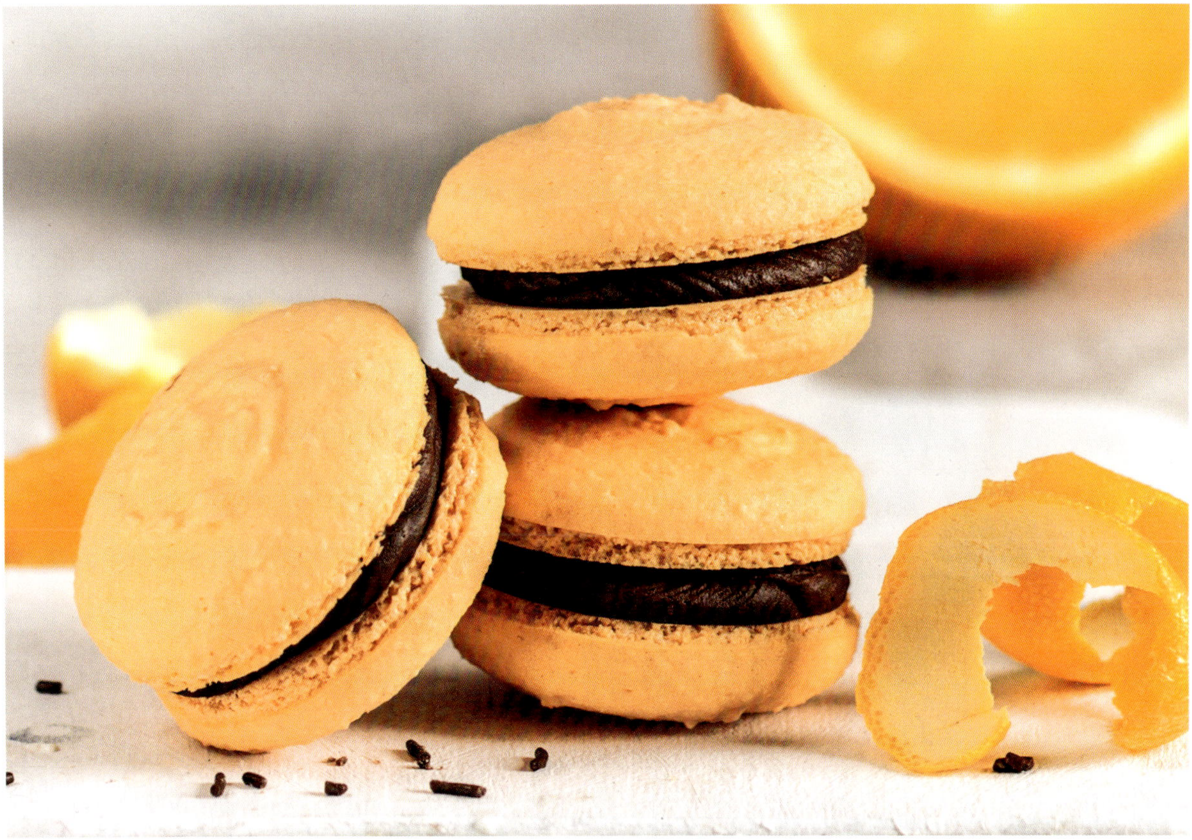

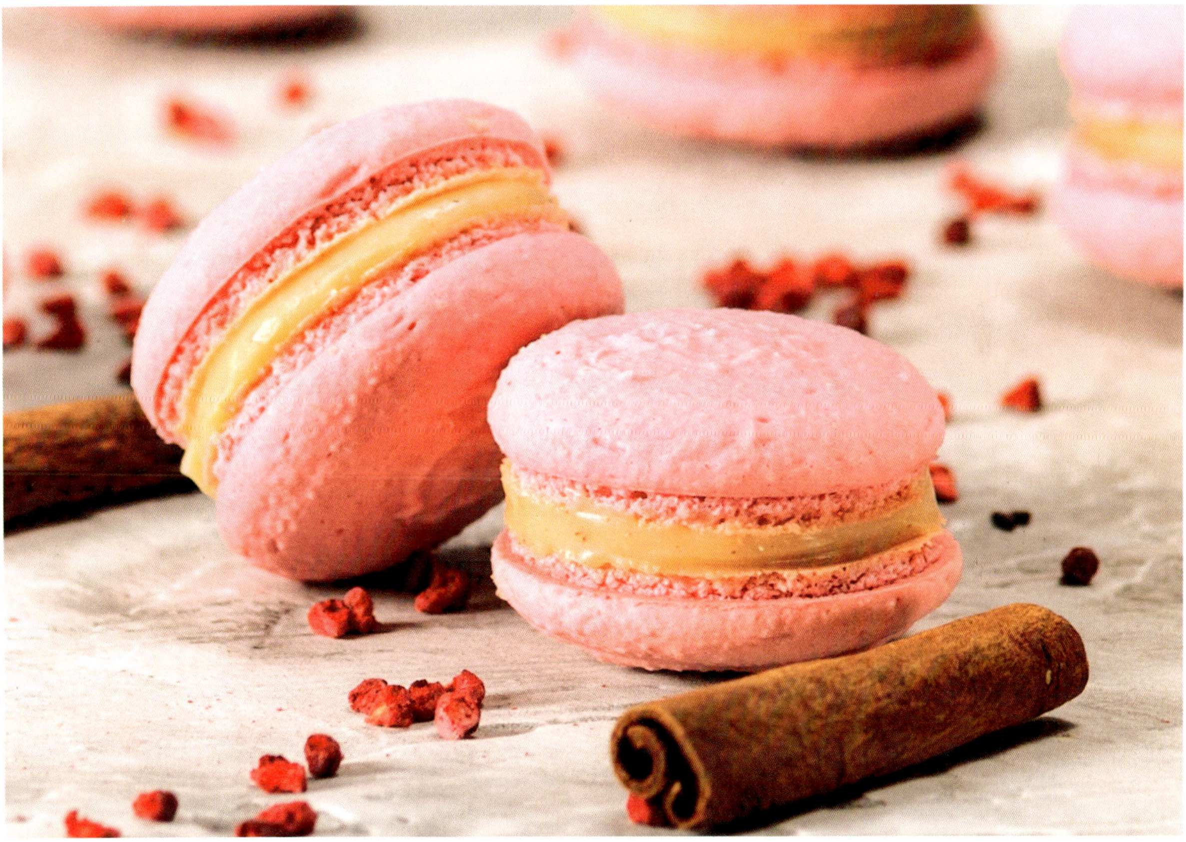

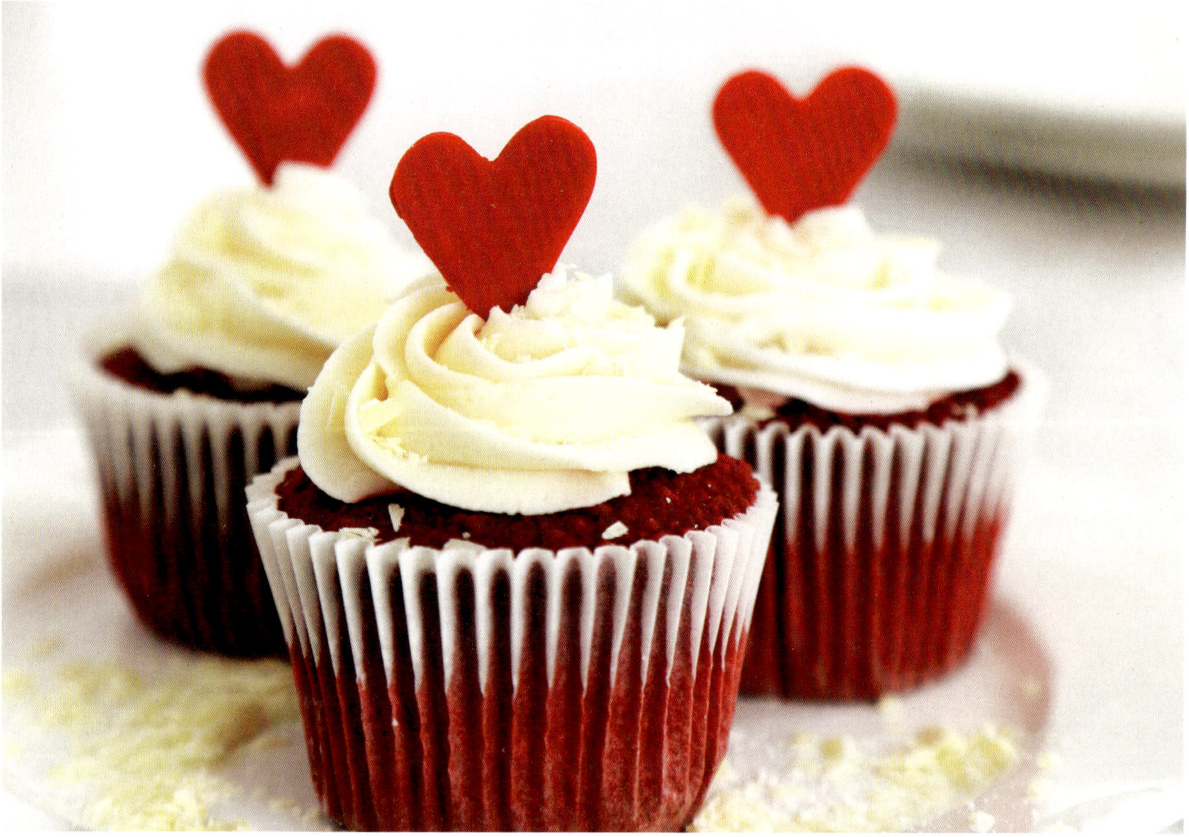

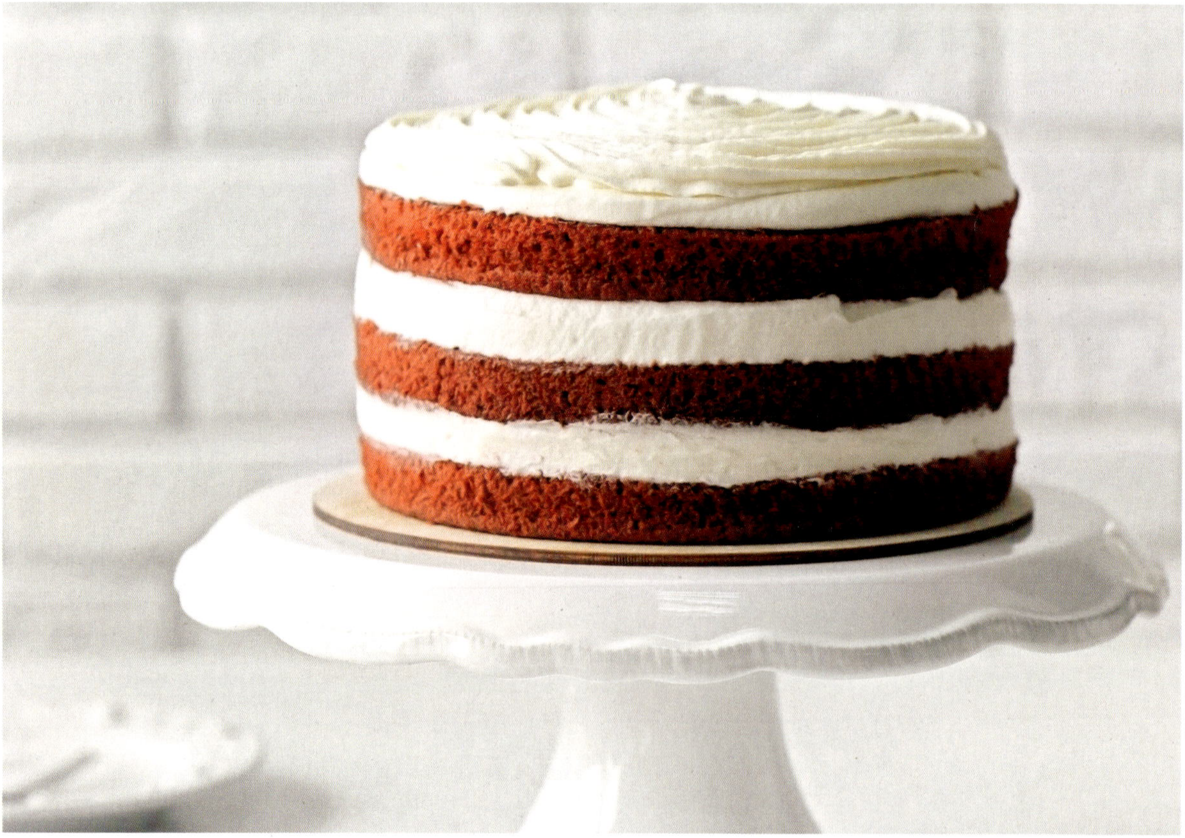

Valentine Cupcakes

MAKES 12

PREP + COOK TIME: 40 MINS + COOLING

CUPCAKES

1⅓ cups (290g) sugar

1¼ cups (325ml) vegetable oil

2 eggs

1 tsp vanilla extract

2 tbsps red food colouring

2 cups (250g) plain flour

2 tbsps cocoa powder

½ tsp salt

1 cup (250ml) buttermilk

2 tbsps white vinegar

1½ tsps bicarbonate of soda

CREAM CHEESE FROSTING

230g cream cheese, room temperature

115g butter, room temperature

¾ cup (120g) icing sugar

Heart decorations

Preheat oven to 180°C and line 12 muffin cups with paper liners.

Using an electric mixer beat together sugar and vegetable oil. Add eggs one at a time, mixing well after each addition. Add vanilla extract and red food colouring and mix to combine. Gradually add dry ingredients to the bowl, alternating with the buttermilk. Mix well after each addition.

Combine vinegar and bicarb of soda in a small bowl. Stir well then add to the batter and stir to combine.

Divide mixture between muffin cups and bake for 20 minutes or until a skewer inserted into the centre comes out clean. Cool on a wire rack before frosting.

Using an electric mixer, combine the cream cheese and butter until light and fluffy. Slowly add the icing sugar until incorporated.

Pipe the frosting on top of the cupcakes and decorate with heart shaped decorations.

Red Velvet Cake

SERVES 12

PREP + COOK TIME: 45 MINS + COOLING

1½ cups (375ml) vegetable oil

2 eggs

1 cup (250ml) buttermilk

1 tbsp white vinegar

1 tsp vanilla extract

2 cups (440g) sugar

1 tbsp cocoa powder

1 tsp salt

1 tsp bicarbonate of soda

2½ cups (310g) plain flour

1 tbsp red food colouring

CREAM CHEESE FROSTING

400g cream cheese, room temperature

120g unsalted butter, room temperature

2 tsps vanilla extract

4 cups (620g) icing sugar

Preheat oven to 175°C. Grease and line three 20cm round cake tins with greaseproof paper.

Using an electric mixer beat together the oil, eggs, buttermilk, vinegar and vanilla. Add in the sugar and mix to incorporate. Add the cocoa powder, salt and bicarb. Beat until smooth. With the mixer on low add the flour and red food colouring and beat to incorporate.

Divide the batter equally between the three prepared tins. Bake for 25-30 minutes or until a toothpick inserted in the centre comes out clean.

Cool in the pan for 10 minutes and then turn the cakes out onto a wire rack to cool completely before frosting.

Beat together cream cheese, butter and vanilla with an electric mixer, until smooth Beat in icing sugar until light and fluffy.

Transfer the frosting to a piping bag with a star shaped nozzle. Pipe the frosting on top of each cake then sandwich the three cakes together.

Panforte

SERVES 10
PREP + COOK TIME: 1 HOUR 10 MINS
DAIRY FREE

5 tbsps unsweetened cocoa powder + more for dusting

2½ cups (325g) mixed nuts (pistachios, almonds, hazelnuts), toasted

1 cup (125g) plain flour

1 cup (170g) dried cranberries, chopped

1 cup (170g) dried figs, chopped

1 tbsp cinnamon

2 tsps ground ginger

Pinch of grated nutmeg

½ tsp chilli powder (optional)

90g dark chocolate, chopped

1 cup (220g) sugar

¾ cup (260g) honey

Preheat the oven to 160°C. Grease and line a large rectangular baking tin. Dust the inside (base and sides) with cocoa powder.

In a large bowl, mix together the cocoa powder, nuts, flour, dried fruit, cinnamon, ginger, nutmeg and chilli powder, if using.

Melt the chocolate in a small, heatproof bowl set over a pan of simmering water. Set aside when just melted.

Heat the sugar and honey in a saucepan over a medium-high heat until the sugar is completely dissolved and the syrup is thickened. Pour the hot syrup over the nut mixture. Add the melted chocolate, and stir to combine. Scrape the batter into the prepared tin and carefully smooth with a spatula.

Transfer to the oven and bake for 40 minutes until set but still just soft in the centre.

Transfer to a wire rack to cool for 15 minutes, then remove from the tin to cool completely. Dust with cocoa powder to serve.

Rum Baba

SERVES 6
PREP + COOK TIME: 45 MINS + 1 HOUR PROVING

3 eggs

5g dried yeast

Pinch of salt

1 tsp honey

1 cup (125g) flour

75g unsalted butter, melted

½ cup (125g) caster sugar

2 cups (500ml) water

½ cup (125ml) dark rum

Peeled zest of 1 orange

6 fresh raspberries to serve

In a large mixing bowl, mix together the eggs, yeast, salt and honey. Set aside for 10 minutes until frothy.

Gradually sift in the flour and stir to create a smooth batter. Pour in the melted butter and mix to incorporate.

Divide the batter between six nonstick baba or dariole moulds and leave to prove in a warm place for 1 hour until the dough has doubled in size.

Preheat the oven to 180°C.

Bake for 10-12 minutes until the babas are golden brown. Remove from the moulds and leave to cool.

Place the sugar, water, rum and orange zest in a medium saucepan and bring to the boil.

Reduce the heat to a gentle simmer, add the babas and soak for 30-60 seconds.

Remove with a slotted spoon. Top with fresh raspberries to serve.

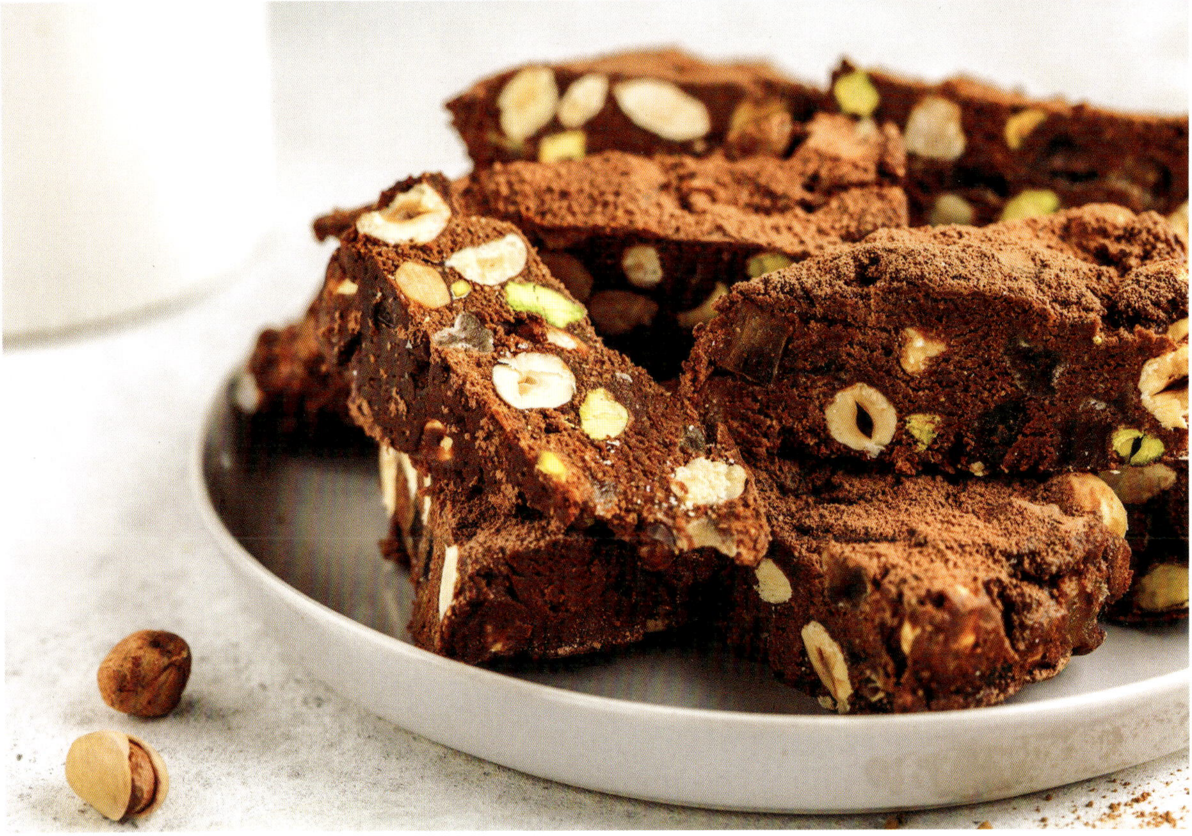

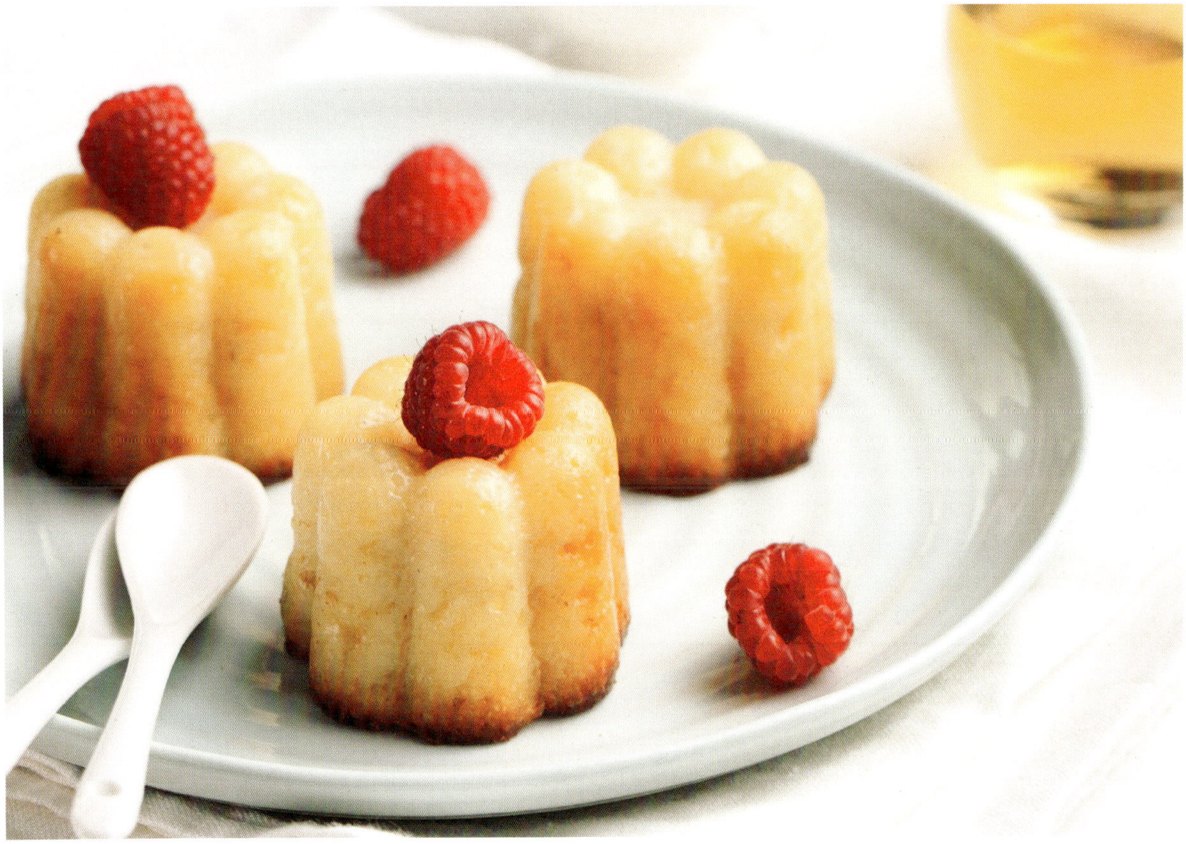

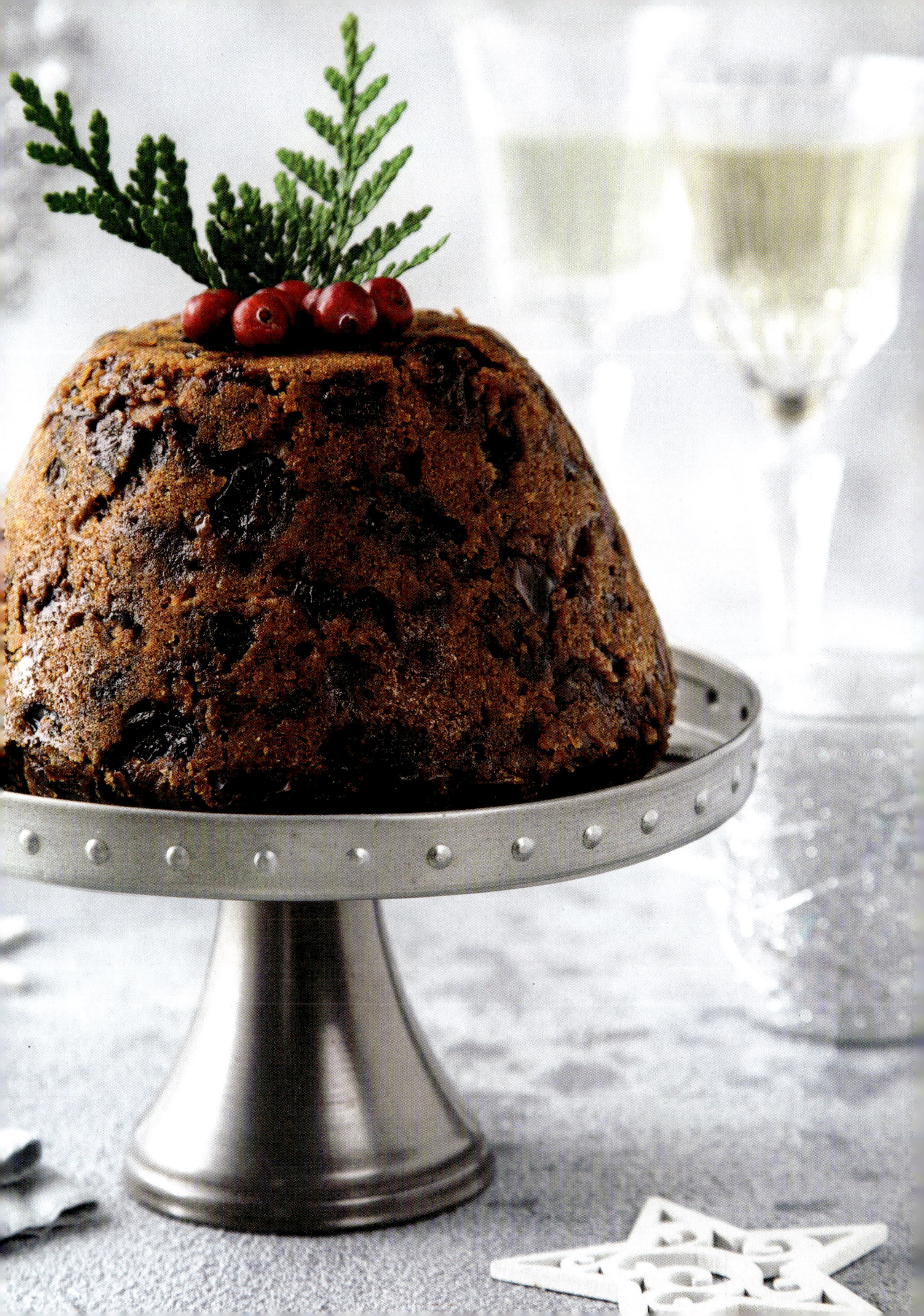

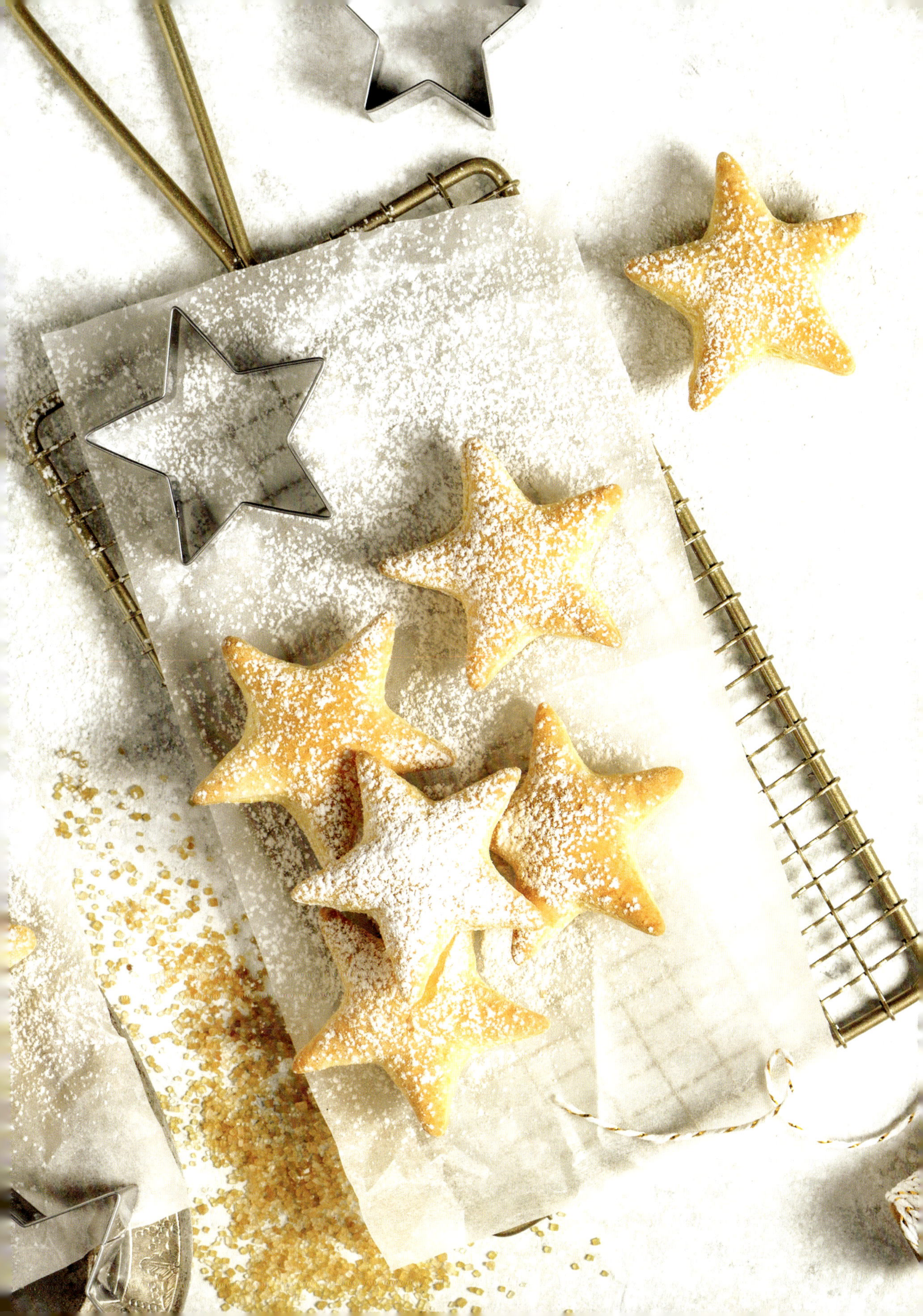

Christmas Pudding

SERVES 10
PREP + COOK TIME: 6 HOURS 30 MINS

3 eggs

1 cup (220g) firmly packed brown sugar

4½ cups (720g) mixed dried fruit (any combination of raisins, sultanas, dried cherries, dried cranberries, dried figs)

¼ cup (20g) candied peel

1¼ cups (300ml) sour cream

2¼ cups (335g) plain flour

1 tsp ground nutmeg

1 tsp bicarbonate of soda

Grease a 7-cup pudding basin and line base with greaseproof paper.

Beat eggs and sugar in a large bowl with an electric mixer until thick and creamy. Add dried fruit, candied peel and sour cream and stir to combine. Sift in the flour, nutmeg and bicarb. Stir to combine. Spoon into the prepared basin.

Grease a 30 x 40cm sheet of foil and top with a sheet of greaseproof paper. Fold a 5cm pleat crossways through the centre of both sheets. Place sheets, greaseproof paper side down, over the basin and secure with string. Make a handle with additional string. Press foil and baking paper firmly around rim to seal.

Place the pudding in a large saucepan with enough boiling water to come halfway up the side of the basin. Cover pan with a tight-fitting lid and steam for 5 hours. Add more boiling water as necessary.

Stand the pudding for 15 minutes before turning out. Allow to cool completely, then wrap in greaseproof paper and store in a cool dry place.

When ready to eat, return to the basin, cover in the same way with foil and greaseproof paper and steam for 1 hour.

Pastry Stars

MAKES APPROX 16
PREP + COOK TIME: 25 MINS

1 sheet puff pastry, defrosted

1 tbsp milk

2 tbsps sugar

Icing sugar for dusting

Preheat oven to 200°C. Line a baking tray with greaseproof paper.

Place pastry on a lightly floured work surface. Cut out star shapes with a pastry cutter. Brush the stars with milk and sprinkle with sugar. Bake for 15 minutes until golden brown. Dust with icing sugar to serve.

Dried Orange Slices

MAKES APPROX 32 SLICES
PREP + COOK TIME: 6 HOURS 10 MINUTES
GLUTEN FREE • DAIRY FREE

4 oranges

Preheat oven to 175°C.

Cut oranges crosswise into ½cm-thick slices.

Arrange orange slices in a single layer on baking trays topped with wire racks.

Cook for 4-6 hours, until dry to the touch, rotating every few hours for even cooking.

Cool completely before storing or using to decorate cakes or cocktails. Store in an airtight container at room temperature for up to 1 month.

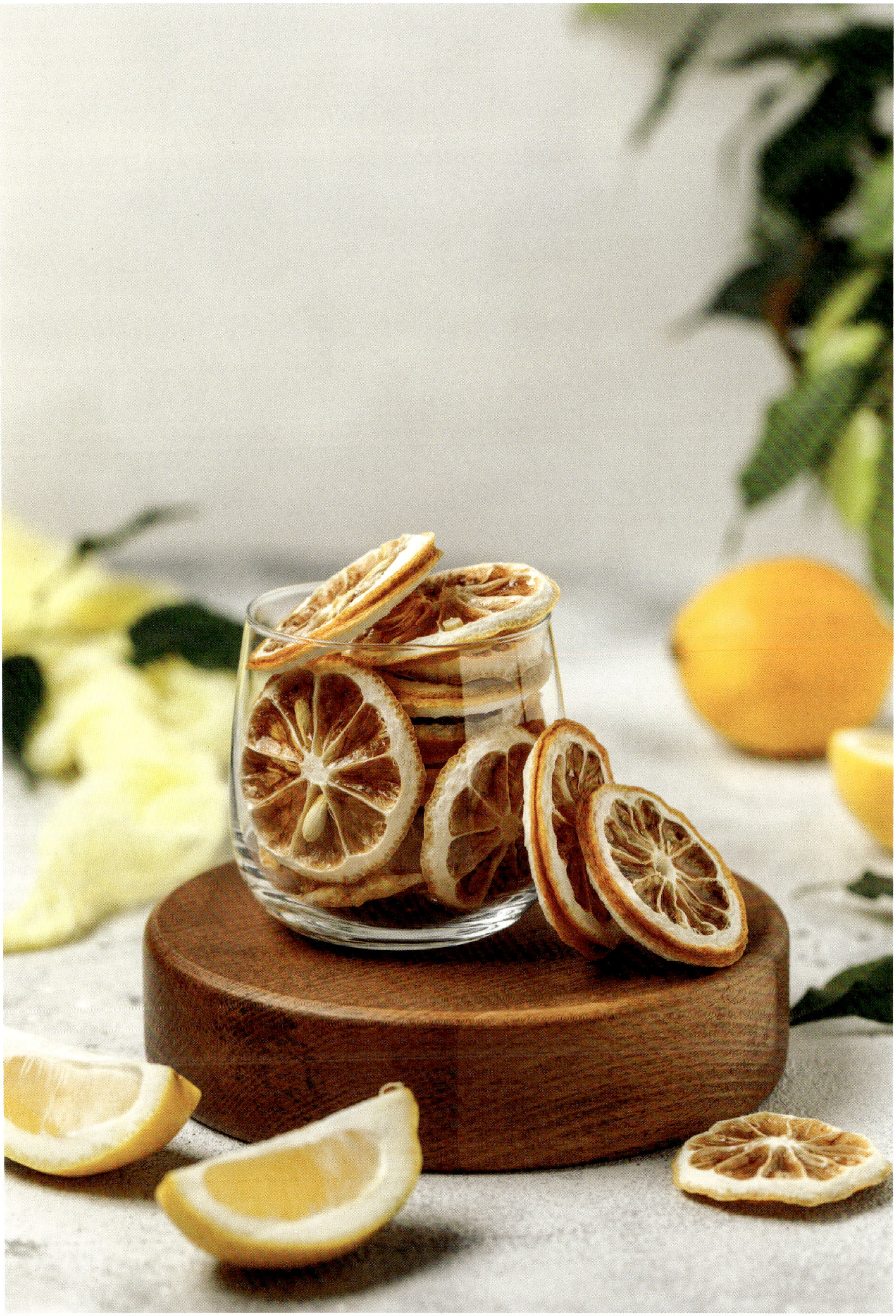

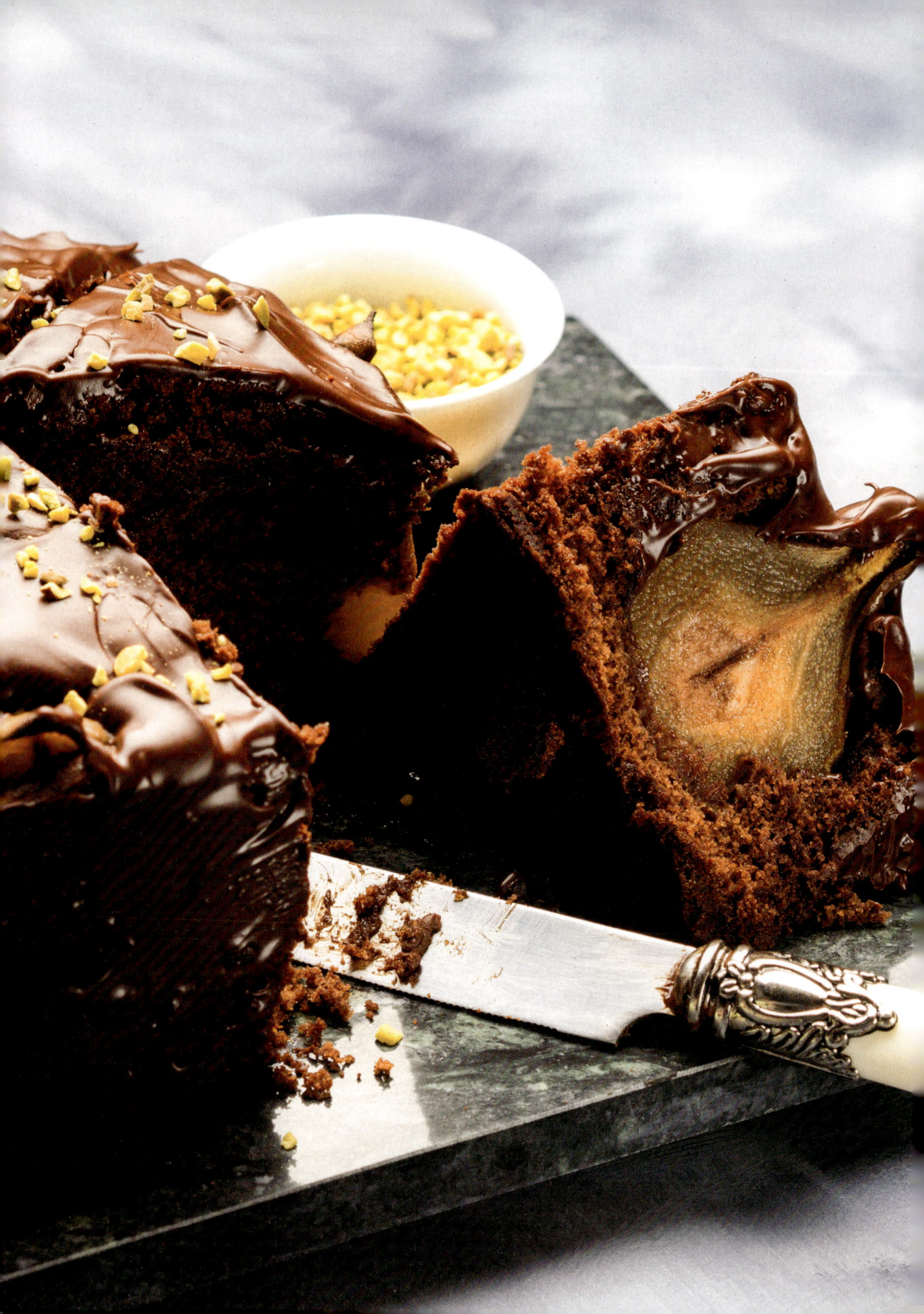

Poached Pear Chocolate Cake

SERVES 8
PREP + COOK TIME: 1 HOUR 30 MINS + COOLING

PEARS

6-8 Beurre Bosc pears, depending on how many can fit in your cake tin

4 cups (1L) water

1½ cups (330g) sugar

1 tsp cinnamon

1 tsp ground nutmeg

2 cardamon pods, crushed

1 tsp vanilla extract

CAKE

1¼ cups (155g) plain flour

⅓ cup (35g) cocoa powder

1 tsp bicarbonate of soda

½ tsp salt

⅔ cup (140g) sugar

1 large egg, room temperature

115g unsalted butter, melted

1 tsp pure vanilla extract

CHOCOLATE GANACHE

¾ cup (125g) dark chocolate chips

⅓ cup (80ml) thickened cream

2 tbsps chopped pistachios

Peel the pears and keep them whole. Place them straight into a large pan with water, sugar, cinnamon, nutmeg, cardamon and vanilla. Bring to a boil and simmer for about 20 minutes until soft. Remove the pears with a slotted spoon and set aside.

Bring the liquid to a boil. Cook until reduced by about a third, leaving at least 1¼ cups. Set aside.

Preheat oven to 175°C. Grease and line a 23cm round cake tin with greaseproof paper.

Whisk together flour, cocoa powder, bicarb and salt in a medium bowl.

Whisk together sugar, egg and melted butter in a large bowl until pale. Add 1 cup of reserved poaching liquid. Whisk to combine. Whisk in vanilla and flour mixture until combined. Pour batter into prepared tin, smooth top then place the pears bottom-side down in the batter.

Bake for 45-50 minutes until a toothpick inserted in the centre comes out clean. Set aside to cool.

To make the ganache, place chocolate into a bowl. Warm up the cream and 1 tablespoon poaching liquid in a small saucepan on the stove until simmering. Pour hot cream mixture over chocolate and let it sit for a minute. Stir until the chocolate is melted and the mixture is smooth.

Spread ganache on top of cake, letting it drip down the sides. Sprinkle with chopped pistachios and let stand for 30 minutes until ganache is set,

Christmas Fruit Cake

SERVES 10-12
PREP + COOK TIME: 3 HOURS 15 MINS + COOLING

250g butter
1kg mixed dried fruit
1½ cups (330g) firmly packed brown sugar
½ cup (125ml) brandy
½ cup (125ml) water
½ tsp bicarbonate of soda
2 tsps orange zest
1 tsp lemon zest
⅓ cup (40g) walnuts, chopped
450g treacle
5 eggs, beaten
2 cups (250g) plain flour
½ cup (60g) self-raising flour

Preheat oven to 140°C. Grease and line the base and sides of a deep 23cm round cake tin, to 5cm above edge of tin.

Place butter, fruit, sugar, brandy and water in a large saucepan over a high heat and bring to the boil. Stir well and then reduce heat and simmer, covered, for 10 minutes. Add bicarb then stir, cover and allow to cool.

Add orange and lemon zest, walnuts, treacle, eggs and flours to cooled mixture and stir well to combine. Spread evenly into prepared tin.

Place in the oven and bake for 2¾ hours.

When cooked remove from the oven and cover tightly with foil. Allow to cool in tin.

Gingerbread Shapes

MAKES 20
PREP + COOK TIME: 35 MINS PLUS CHILLING

110g butter
½ cup (100g) dark brown sugar
¼ cup (90g) honey
1 tsp vanilla extract
1 egg
2½ cups (315g) flour
½ tsp salt
½ tsp cinnamon
1 tsp ground ginger
¼ tsp ground cloves
1 tsp bicarbonate of soda

ICING
1 cup (155g) icing sugar
1-2 tbsps milk

In a large bowl cream together butter, sugar, honey and vanilla extract. Add the egg and mix to combine.

In another bowl whisk together flour, salt, spices and bicarb. Add to the butter and sugar mixture and stir until the dough comes together to form a ball. Cover with plastic wrap and refrigerate for 30 minutes.

Preheat oven to 180°C. Line two baking trays with greaseproof paper.

Roll out the dough between two sheets of greaseproof paper to 3mm thickness. Cut the dough into various shapes using cookie cutters. Re-roll the scraps and cut out more shapes.

Place the gingerbread onto the prepared baking trays, leaving a little space between each one. Bake for 7-10 minutes until darker and crisp around the edges. Allow to cool completely.

Combine icing sugar with milk. Spoon the icing into a piping bag and decorate the gingerbread shapes.

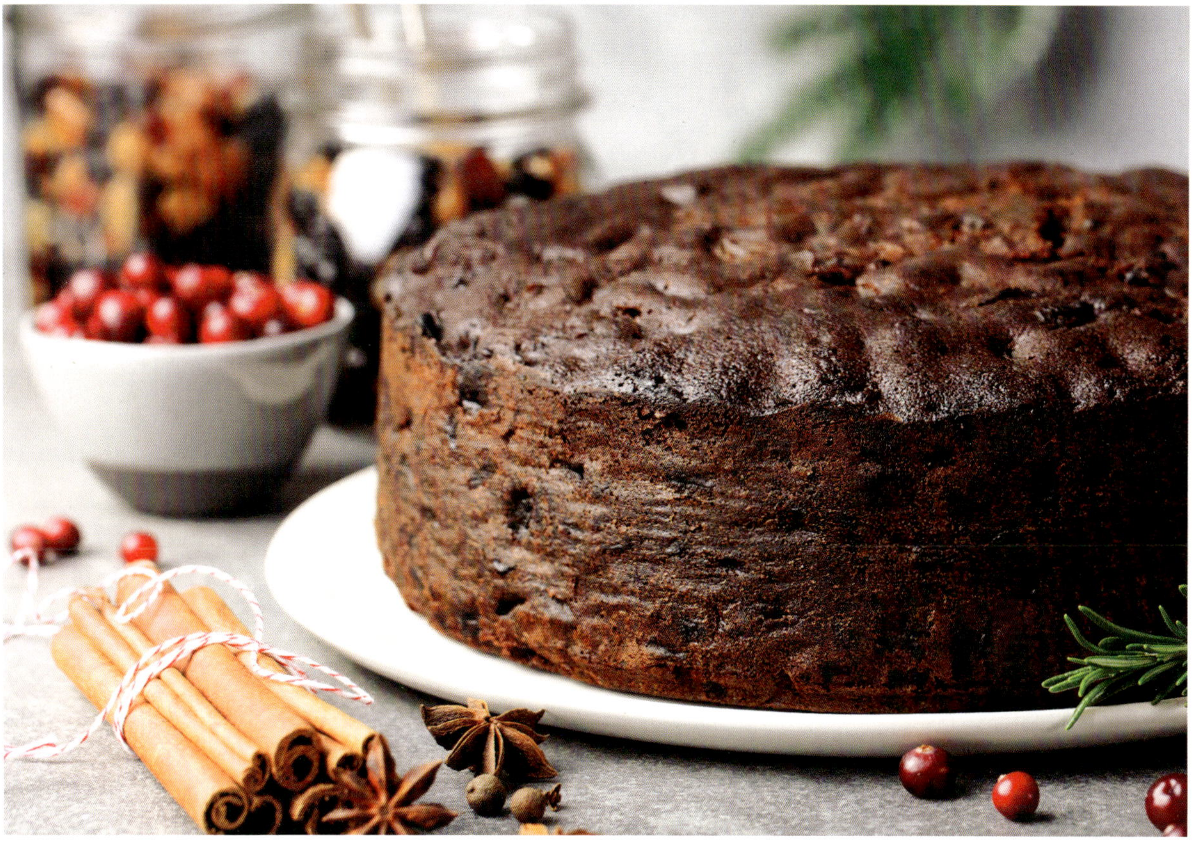

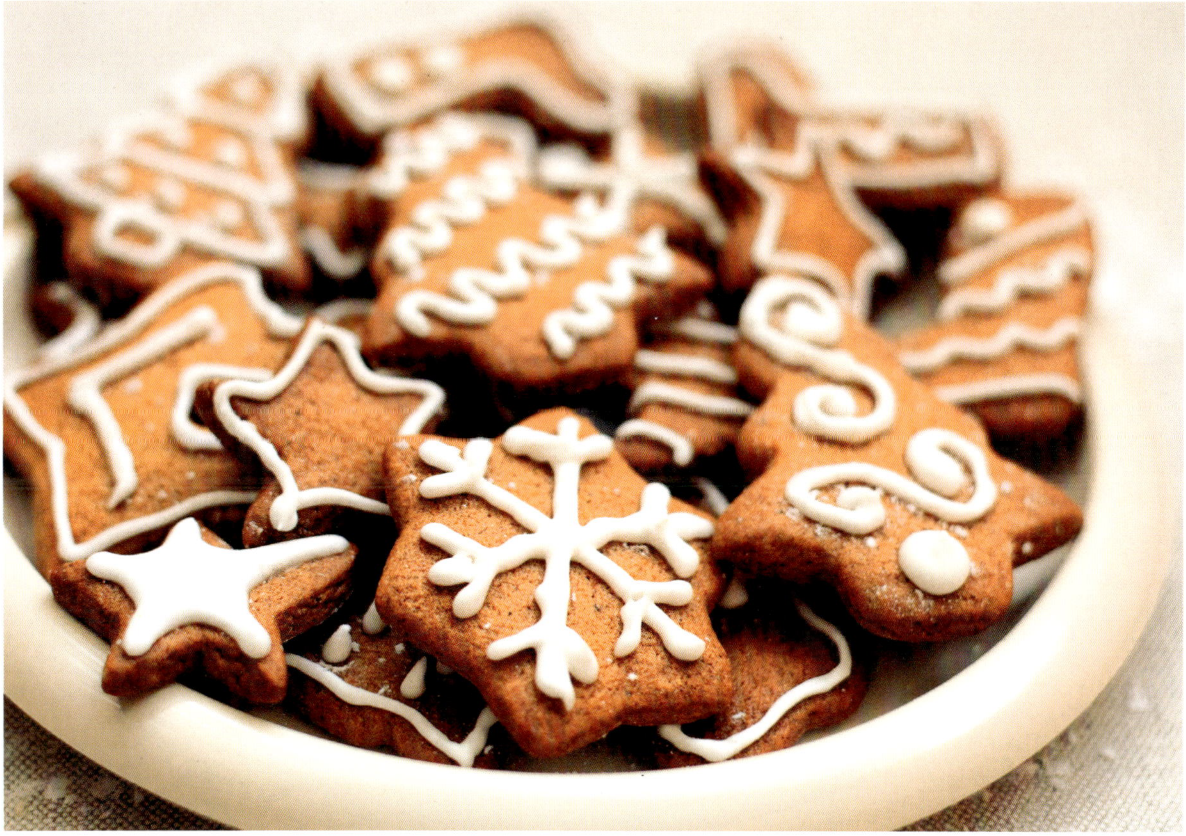

8

Savoury

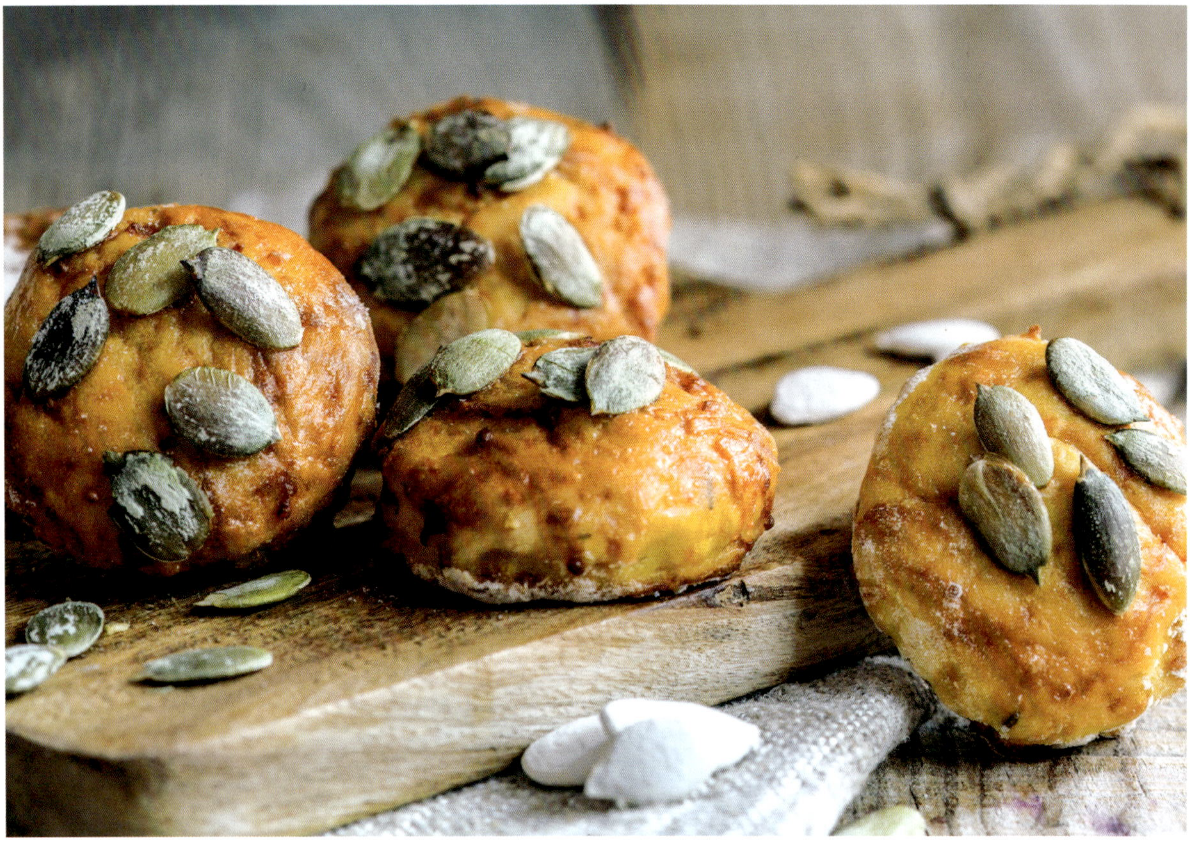

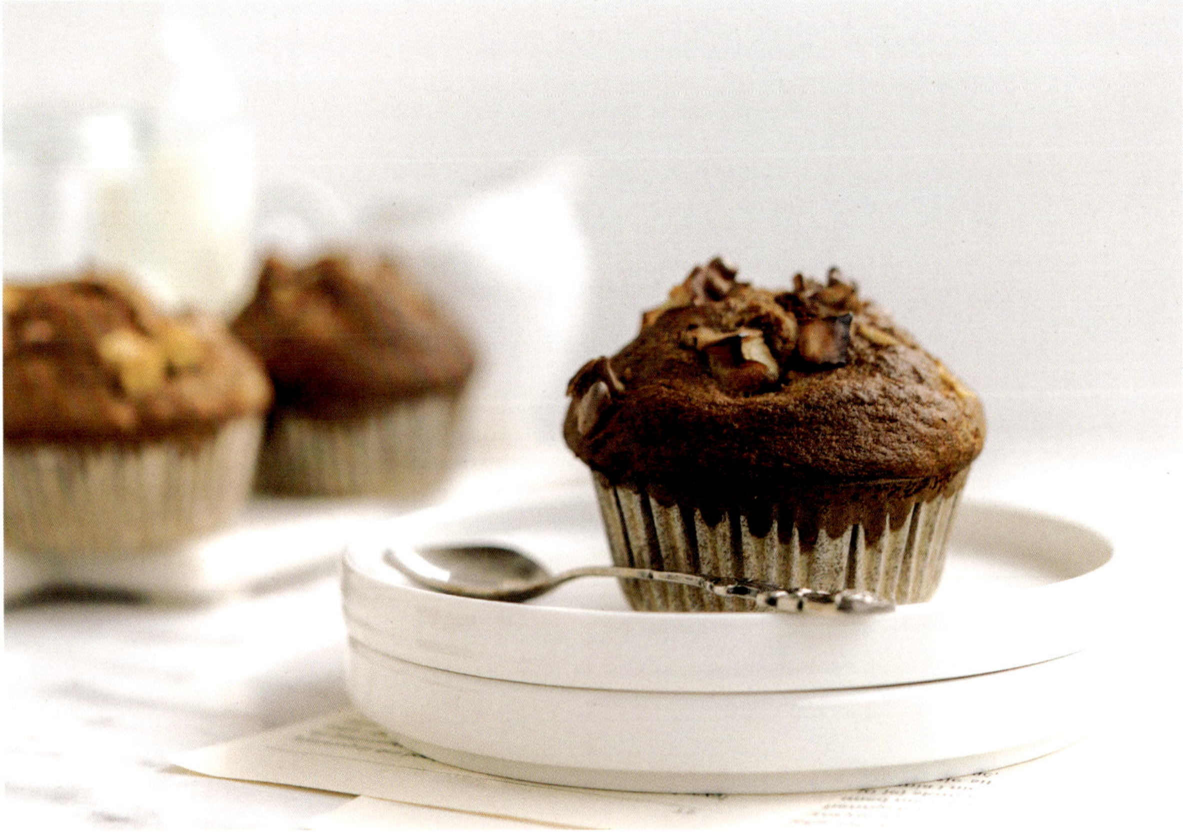

Pumpkin Rolls

MAKES 15
PREP + COOK TIME: 50 MINS + 2 HOURS PROVING

½ cup (110g) mashed cooked pumpkin
½ cup (125ml) full-cream milk, room temperature
60g butter, softened
1 large egg
2 tsps instant yeast
1 tsp salt
2½ cups (310g) plain flour
1 tbsp melted butter
¼ cup (30g) toasted pumpkin seeds (optional)

In a large bowl, add mashed pumpkin, milk, butter, egg, yeast and salt and whisk to combine. Add flour and stir well to combine until there is no dry flour visible in the bowl.

Transfer the dough onto a clean and lightly greased surface. The oil will help keep the dough from sticking. Knead the dough until it is smooth and not sticky.

Transfer the kneaded dough back into the bowl. Lightly brush the dough with oil and cover the bowl with a tea towel. Let it rise for 1 hour or until it has doubled in size.

Transfer the dough onto a clean surface and deflate by punching the air out. Roll the dough into a log and divide it into 15 equal pieces with a knife. Cover the dough with a damp cloth or plastic wrap to prevent it from drying out. Take one piece at a time and shape each piece into a smooth ball.

Transfer the dough balls to a baking tray lined with greaseproof paper. Cover the baking tray with aluminium foil and let the rolls rise for 1 hour. The rolls should almost double in size.

Preheat the oven to 190°C. Bake for 20 minutes, or until the tops are golden brown. Lightly brush with melted butter and top with toasted pumpkin seeds, if desired. Let the rolls cool on a wire rack for 15 minutes before serving.

Pumpkin Carrot Muffins

MAKES 12
PREP + COOK TIME: 35 MINS

1½ cups (185g) plain flour
1 tsp bicarbonate of soda
1 tsp cinnamon
½ tsp salt
2 eggs
½ cup (125ml) milk
1 cup (225g) mashed cooked pumpkin
⅓ cup (80ml) oil
½ cup (110g) sugar
¼ cup (50g) brown sugar
1 tsp vanilla
1 cup (110g) grated carrot
½ cup (60g) chopped walnuts + extra for topping
½ cup (60g) chopped apple for topping

Preheat oven to 180°C and line a 12-hole muffin tin with paper cases. In a medium bowl, whisk together flour, bicarb, cinnamon and salt. Set aside.

In another bowl, whisk together eggs, milk, pumpkin, oil, sugars and vanilla. Pour wet ingredients into dry ingredients. Fold in carrots and walnuts.

Spoon batter into muffin tin and fill each case almost to the top. Top with extra walnuts and apple pieces.

Bake for 22-25 minutes or until a toothpick comes out clean. Allow to cool before serving.

Zucchini Cheese Loaf

SERVES 10
PREP + COOK TIME: 1 HOUR 15 MINS

1½ cups (340g) zucchini, grated
2 cups (250g) plain flour
2 tsps baking powder
½ tsp bicarbonate of soda
½ tsp salt
1 cup (250ml) milk
1 tbsp apple cider vinegar
3 tbsps butter, melted
1 egg
1 cup (125g) grated Cheddar cheese
½ cup (50g) grated Parmesan cheese
½ cup (20g) chopped basil leaves

Preheat oven to 175°C. Grease and line a 23cm loaf tin with greaseproof paper.

Wrap grated zucchini in a clean tea towel and squeeze out excess liquid.

In a large bowl, combine flour, baking powder, bicarb and salt.

In a small bowl, combine milk and vinegar. Stir together until the milk curdles slightly. Mix in melted butter and egg.

Add milk mixture to dry mixture and stir until just combined. Add grated zucchini, cheeses and basil. Fold to combine.

Pour batter into prepared tin and bake for 1 hour until a skewer inserted in the centre comes out clean.

Cool for 10 minutes in the pan before transferring to a wire rack to cool completely.

Walnut & Carrot Loaf

SERVES 10
PREP + COOK TIME: 1 HOUR 30 MINS

1¼ cups (155g) + 1 tbsp plain flour
1½ tsps baking powder
1½ tsps cinnamon
½ tsp salt
½ cup (80g) golden raisins
½ cup (60g) walnuts, coarsely chopped
3 large eggs
1 cup (220g) sugar
1 cup (250ml) vegetable oil
2 tsps vanilla extract
2 cups (220g) coarsely grated carrot

Preheat oven to 175°C. Grease and line a 23cm loaf tin.

Whisk 1¼ cups flour, baking powder, cinnamon, and salt in a small bowl.

In another bowl toss raisins and walnuts with remaining 1 tablespoon flour.

Using an electric mixer, beat eggs and sugar in a medium bowl until light and fluffy. With mixer running, gradually drizzle in the oil, then add vanilla. Fold in dry ingredients, raisin mixture and carrots. Scrape batter into prepared pan.

Bake for 65-75 minutes until a skewer inserted in the centre of the cake comes out clean.

Let cool in pan for 10 minutes before turning out onto a wire rack to cool completely.

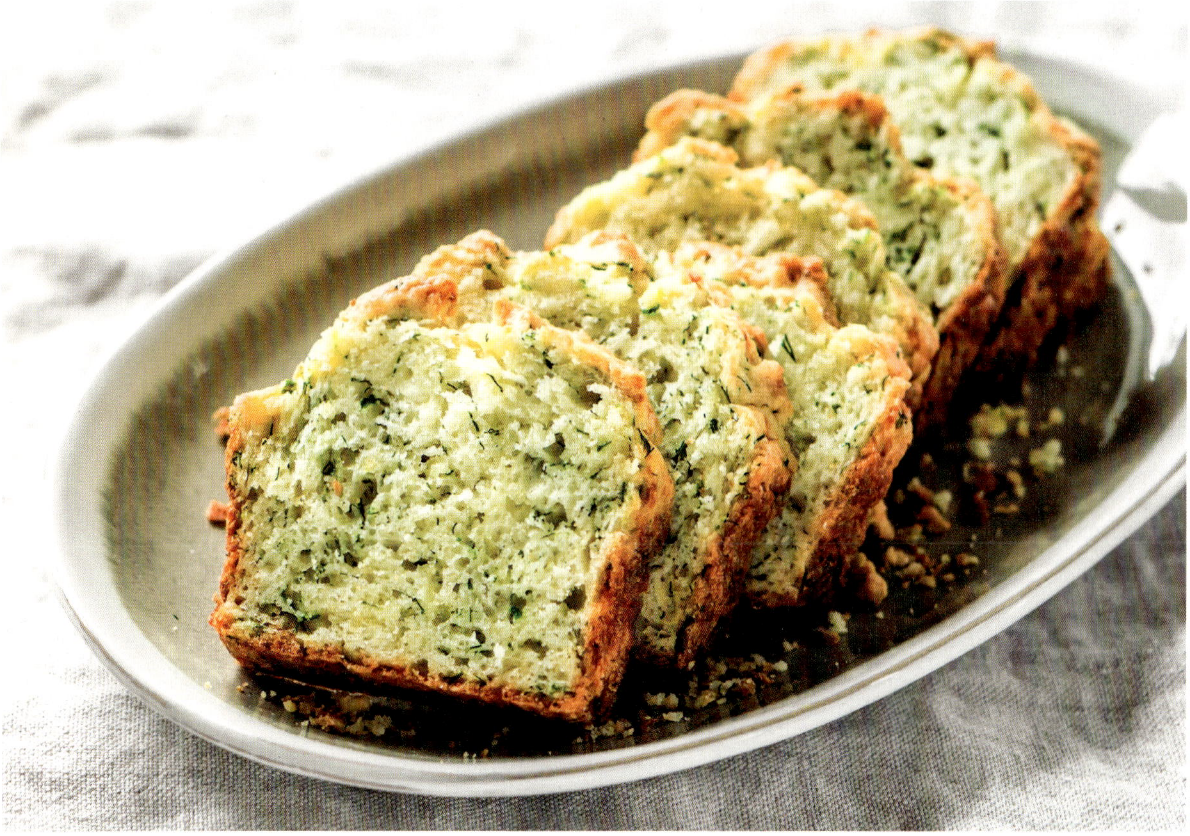

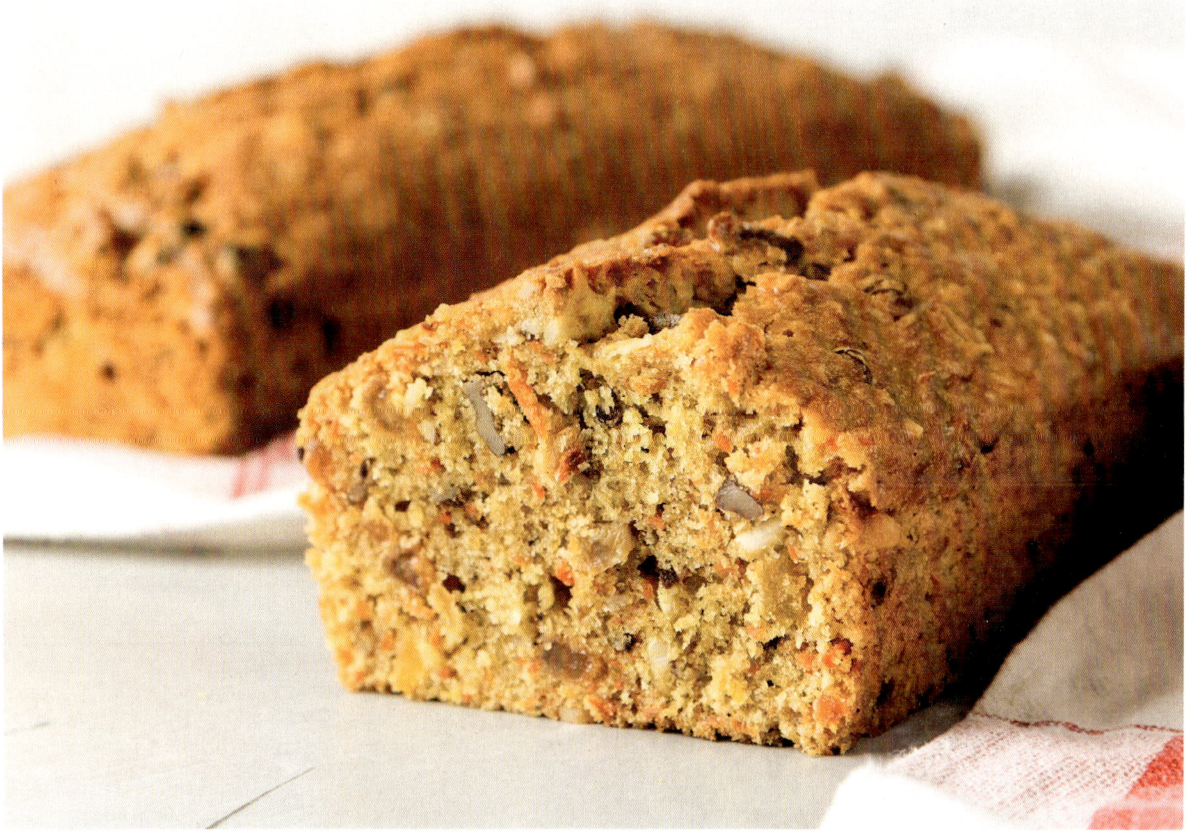

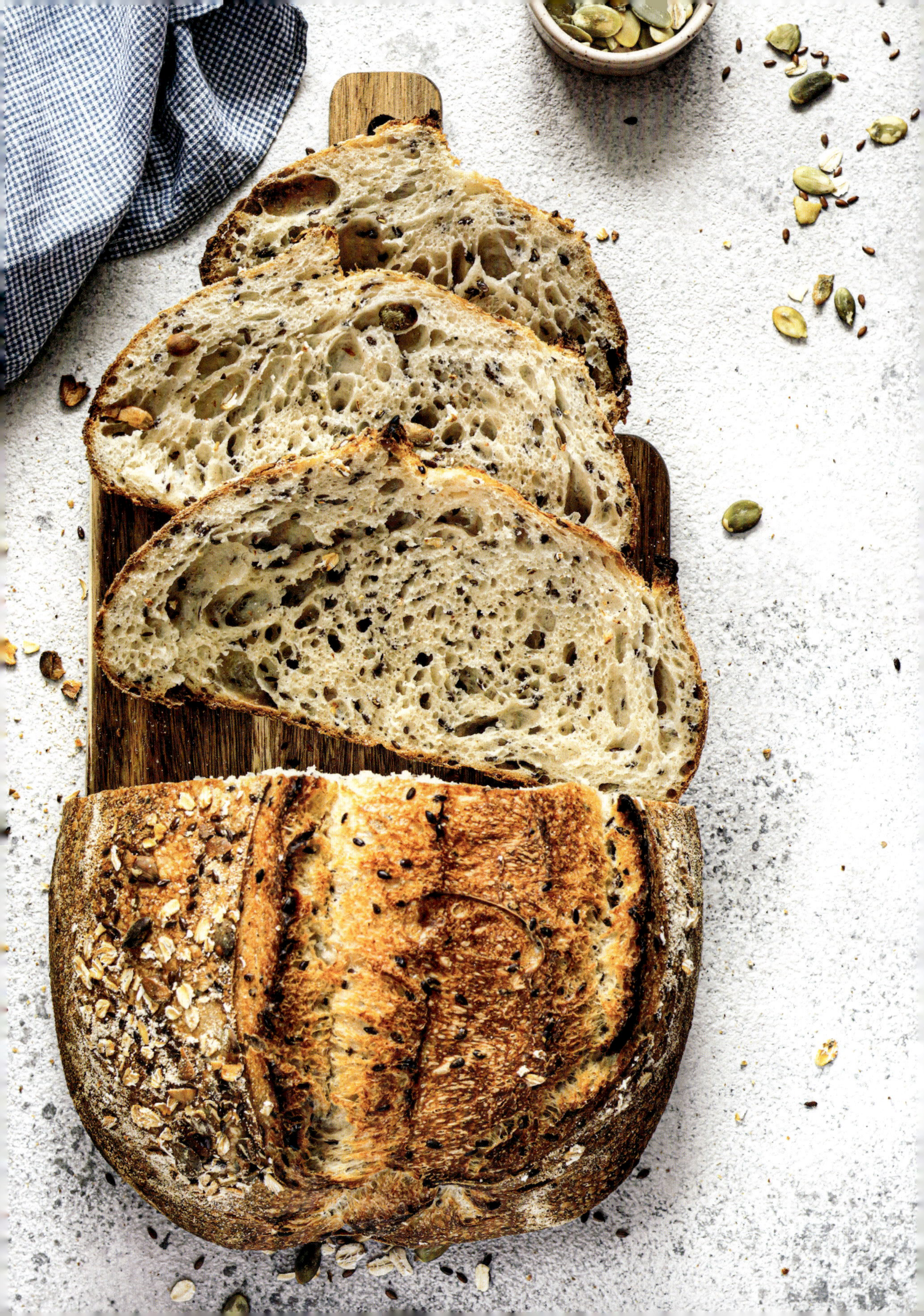

Seeded Sourdough Bread

MAKES 2 LOAVES
PREP + COOK TIME: 1 HOUR + FERMENTATION + OVERNIGHT PROVING
DAIRY FREE

SEED MIX

3 tbsps pumpkin seeds
3 tbsps sunflower seeds
3 tbsps rolled oats
2 tbsps red quinoa, rinsed
2 tbsps flaxseed
¾ cup (185ml) hot water at about 65°C

DOUGH

¼ cup (60ml) sourdough starter, previously fed, bubbly and active (see recipe on page 218)
1⅓ cups (330ml) lukewarm water
2½ tbsps maple syrup
3 cups (375g) bread flour
½ cup (60g) + 1 tbsp whole wheat flour
2 tsps fine sea salt

Add the seed mix to a bowl with the hot water and set aside.

In the evening, whisk the starter, water and maple syrup together in a large bowl with a fork. Add the flours and salt. Mix with a fork until a shaggy dough forms, then use your hands to fold and push the dough until the flour is fully incorporated.

Cover bowl with a damp tea towel and set aside for 30 minutes.

Add the soaked seed mix to the dough. Knead and fold the dough to incorporate.

Cover bowl with a damp tea towel and set aside for 30 minutes.

Grab a portion of the dough while it remains in the bowl, stretch it up and fold it over, pressing your fingertips into the centre of the dough. Turn the bowl a quarter turn and repeat the stretch and fold. Repeat twice more, turning the bowl a quarter turn before stretching and folding.

Cover bowl with a damp tea towel and set aside for 30 minutes. Repeat the whole stretch and fold process, turning the bowl between each stretch. Then rest for another 30 minutes before stretching for a final four times.

Cover the bowl with a damp tea towel and allow to rise overnight at room temperature until doubled in size.

In the morning, transfer the dough onto a floured work surface.

Gently stretch the dough into a circle. Fold over the left side to the middle, then the right side to the middle, overlapping slightly. Gently press the fold down to seal them together to make a long oval shape.

Meanwhile, line an oval proving basket with a floured tea towel. Alternatively shape the dough into a large ball and line a large bowl with a floured tea towel. Scoop the dough up and place into the bowl or basket, bottom-side up. Sprinkle the bottom of the dough with a dusting of flour.

Cover with a damp tea towel and set aside for 30-45 minutes until puffy and risen slightly.

Preheat the oven to 260°C.

Line a Dutch oven big enough to fit your loaf with greaseproof paper.

Turn the dough out of the bowl or basket and place in the Dutch oven. Score the dough about 1cm deep and about 7cm long on the top. Cover with a lid and transfer to the oven. Reduce heat to 230°C. Bake for 20 minutes. Remove the lid and continue to bake for 30-35 minutes until dark golden brown.

Allow to cool on a wire rack for 1 hour before slicing.

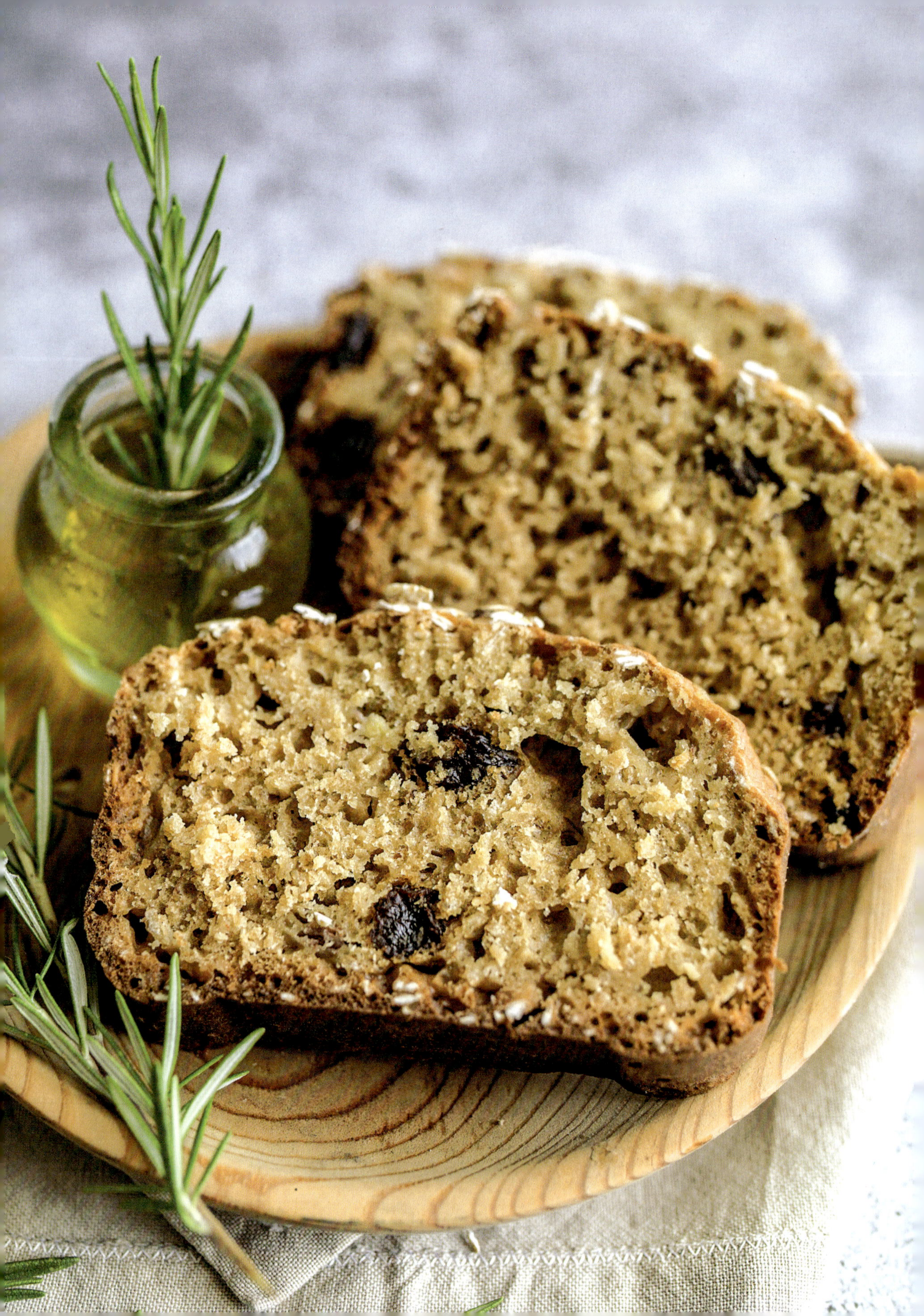

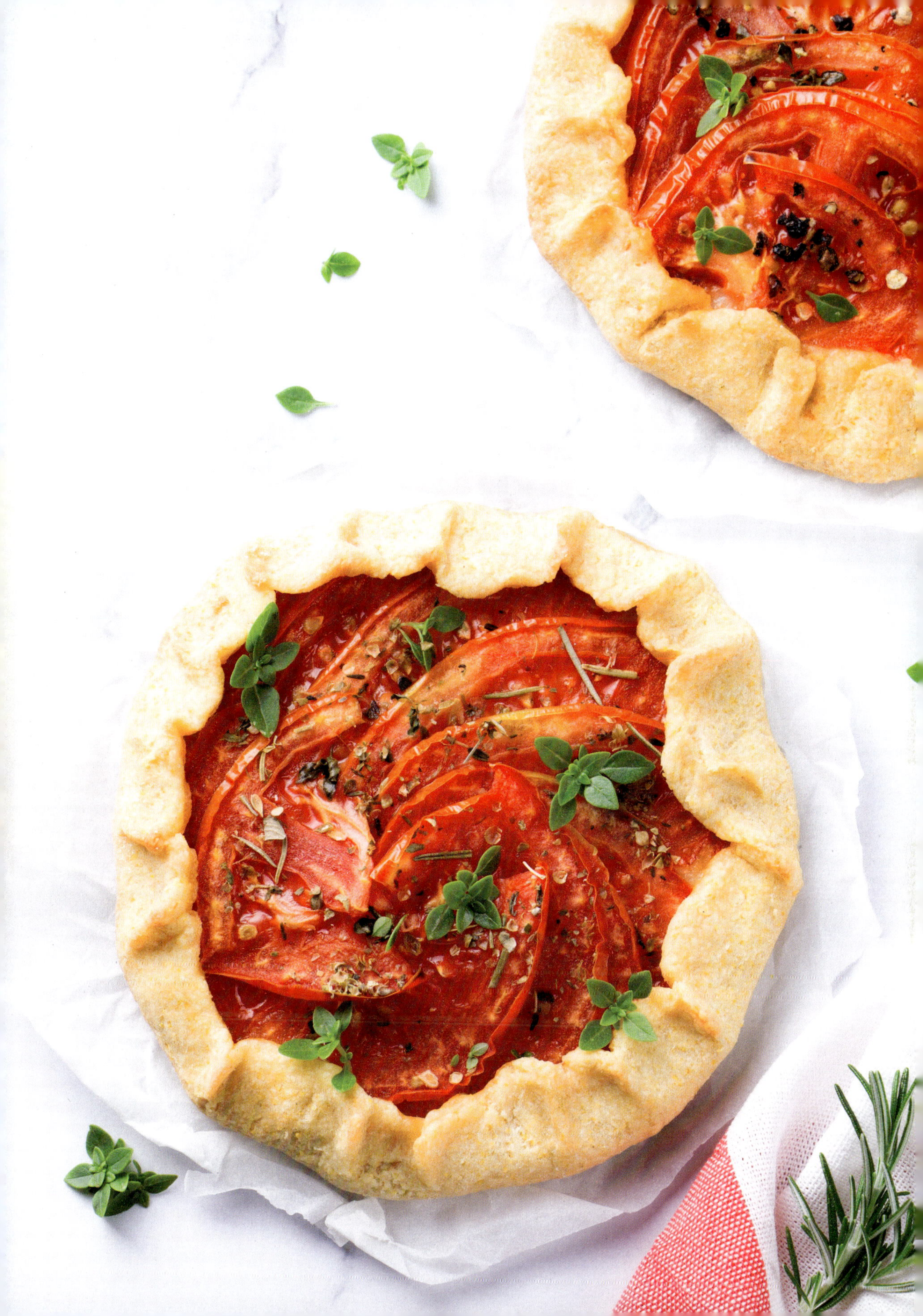

Oat & Raisin Loaf

SERVES 10
PREP + COOK TIME: 1 HOUR 15 MINS

1 cup (160g) raisins
1 cup (250ml) water
2 tbsps butter
1 cup (125g) plain flour
3 tsps baking powder
¼ cup (55g) sugar
¼ tsp salt
1 cup (90g) + 1 tbsps rolled oats
2 large eggs

Preheat the oven to 190°C. Grease and line a loaf tin with greaseproof paper.

Combine the raisins and water in a small saucepan. Place over medium heat for 3 minutes, or until the raisins are plump. Remove from the heat and stir in the butter until melted. Set aside to cool.

In a large bowl, sift together the flour, baking powder, sugar and salt. Add 1 cup oats and stir to combine together.

Add the eggs to the cooled raisin mixture and whisk to combine. Pour the raisin mixture into the dry ingredients and stir to incorporate.

Pour the mixture into the loaf tin and sprinkle with the remaining tablespoon of oats. Bake for 45-55 minutes or until a skewer inserted in the centre comes out mostly clean. Cool in the tin for 10 minutes before transferring to a wire rack to cool completely.

Tomato Galette

SERVES 2-4
PREP + COOK TIME: 1 HOUR 10 MINS

500g beef tomatoes, sliced ½cm thick
2 cloves garlic, thinly sliced
Flaky salt and pepper
2 sheets frozen shortcrust pastry, defrosted
1 cup (125g) grated mature Cheddar cheese
1 tsp dried Italian herbs

Preheat oven to 200°C. Line two baking trays with greaseproof paper. Toss tomatoes, garlic and 1 teaspoon salt in a bowl. Let sit 5 minutes, then drain off liquid. Cut a 24cm circle out of each sheet of pastry. Scatter cheese over pastry circles, leaving a 3cm border on each. Arrange tomatoes and garlic over cheese. Scatter with dried herbs. Fold edges of pastry up and over filling, overlapping as needed. Season with salt and pepper. Bake for 50-60 minutes until golden brown.

Sourdough Starter

MAKES 1 CUP
PREP + COOK TIME: 6 DAYS
DAIRY FREE

1 cup (125g) whole wheat flour or rye flour
½ cup (125ml) filtered water per feeding
½ cup (60g) organic white bread flour per feeding

Place whole wheat flour and ½ cup water in a large jar. Mix well and cover loosely with a lid. Sit at room temperature for 24-48 hours until bubbles appear. Discard all but ½ cup mixture. Feed with ½ cup organic white bread flour and ½ cup filtered water.

Cover loosely with a lid and set at room temperature for 24 hours. Repeat the process of discarding, feeding and resting each day for the next 4 days. After the fifth feeding, rest for 12 hours before discarding and feeding once more, then rest just until very bubbly, then use.

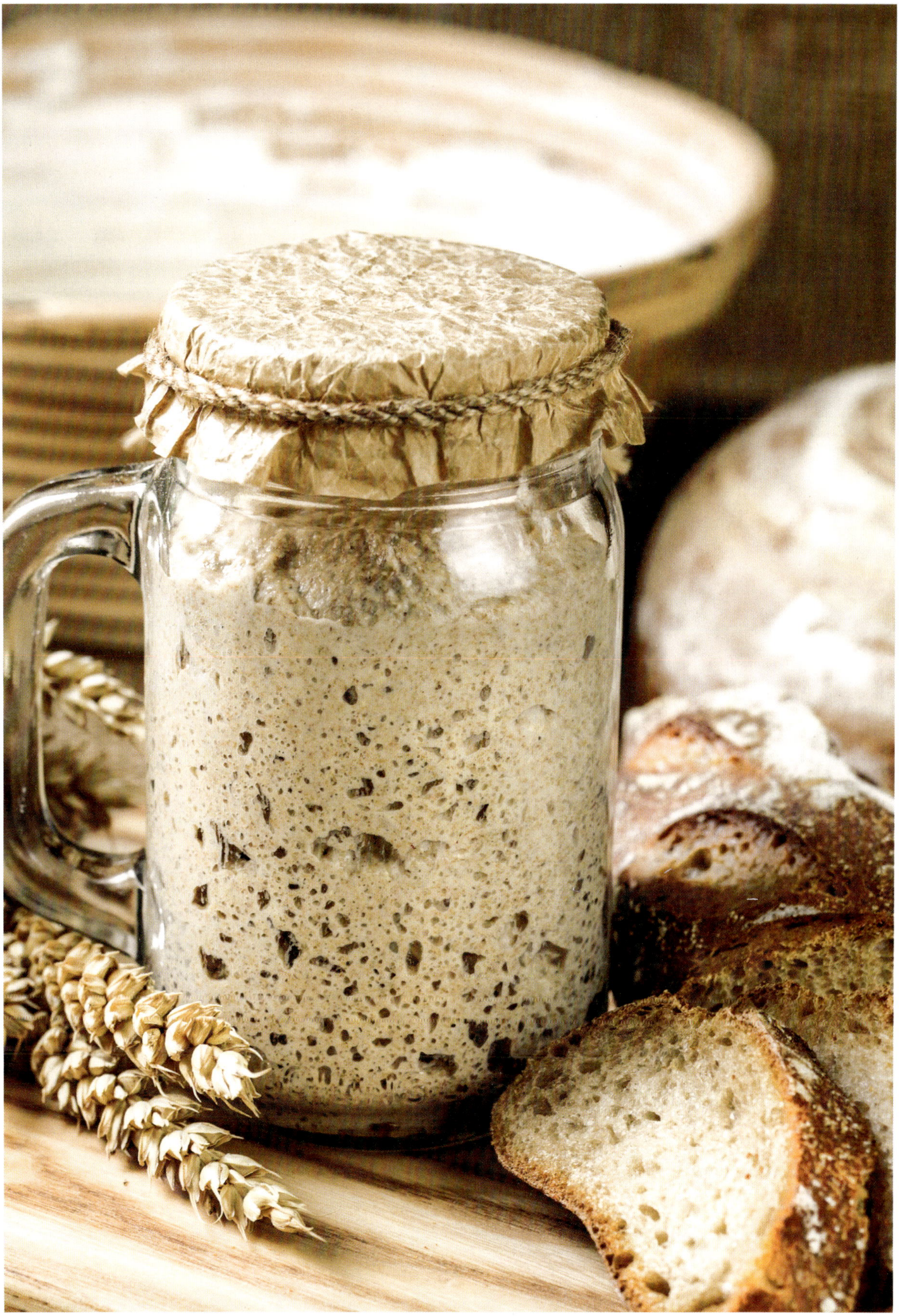

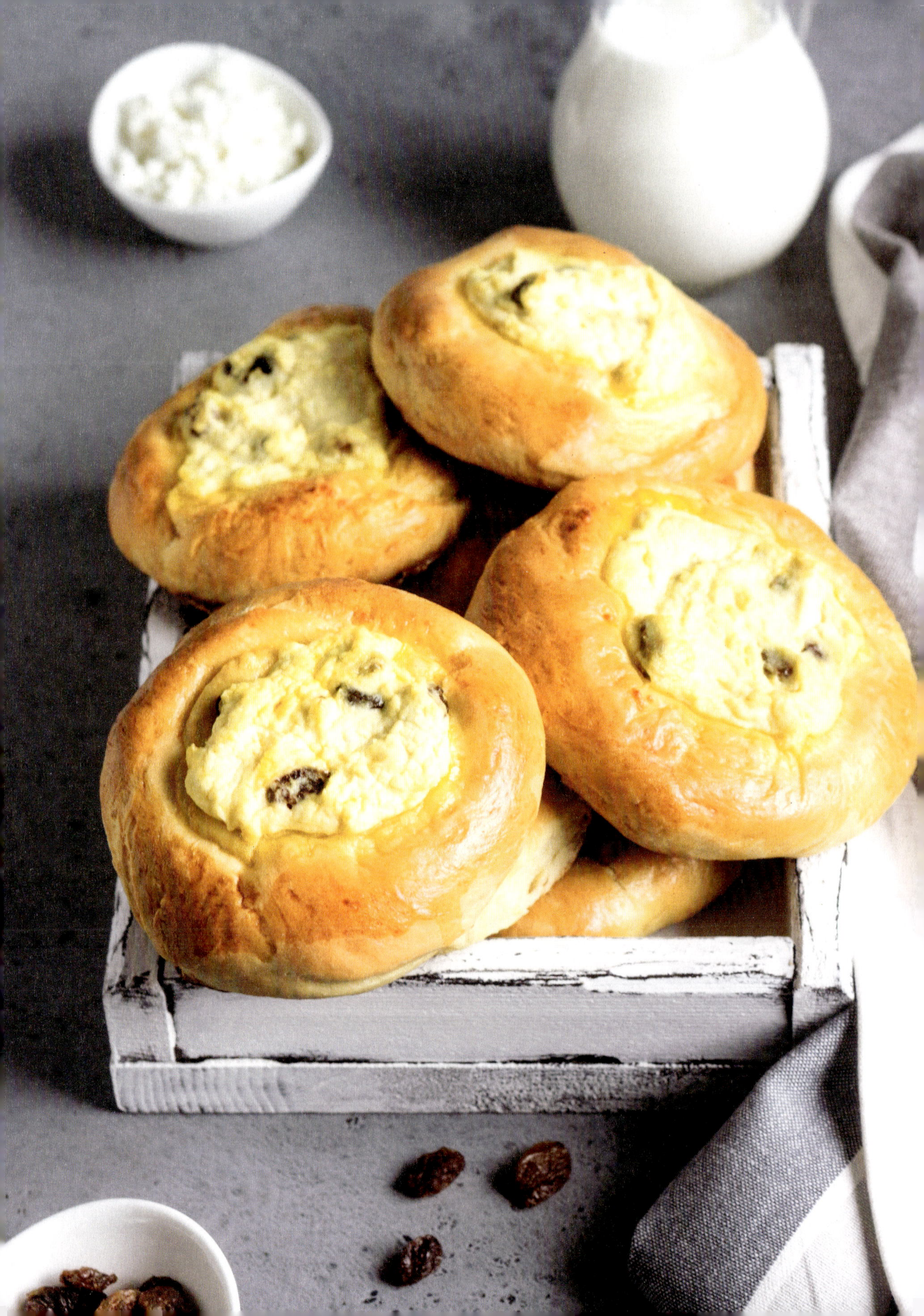

Cottage Cheese Yeast Buns

MAKES 12
PREP + COOK TIME: 1 HOUR + 1 HOUR PROVING

21g fresh yeast, crumbled
¾ cup (175g) sugar
¾ cup (200ml) milk, lukewarm
3⅔ cups (450g) plain flour, sifted
2 eggs
50g butter, melted
1 tbsp sunflower oil

FILLING
400g cottage cheese
⅓ cup (75g) sugar
⅓ cup (50g) raisins
2 tsps vanilla extract
1 egg
¼ tsp salt

In a large bowl combine fresh yeast, 1 tablespoon of sugar, warm milk and 2 tablespoons of flour. Mix thoroughly. Set aside for 15 minutes in a warm place.

In another large bowl combine the remaining sugar and one egg. Beat with an electric mixer until light and fluffy. Add the butter and oil and beat to combine. Add the yeast mixture and stir with a wooden spoon to combine. Add the remaining flour a little at a time, stirring between each addition.

Transfer the dough to a lightly floured work surface and knead for 5-7 minutes until smooth and elastic. Transfer to a lightly greased bowl and cover with a tea towel. Set aside in a warm place for 60-90 minutes until doubled in size.

Preheat the oven to 180°C. Line two baking trays with greaseproof paper.

Punch the dough down then divide the dough into 12 equal pieces. Roll each piece of dough into a ball. Transfer balls to lined baking trays leaving 5cm between each one. Use the bottom of a bowl or cup to slightly indent the centre of each bun. Cover with a tea towel and set aside for 10 minutes.

Meanwhile combine cottage cheese, sugar, raisins, vanilla, egg and salt. Mix thoroughly.

Fill each bun with approximately 2 tablespoons of cottage cheese mixture. Brush the buns with beaten egg.

Transfer to the oven and bake for 20-25 minutes until golden brown.

Brazilian Cheese Bread

SERVES 6
PREP + COOK TIME: 40 MINS
GLUTEN FREE

- ⅓ cup (80ml) olive oil
- ½ cup (125ml) water
- ⅓ cup (80ml) milk
- 1 tsp salt
- 2 cups (230g) tapioca flour
- 1 cup (100g) grated Parmesan cheese
- 2 eggs, beaten

Preheat the oven to 190°C. Line a baking tray with greaseproof paper.

Combine olive oil, water, milk and salt in a large saucepan and place over high heat. Bring to a boil and immediately remove from the heat.

Stir in tapioca flour straight away, stirring until smooth. Set aside to rest for 10-15 minutes.

Stir cheese and eggs into tapioca mixture until combined; the dough will be chunky, like cottage cheese.

Drop dough in ¼ cup-size balls onto the baking tray.

Bake in the oven until the tops are lightly browned, 15-20 minutes.

Cheese & Herb Soft Bread

SERVES 12
PREP + COOK TIME: 1 HOUR 10 MINS + PROVING

- 3¼ cups (400g) plain flour + more as needed
- 1 tsp salt
- 2½ tbsps sugar
- ½ cup (125ml) water, lukewarm
- ½ cup (125ml) + 1 tbsp milk, room temperature
- ¾ tbsp instant yeast
- 60g unsalted butter, melted + 2 tbsps butter, room temperature
- 1½ cups (150g) grated Parmesan cheese
- ½ tsp garlic powder, or 2 tsps fresh garlic
- ¼ cup (10g) chopped fresh herbs or 1 tbsp dried herbs
- Sesame seeds for topping

In a mixing bowl combine flour, salt and sugar. In a large measuring jug, combine water and milk and whisk in yeast until dissolved. Add this mixture, along with the melted butter, to the dry ingredients. Mix until combined. Let dough rest for 5 minutes.

Transfer dough to a lightly floured surface and knead for a couple of minutes, adding more flour only if the dough is sticking, then form dough into a ball. Place dough in a lightly oiled bowl, cover with plastic wrap and allow to sit at room temperature until doubled in size.

Grease a 20 x 10cm loaf tin and set aside. Dust dough with flour and roll out into a rectangle 25 x 40cm in size. Spread the softened butter over the surface of the dough. Sprinkle evenly with Parmesan, garlic and herbs. Press lightly to press the toppings into the butter. Starting with the shortest side, roll dough up and pinch the seam together.

Lift dough into the loaf tin, cover with greased plastic wrap and allow to rise until the dough is about 2½cm above the side of the tin. Preheat oven to 180°C. Bake for 45-50 minutes (cover with foil if browning too quickly).

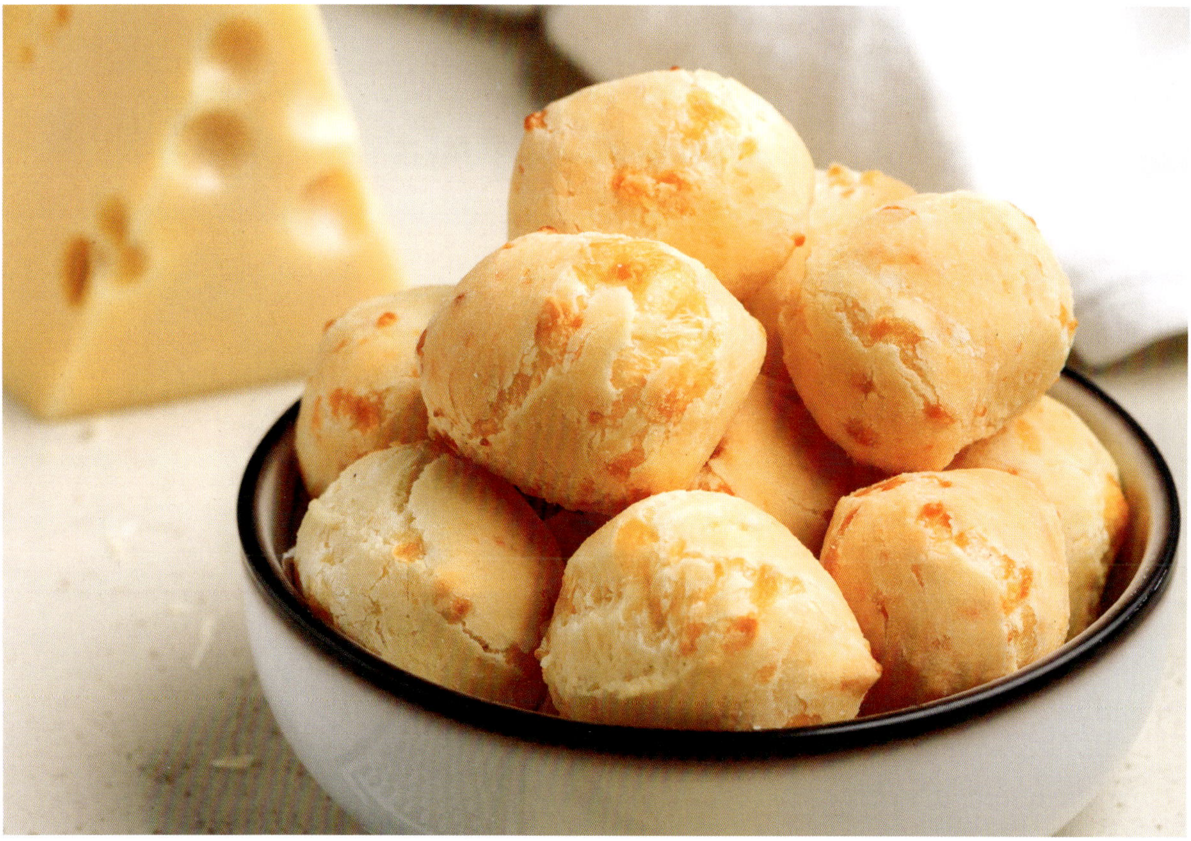

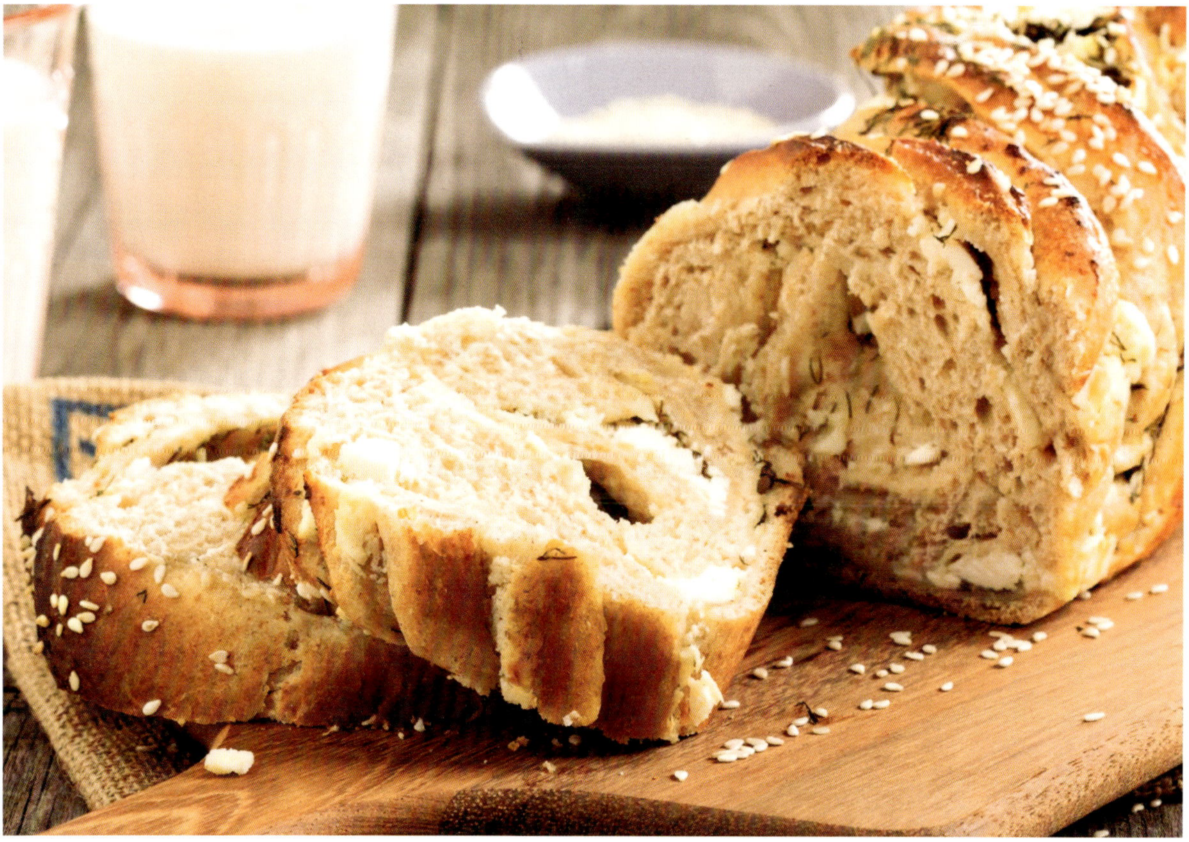

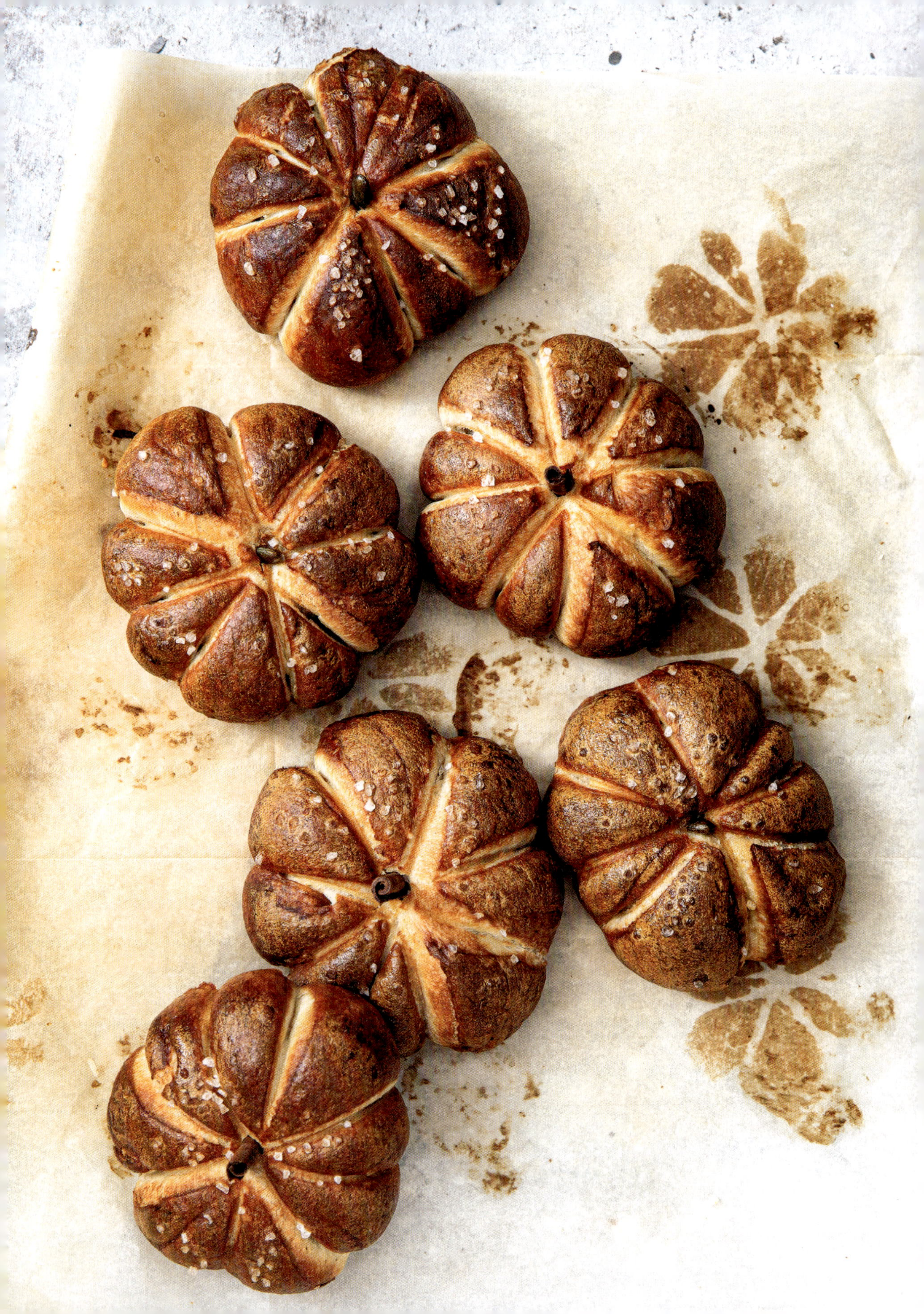

Pumpkin-Shaped Dinner Rolls

MAKES 12
PREP + COOK TIME: 2 HOURS 20 MINS + PROVING

1 cup (250ml) milk, warmed
2¼ tsps (1 packet) active dry yeast
1 tbsp honey + more to taste
4 tbsps melted butter
1 tsp fine salt
3 cups (375g) plain flour + more as needed
Kitchen string
Vegetable oil
Flaky salt
12 x 3cm pieces of cinnamon stick, 12 pumpkin seeds or 12 x 3cm pieces of pretzel stick (for stalks)

Place warm milk, yeast, honey and melted butter in a bowl. Stir to combine. Add fine salt and flour. Stir using a wooden spoon until a sticky dough forms.

Transfer to a floured work surface. Knead the dough until smooth and elastic, adding more flour if needed. Form dough into a ball and place in a lightly greased bowl, cover with a tea towel and let rise in a warm place for 60-90 minutes until doubled in size.

Meanwhile, cut some kitchen string into 48 strands, each 20cm long. Place strings in a bowl and toss with vegetable oil to coat. Set aside.

Punch dough down then transfer to a floured work surface. Cut dough in half and cut each half into six wedges. Roll each wedge into a round ball. Cover with a tea towel and let rest for 15 minutes.

Preheat the oven to 190°C. Line two baking trays with greaseproof paper.

Place four pieces of string on your work surface. Criss-cross strings over a centre point into a star formation. Place a dough ball, smooth-side down, onto the centre point. Firmly tie each string into a knot over the centre of the roll. Snip off excess string with kitchen scissors.

Place tied roll onto a prepared baking tray knot-side up. Repeat with remaining strings and dough balls. Let rolls rise for 30 minutes.

Sprinkle the rolls with flaky salt then transfer to the oven. Bake for 20-25 minutes until dark golden brown.

Remove from the oven and let cool until safe to handle. Cut strings off each roll at the tops then peel down slowly and carefully to remove the string. Cut a small hole in the tops of each roll with a small sharp knife. Press a cinnamon quill, pumpkin seed or pretzel stick into each hole to make the stems.

Serve warm or cold.

Parmesan & Herb Popovers

MAKES 12
PREP + COOK TIME: 45 MINS

1 cup (250ml) milk

2 large eggs

2 tbsps butter, melted

1 cup (125g) plain flour

¼ tsp salt

½ cup (50g) grated Parmesan cheese

1 tsp finely chopped thyme

1 tsp finely chopped rosemary

Preheat oven to 230°C. Grease a 12-hole muffin tin with butter. When the oven is fully heated, place the muffin tin in the oven for 10 minutes.

In a medium bowl, whisk together the milk, eggs, melted butter, flour and salt until well combined. Add Parmesan and herbs and stir to incorporate.

Scrape the batter into a jug. Remove the tin from the oven and carefully pour the batter evenly among the prepared muffin cups, filling the cups about half full. Remember the tin is hot.

Return the tin to the oven and bake for about 15 minutes. Reduce the oven temperature to 200°C and continue baking for 15 minutes more, or until popovers are puffed and browned. Remove from pan immediately and serve hot.

Spinach & Cheese Parcels

MAKES 8
PREP + COOK TIME: 50 MINS

250g cream cheese, cut into 3cm pieces

2 large eggs

2 cloves garlic, chopped

¼ tsp dried oregano

Salt and pepper to taste

300g frozen spinach, thawed and thoroughly pressed dry

½ cup (120g) crumbled feta

¼ cup (25g) finely grated Parmesan cheese

2 sheets frozen puff pastry, thawed

Preheat oven to 200°C. Line two baking trays with greaseproof paper.

Place the cream cheese pieces in a wide, microwave-safe bowl. Microwave in 10-second bursts until the cream cheese is very soft and melty but not steaming hot. Stir in 1 egg, garlic and oregano and season with salt and pepper.

In a separate bowl, combine the spinach, feta and Parmesan with a fork. Add the cream cheese mixture and stir well to combine.

Cut each pastry sheet into four squares. Place 2 tablespoons of the spinach mixture onto the centre of each square. Brush edges with water. Bring the four points of each puff pastry square together towards the centre so that they cover the filling, then lightly press them together in the middle.

Beat the remaining egg in a small bowl. Brush pastry with egg.

Place the parcels on the baking trays and bake for 25-30 minutes or until golden and cooked through.

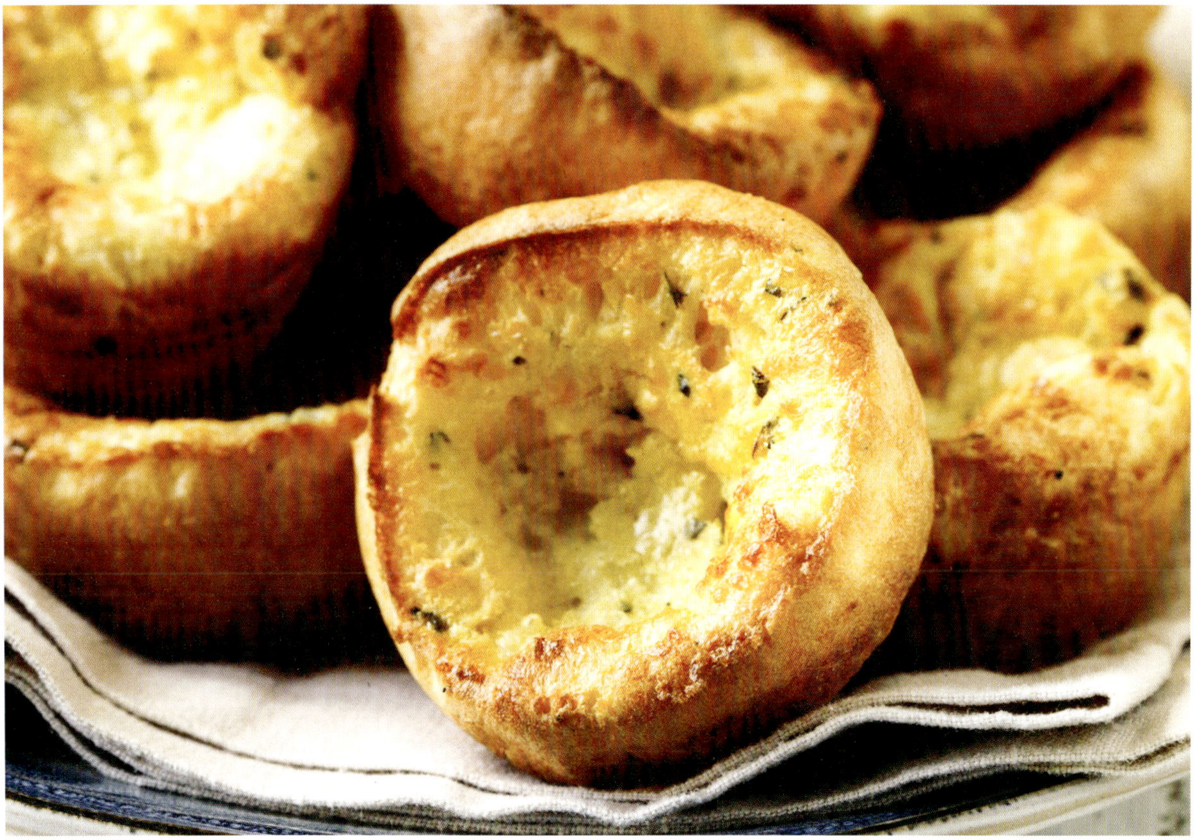

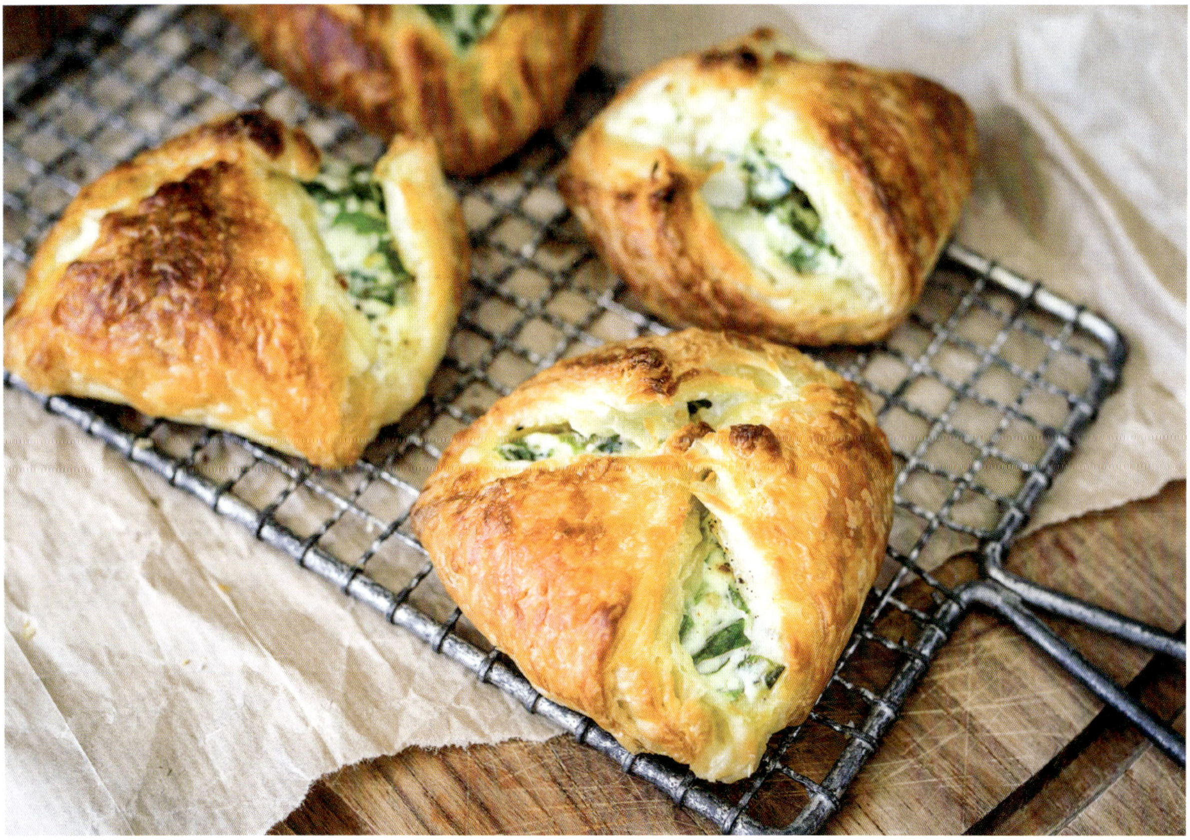

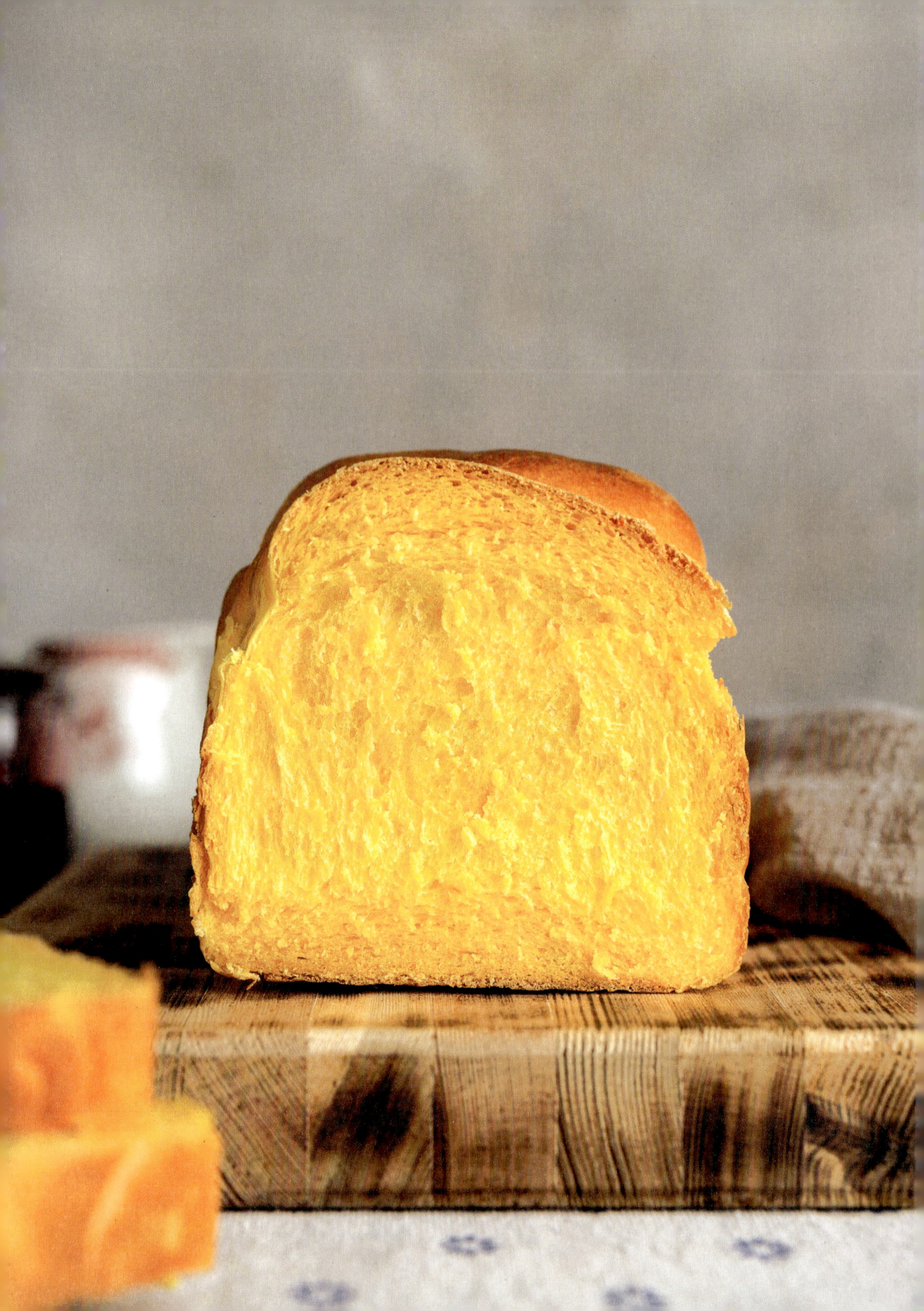

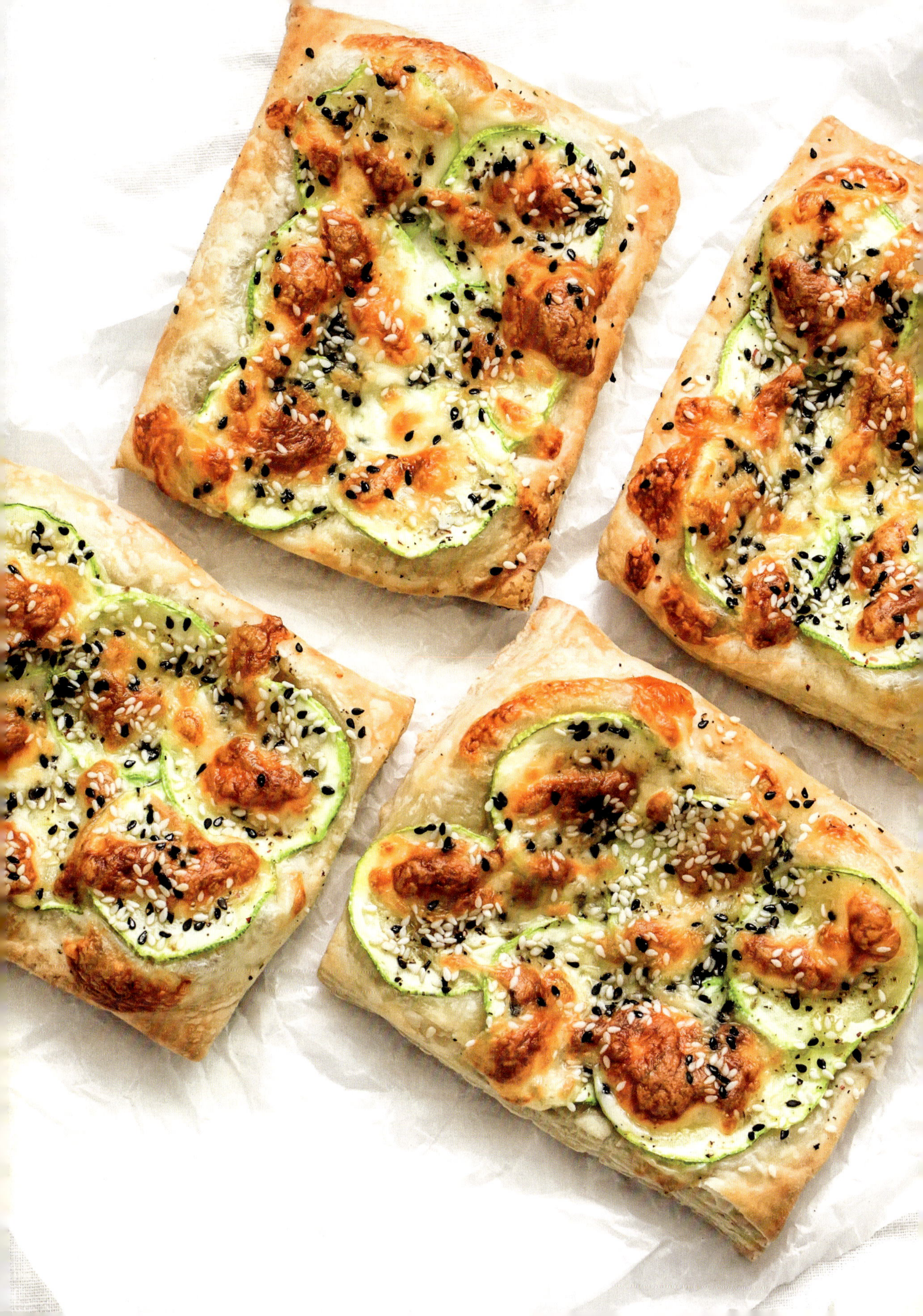

Carrot Bread

SERVES 10
PREP + COOK TIME: 1 HOUR 30 MINS + 2 HOURS PROVING
DAIRY FREE

1¾ cups + 3 tbsps (480g) bread flour, sifted
2 tsps instant yeast
4 tbsps sugar
1½ tsps salt
2 cups (220g) finely grated carrots
½ cup (125ml) water
2 tbsps light olive oil, melted coconut oil or avocado oil
1 egg, beaten

Mix the flour and yeast into the bowl of a stand mixer with dough hooks attached. Add sugar and salt then the finely grated carrots. Mix to combine. Add water a little at a time, mixing as you do so, until all the ingredients are just combined. Add the oil and continue to knead for 8-10 minutes, or until the dough pulls away from the bowl and forms a smooth, supple ball.

If you don't have a stand mixer you can mix by hand then knead for 8-10 minutes.

Transfer the dough to a lightly greased bowl. Cover and set in a warm place for about an hour until doubled in size.

Punch down the dough, then remove from bowl. Flatten into a rectangle then roll up into a loaf shape and place into a well-oiled loaf tin. Set aside in a warm place for another 40-60 minutes until puffy.

Preheat the oven to 180°C.

Brush the top of the loaf with beaten egg and bake for 15 minutes, then cover the bread with aluminium foil to prevent over-browning, and bake for an additional 10-15 minutes.

Allow the bread to cool in the tin for 10 minutes then turn out onto a wire rack to cool completely, before slicing and serving.

Zucchini Pizzas

SERVES 4
PREP + COOK TIME: 35 MINS

1 sheet frozen puff pastry, thawed
1 cup (125g) freshly grated mozzarella cheese
1 zucchini, very thinly sliced
Salt and pepper to taste
½ tsp garlic powder
¼ tsp dried chilli flakes
Zest of 1 lemon
2 tsps black and white sesame seeds

Preheat the oven to 220°C. Line a baking tray with greaseproof paper.

Cut the puff pastry sheet into four equal pieces and place on prepared baking tray. Cover pastry with half the mozzarella cheese then arrange the zucchini slices on top. Season with salt and pepper and sprinkle over garlic powder, chilli flakes and lemon zest. Cover with the remaining mozzarella. Scatter over the sesame seeds. Bake for 20-25 minutes until golden.

Spiced Almonds

SERVES 20
PREP + COOK TIME: 45 MINS
GLUTEN FREE

5 cups (625g) unsalted almonds
2 tbsps olive oil
¼ tsp chilli flakes
2 tsps dried rosemary
2 tsps smoked paprika
1 tsp pepper
½ tsp salt

Preheat oven to 150°C.

Place ingredients in a bowl and toss to coat. Spread in a single layer on a baking tray. Bake, stirring occasionally, for 30-40 minutes, until golden brown.

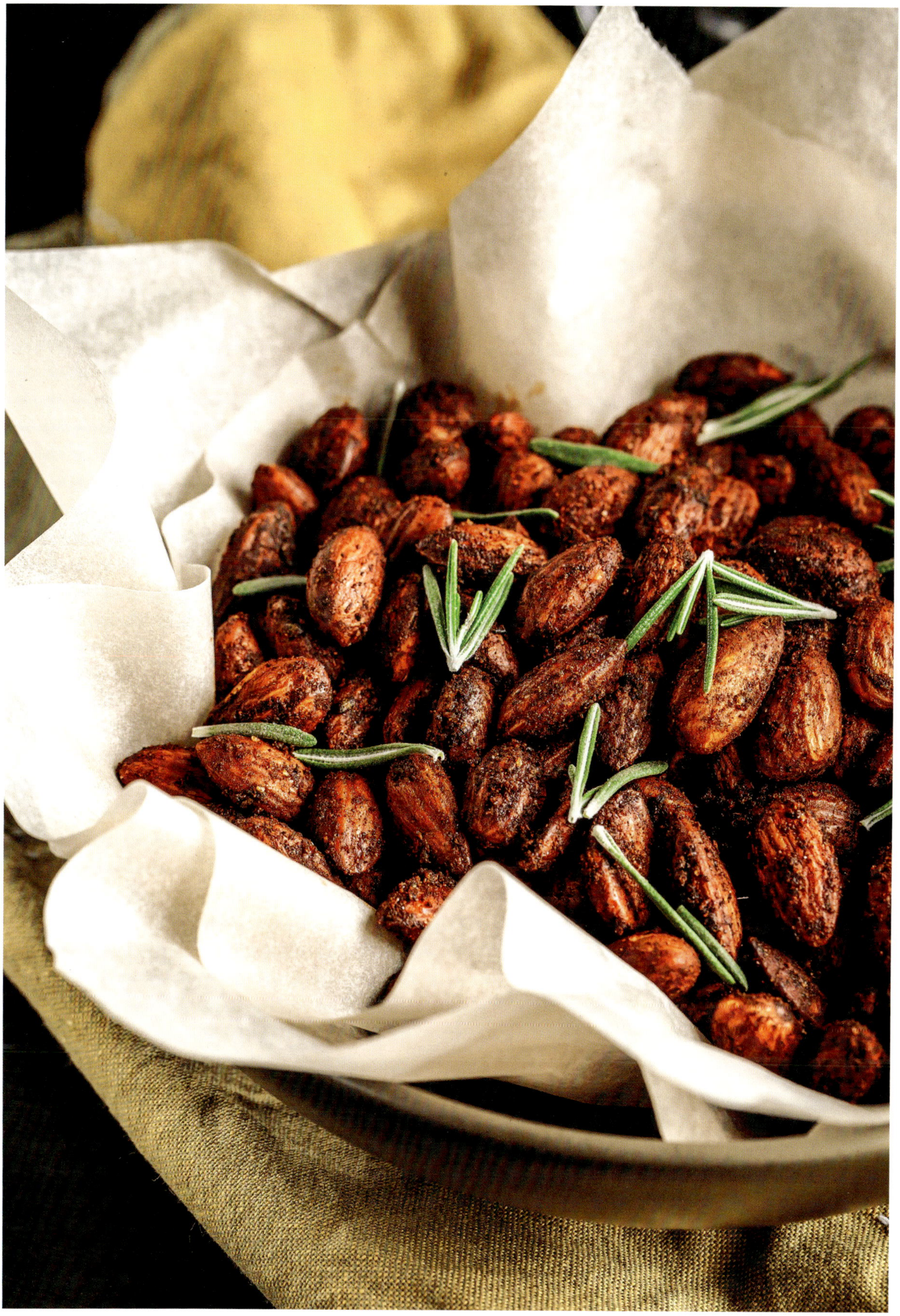

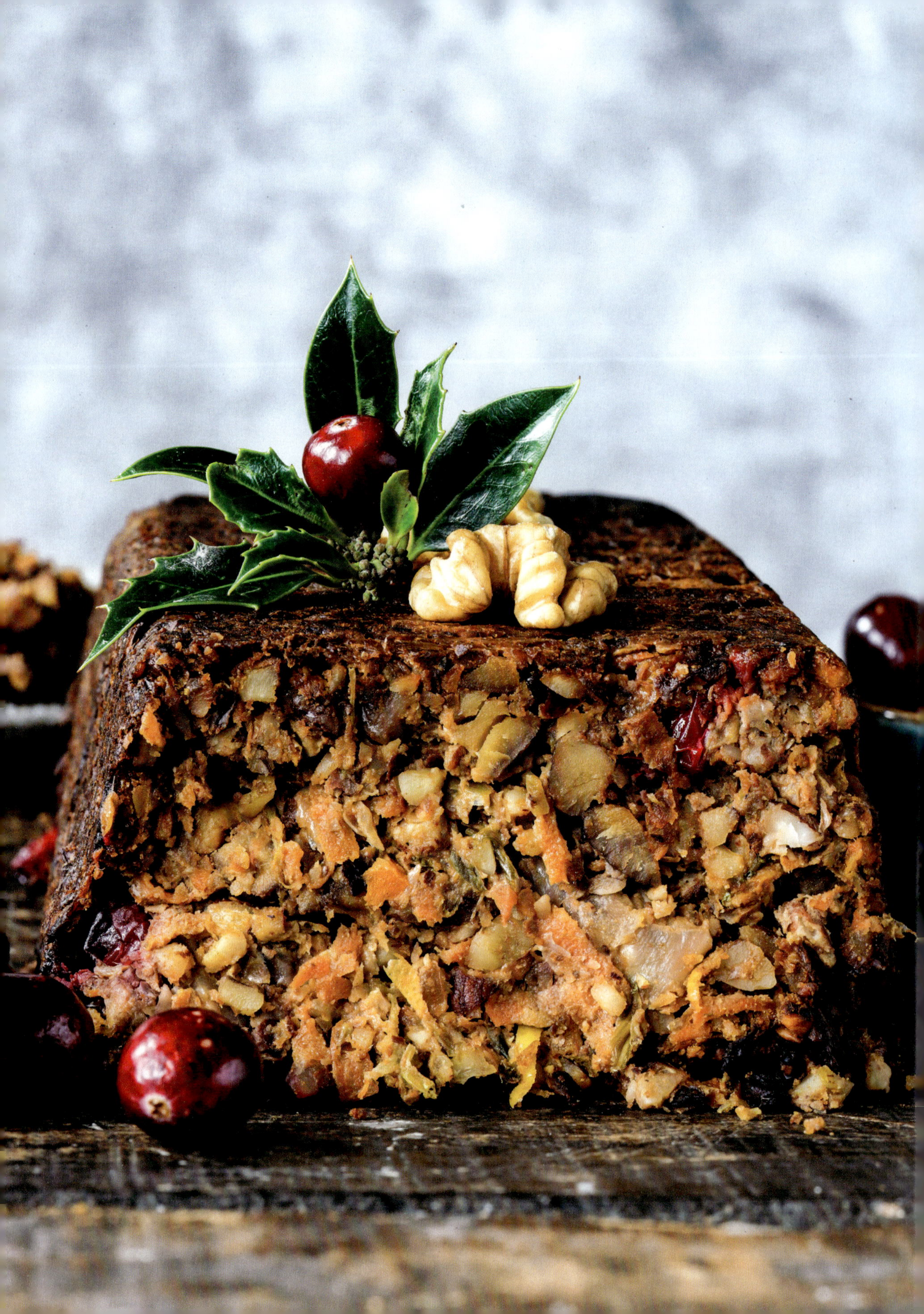

Lentil & Cranberry Nut Loaf

SERVES 8
PREP + COOK TIME: 1 HOUR 30 MINS
GLUTEN FREE

1 cup (200g) green or brown lentils, picked over and rinsed

4 cups (1L) water

Salt and pepper to taste

2 tbsps olive oil

1 small onion, peeled and diced

2 carrots, grated

300g baby bella mushrooms, finely chopped

5 cloves garlic, minced

3 tbsps chopped fresh sage

2 tbsps chopped fresh rosemary

1 tsp paprika

1 tsp dried thyme

300g mixed nuts, finely chopped

1 cup (140g) dried cranberries

Zest and juice (about ¼ cup) of 1 small orange

Zest of ½ a lemon

3 eggs, beaten

Combine the lentils, water and ½ teaspoon salt in a medium saucepan over medium-high heat. Bring to a vigorous simmer then reduce heat, cover and simmer gently for 20-30 minutes, until the lentils are completely tender. Drain and set aside.

Preheat the oven to 190°C. Line a 23cm loaf tin with enough greaseproof paper to overhang the sides by about 3cm.

Heat the olive oil in large frying pan over medium-high heat. Add the onion and carrot and saute for 7 minutes, stirring occasionally, until soft. Add the mushrooms and garlic and saute for 5 minutes, stirring occasionally, until the mushrooms soften and most of the liquid in the pan evaporates. Add the sage, rosemary, paprika and thyme. Cook for 1 minute, stirring frequently, until fragrant. Remove pan from heat.

In a large mixing bowl, add the cooked lentils, cooked vegetables, nuts, cranberries, orange zest and juice and lemon zest. Stir well to combine. Season to taste with salt and pepper.

Transfer about one-third of the mixture to a food processor and pulse a few times until the mixture forms a rough puree. Stir the pureed mixture back into the bowl with the remaining mixture. Add the eggs and stir well to combine.

Press the mixture into the prepared tin, packing it down quite firmly.

Bake uncovered for about 45 minutes, or until the top is lightly browned and the loaf is cooked through.

Transfer the tin to a wire rack and let the loaf rest for 15-20 minutes. Carefully lift the edges of the greaseproof paper to remove the loaf from the tin. Slice with a sharp knife to serve.

Olive & Sun-Dried Tomato Muffins

MAKES 12
PREP + COOK TIME: 40 MINS

2 cups (250g) plain flour
1½ tsps baking powder
½ tsp bicarbonate of soda
½ tsp salt
1 large egg
1 cup (250ml) milk
¼ cup (60ml) sour cream
¼ cup (60ml) olive oil
1 clove garlic, minced
2 cups (250g) grated Cheddar cheese
75g feta, crumbled
⅔ cup (95g) pitted black olives, sliced
½ cup (30g) sun-dried tomatoes, sliced

Preheat oven to 180°C. Line a 12-hole muffin tin with paper liners.

Whisk flour, baking powder, bicarb and salt in a bowl.

In a separate bowl whisk together the egg, milk, sour cream, oil and garlic. Pour the wet ingredients into the dry ingredients and stir to incorporate. Fold in the grated cheese, feta, olives and sun-dried tomatoes.

Divide evenly between the muffin cups.

Bake for 25 minutes or until the muffins are golden and firm on top and spring back when pressed in the centre.

Cool in the tin for 10 minutes before transferring to a wire rack. Serve warm or cold.

Garlic & Rosemary Focaccia

SERVES 12
PREP + COOK TIME: 1 HOUR + 1 HOUR PROVING
DAIRY FREE

½ cup (120ml) olive oil
2 cloves garlic, finely minced
1 tbsp chopped fresh thyme
1 tbsp chopped fresh rosemary
¼ tsp pepper
1 cup (235ml) water, warm
2¼ tsps active dry yeast (1 packet)
¼ tsp honey
2½ cups (325g) plain flour
½ tsp fine salt

Combine olive oil, garlic, thyme, rosemary and pepper in a small pan and place over low heat. Cook, stirring occasionally, for 5 minutes until fragrant. Remove from heat and set aside.

In a large bowl, combine the warm water, yeast and honey. Let sit for 5 minutes until frothy. Add 1 cup of flour and a ¼ cup of the garlic olive oil mixture. Stir to combine then let sit for another 5 minutes.

Stir in the remaining 1½ cups of flour and salt. Transfer to a floured work surface and knead until smooth.

Transfer dough to an oiled bowl, cover with a damp towel and set aside in a warm place for 1 hour to double in size.

Preheat oven to 230°C. Grease a large baking tray with a little of the garlic olive oil mixture.

Transfer the dough to the baking tray and shape into a large, flat oval. Use your fingers to dimple the dough then drizzle the top with the remaining garlic olive oil mixture. Let the dough rise for 20 minutes until it puffs slightly.

Bake for 15-20 minutes until golden brown. Serve warm or cold.

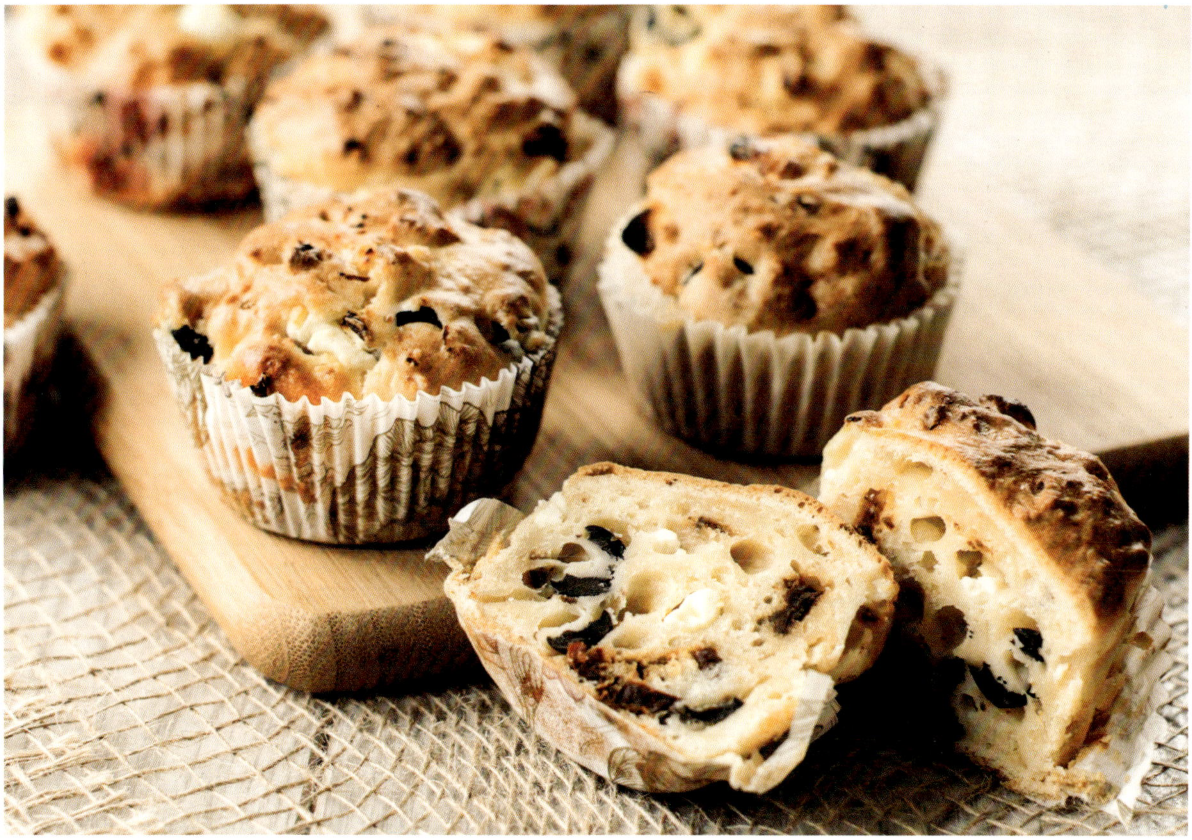

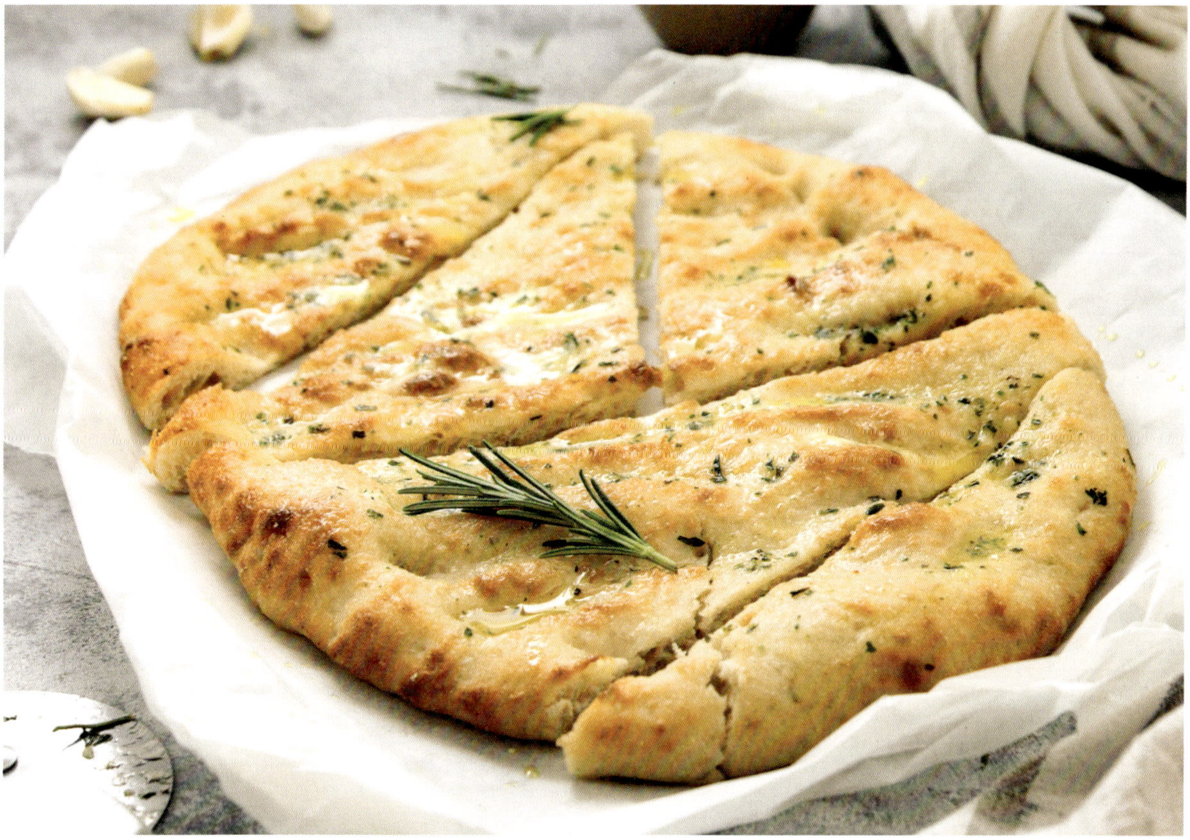

Index

accompaniments

biscuits

breads

brownies

buns

cakes

cheesecakes

Index cont.

HERRON
First Published in 2023 by Herron Book Distributors Pty Ltd
14 Manton St
Morningside
QLD 4170
www.herronbooks.com

Captain Honey
WWW.CAPTAINHONEY.COM.AU

Custom book production by Captain Honey Pty Ltd
12 Station St
Bangalow
NSW 2479
www.captainhoney.com.au

Cataloguing-in-Publication. A catalogue record for this book is available from the National Library of Australia.

ISBN 978-1-922944-08-5

Printed and bound in China.

5 4 3 2 1 23 24 25 26 27